WAY KNOWING ABOUT BIRTH

MOTHERS, MIDWIVES, MEDICINE, & BIRTH ACTIVISM

SELECTED WRITINGS BY

ROBBIE DAVIS-FLOYD

AND COLLEAGUES

WAVELAND PRESS, INC.

Long Grove, Illinois

For information about this book, contact:
Waveland Press, Inc.
4180 IL Route 83, Suite 101
Long Grove, IL 60047-9580
(847) 634-0081
info@waveland.com
www.waveland.com

Cover photo: Drawn together at a midwifery conference in Mexico, Mexican traditional and professional midwives, two American midwives, and three obstetricians—one Brazilian, one Venezuelan, and one Mexican—join the hands that catch the babies, in a spontaneous moment of solidarity around sharing knowledge systems and working together in support of woman-centered maternity care around the world.

Unless otherwise indicated, all photos were taken by the author and used with permission from the people in them.

10-digit ISBN 1-4786-3362-X
13-digit ISBN 978-1-4786-3362-4

Printed in the United States of America

7 6 5 4 3 2 1

WAYS OF KNOWING ABOUT BIRTH

I dedicate this, my legacy book,
to my three living human legacies—
my son Jason, and his sons/my grandsons
Jaxon and Grayson—
two amazing boys who are the joyous lights of my life.
May they live long and prosper!

Contents

Foreword by Lisa Kane Low xiii
Preface xvii

PART ONE
Ritual, Paradigms, Medicine, and Mothers

1 The Technocratic, Humanistic, and Holistic Paradigms of Birth and Health Care **3**

The 12 Tenets of the Technocratic Model of Medicine and Birth 4
The 12 Tenets of the Humanistic Model of Medicine and Birth 14
The 12 Tenets of the Holistic Model of Medicine and Birth 27
Stratified Holism and the Limitations of a Focus on the Individual 38
Functional Medicine: A Brief Note 40
The Importance of Ideology: Why Paradigms Matter 41

2 The Rituals of Hospital Birth: Enacting and Transmitting the Technocratic Model **45**

Rites of Passage 46
The Characteristics of Ritual and Obstetric "Routines": Hospital Birth as a Technocratic Rite of Passage 49

Mutilation and Prosthesis: The One-Two Punch of Technocratic Birth 66
Conclusion: Ritual Socialization 69

3 The Technocratic Body and the Organic Body: Hegemony and Heresy in Women's Birth Choices **71**

Women's Agency in Birth: Body Image as Microcosmic Mirror of Worldview 71
Women's Body Models: Technocratic and Holistic 73
Women's Perceptions of the Technocratic and Holistic Models of Birth and the Body Compared 97
Body Image as a Template for the Future? 99

4 Medical Training as Technocratic Initiation **107**

Ritual and Rite in Medical Training 108
Psychological Transformation in Medical School and Residency: Medical Training and Cognitive Narrowing 109
Trends in Medical Education: "Walking between the Worlds" 132
Conclusion: Hope for the Future? 138

5 The Paradigm Shift of Humanistic and Holistic Obstetricians: The "Good Guys and Girls" of Brazil **141**
with Eugenia Georges

Humanizing Self and Practice: Becoming a "Good Guy or Girl" 143
The Process of Transformation 154
Conclusion: The Obstetric Backlash and Positive Change 158

PART TWO
Midwives, Culture, Ideologies, and Birth

6 **American Midwifery: A Brief Anthropological Overview** **165**

Why I Wrote This Chapter: A Public Lack of Understanding of the Complexities of American Midwifery 165

A Short History of American Midwifery 166

The Development and Growth of Nurse-Midwifery 167

The Lay Midwifery Movement and the Creation of the CPM 169

Two Direct-Entry Certifications: The Creation of the CM 173

National Recognition: Certification, Accreditation, and the ICM Standards 173

Midwifery Differences and Commonalities: Working towards a More Unified Future? 176

Appendix: The Collaborative Work of US MERA 183 by Ida Darragh

7 **Intuition as Authoritative Knowledge in Midwifery and Homebirth** **189**
with Elizabeth Davis

On the Nature of Intuition: Theoretical Perspectives 191

Background and Context: Midwifery as Radical Cultural Critique 195

Methods and Collaboration: How an Anthropologist and a Midwife Came to Co-Create This Study 196

Midwives and Intuition 198

Normalizing Uniqueness 212

Conclusion: The "Connective Dance" 215

Appendix: Items that a Typical American Homebirth Midwife Carries with Her to a Homebirth 217

8 Daughter of Time: The Postmodern Midwife 221
with Etsuko Matsuoka, Holly Horan, Bonnie Ruder, and Courtney L. Everson

The Transnational Nature of Midwifery Knowledge: A Contemporary Exemplar 221
Back to the Future: Premodern, Modern, and Postmodern 222
Informed Relativism: The Characteristics of the Postmodern Midwife 225
A Short Story: How I Came to Identify and Understand "The Postmodern Midwife" 226
Postmodern Traditional Midwives 228
Postmodern Professional Midwives 242
Professional vs. Traditional Midwives: The Ramifications of Definition 258
Conclusion: Daughters of the Past Redefining Themselves in the Present 263

9 Mutual Accommodation or Biomedical Hegemony? A Brief Anthropological Overview of Global Issues in Midwifery 265

A Dysfunctional Maternity Care System 265
Achieving Functionality: Examples of Mutual Accommodation 275
Biomedical Hegemony: Examples of Its Consequences 277
"Midwifery Hegemony": What Happens When Professional Midwives Buy into the Biomedical Hierarchy? 280
Conclusion: Midwives and the Possible Future 281

10 Homebirth Emergencies in the US and Mexico: The Trouble with Transport 283

Articulation and Authoritative Knowledge: Biopower Meets the Homebirth Midwife 285
Methodology: Why and How I Chose to Study Midwives' Transport Stories 287
Background and Context: Obstetrics and Midwifery in the US and Mexico 288
Midwives' Transport Stories 295

Cross-Cultural Perspectives on Transport: Biomedicine as the Ultimate Recourse and the Ultimate Enemy 316
Transport Epilogue 2017: Developing Smooth and Seamless Articulations in the United States 319

11 The Midwifery Model of Care: Anthropological Perspectives 323
The Importance of Ideology: What's in a Name? 323
The Midwifery (Humanistic–Holistic) Model of Care 328
Conclusion: The Model behind the Model 336

12 Renegade Midwives: Assets or Liabilities? 339
with Christine Barbara Johnson
Renegade Midwives' Stories 339
Stories from Women Who Chose to Give Birth with Renegade Midwives 342
Normalizing Uniqueness: How Far Should It Go? 344
Hospital Midwives as Renegades 348
Robbie's Story and the Renegade Dilemma 349
Results and Consequences: The Renegade Spectrum 350
The Role of the Stranger 351
Living into the Answers 354

PART THREE
Anthropology and Birth Activism

13 Anthropology and Birth Activism: What Do We Know? 361
Penny's Toast 361
The Fault Line 362
Evidence vs. Practice 363
Ethnography as Activism 365
High Art to Birth Activists 367
Holding Spaces for Informed Choice 370

14 Working with Anthropology in Policy and Practice: An Activist's Experiences **373**

Introduction: My Choices to Study Birth and Midwives, and to Become a Birth Activist and Midwifery Advocate 373

Participant-Observation and Activism in the American Midwifery Movement: Conducting Political Ethnography 375

My Greatest Challenge as a Midwifery Ethnographer 380

Participant-Observation and Activism in the Birth Movement at the International Level 382

Forging My Path and Passing on Gitti's Mantle: An Ongoing Journey 386

15 Creating the International MotherBaby Childbirth Initiative (IMBCI): Anthropologically Informed Activism **389**

The Role of CIMS and the Creation of the IMBCI 389

The MotherBaby, and Women's Rights as Human Rights 392

IMBCO's Ongoing Work 393

The FIGO Initiative and a Possible Merger with the IMBCI 394

Conclusion: The Educational and Instrumental Goals of the IMBCI 395

Epilogue

Inner Space and Outer Space as Cyberspace? Technocratizing Womb and World 397 **397**

The Myth of Technological Transcendence 397

A Vision for Commercializing Outer Space: The SATWG Story 398

Cyborg Birth and a Holistic Story 403

Limitless Possibilities 408

Appendix

Applying Anthropology: What You Can Learn from This Book to Help You Achieve the Birth You Want **413**

References 421

Foreword

It is both an honor and a pleasure to introduce Robbie Davis-Floyd's "legacy book," as she herself calls it, since it contains articles she wrote sometimes decades ago and has fully updated for this anthology. I have had the privilege of engaging with Robbie over many years, as she is the "midwife's midwife," constantly engaging us in challenging conversations, critiquing dominant medical practices during childbirth, and encouraging us, as midwifery students, practitioners, and researchers to do our best and stay passionate. While the broad midwifery community most certainly feels a sense of kinship with Robbie, her contributions and theoretical development extend well beyond. Robbie is widely recognized in the field of reproductive anthropology, most specifically in the anthropologies of childbirth, midwifery, and obstetrics, which she has helped to create and expand. And at various times in her career she has shifted her focus outward to include the study of the psychological aspects of medical training (Chapter 4) and the paradigm shifts of humanistic and holistic physicians of all types (Chapter 5), not to mention her fieldwork with aerospace engineers (see the Epilogue).

Her theoretical contributions include (1) identifying the characteristics of the technocratic, humanistic, and holistic models of birth and health care and placing them on a comparative spectrum (Chapter 1), enabling health practitioners and consumers to understand the profound differences among these three paradigms and to use that knowledge to choose where they wish to place themselves along that spectrum; (2) her meaningful explanation of why non-evidence-based and often downright harmful "standard obstetric procedures" during labor and birth are routinely used anyway; her conclusion has long been that these procedures are rituals designed to display and convey the core values of technocratic societies to care providers and to women-becoming-mothers during their pregnancies and births (Chapter 2). Her work in this area has been extraordinarily valuable to all those trying to understand modern obstetric practice, has served as a call to action for childbirth activists, and has offered new insights for midwives and others engaged in maternity care to make it better.

Perhaps her major theoretical contribution to understanding contemporary midwifery is her notion of "the postmodern midwife"—midwives who are characterized by an approach she calls *informed relativism*—meaning that such midwives have the ability to move fluidly among the knowledge systems of technocratic obstetrics, hospital-based midwifery, home-based midwifery, and the traditional knowledge systems of indigenous cultures, many of whose ancient midwifery skills and techniques are of high value in the contemporary effort to keep normal, healthy physiologic birth alive and well in the 21st century (Chapter 8). As *traditional* midwives (who can be thoroughly postmodern themselves) continue to be phased out of practice in most countries, especially in the low-resource countries where they are often the only access point to care during childbirth, postmodern *professional* midwives make concerted efforts to learn from those traditional midwives still remaining, to bring forward into the future the best of the midwifery traditions and skills of what is rapidly becoming the past.

At literally hundreds of conferences and throughout her fieldwork, Robbie often served as a facilitator or bridge, bringing together old and young, midwife and obstetrician, nurse-midwife and direct-entry midwife, all in the spirit of healthy debate. She often initiated and supported challenging conversations and always encouraged collaboration. I have had the honor of presenting at some of those conferences with Robbie as we explored the process of socialization in the midwifery education, considering ways to grow the profession and enhance collaboration between those holding the varied midwifery credentials that midwives can pursue in the U.S. (Chapter 6).

Robbie is respected by anthropologists and beloved by many midwives. Her work is often taught in midwifery, social science, women's studies and interdisciplinary courses in many countries. Her former pre-med students still today often tell her that they carry her book *From Doctor to Healer: The Transformative Journey* (1998) in their hearts, holding onto her words like a "golden nugget" reminder that there is a better way to practice medicine. Midwives write to tell her how her articles and talks have changed their practices for the better, as do mothers who have advocated for and then had better birthing experiences after reading her works. I still have my first copy of her first book, *Birth as an American Rite of Passage*, with many worn pages; it has served as a constant resource as I teach courses in women's health, women's studies and midwifery, describing the paradigms of birth to develop students' understanding of the ways in which socialization through tightly defined disciplinary perspectives can lead to entrenched approaches to care that seek coherence with their paradigm rather than being informed by evidence.

From the beginning of her career in birth and midwifery research (1983), Robbie has been invited to give talks to practitioners, and their insistent questions about how her work could be made relevant to their daily practices and their own births have kept her trying hard to make her publications accessible and useful both inside and outside of anthropology. Robbie loves anthropology

because it gives students a means of studying, understanding, and explaining to others *any* type of human behavior, past, present, or future, and she believes that asking the key anthropological question—*why*?—has itself provided many keys to understanding sometimes otherwise inexplicable things that humans, in their vast diversity, do. Robbie's anthropological lens and points of analysis offer scholars, students, and practitioners new comprehension of how culture and ritual are embedded in the education/socialization of health care providers, perpetuating their entrenchment in the belief systems of their fields.

During her anthropological research with midwives of all types, she sought to help us as best she could by spreading the word to the public about our value as the practitioners most qualified to attend normal births and to facilitate healthy physiologic approaches. She became a strong midwifery advocate and birth activist, bringing her insights and calls to action to numerous audiences across disciplines (Part 3 of this book). Robbie's midwifery advocacy has always been for *all* types of midwives—traditional and professional, home-, birth-center-, and hospital-based, and across credentials. She is not blind to the potential deficiencies of traditional midwives when their practices are sometimes harmful and ill-informed by tradition, or to those of professional midwives who adopt an attitude of superiority that keeps them from working with the "other" midwives whose educational pathway or training may not be valued, or who internalize the technocratic biomedical model and use far too many interventions in their birth "management" (Chapter 9).

It is my hope that this book will be widely used for teaching in gender studies, social science, obstetric, and midwifery courses, and read by practitioners, global development planners, public health leaders, and the general public for the many wise insights and practical suggestions it provides. I look forward to continuing to use Robbie's work as a critical component of my courses in women's studies, interprofessional education, and midwifery programs. This anthology continues the "rite of passage" that I believe is an essential part of socialization for all who desire to engage as practitioners, activists, scholars, and consumers in understanding the complex context and systems of care surrounding childbirth.

Thank you, Robbie, for continuing our education and offering us analytic tools and understandings. You are making a difference for us, from the individual ways we approach the care we provide to the global development of integrated systems of care that value and support optimal approaches that benefit childbearing families. I know everyone will take away something from this outstanding book, and I look forward to continuing to participate in the challenging conversations Robbie's work often generates, and to advocate for optimal models of care in the tradition of activism that Robbie has inspired in so many of us, her readers.

Lisa Kane Low PhD, CNM, FACNM, FAAN
President, American College of Nurse-Midwives, 2016–2018

Preface

As a cultural, medical, and symbolic anthropologist, midwifery advocate, and birth activist, I have been studying and working in the arenas of childbirth, midwifery, obstetrics, and medicine for over 30 years. During that time, I have authored or coauthored many articles on these topics and others, including 23 encyclopedia articles on birth, midwifery, ritual, and the new reproductive technologies. The advent of ResearchGate has made me aware, on a daily basis, of the fact that many of my publications are still being widely read, and many of my colleagues tell me that they often use my articles for teaching. So I thought it might be a good idea to compile the most popular of my articles into one volume, an anthology designed for teaching in anthropology, midwifery, and obstetric educational programs, as well as for the interested lay reader. I have updated every article included here as a chapter to the best of my ability, adding new material and information in all of them, and have included at the end both questions for thought and discussion, and recommendations for appropriate films and videos to accompany the chapters. Because, for teaching purposes, I wanted each chapter to be able to stand alone—to make sense if it's read by itself and not in the context of the entire anthology—readers will find rather a lot of redundancy in these chapters, for which I hope they will forgive me.

I am happy to provide this compilation of much of my life's work to students, teachers, researchers, practitioners, and others, and hope that its readers will find it useful in their academic or midwifery or medical careers, as well as in their daily lives and the choices they will make around their own pregnancy and birth experiences. I hope you find this book both educational and entertaining, and that its chapters will enhance your knowledge and understanding of these topics in useful ways.

A Note on Gender Terminology

I wish my readers to know that I am aware of the complexities introduced into our language by the calls issued by LGBTQ communities to make the English language fully inclusive of queer and other non-binary gender identities—an enterprise I support and am trying to adapt to. However, most of the chapters in this book were written long before gender inclusive language was applied to birth. In contemplating what to call participants from studies in my past, I have decided to call people what they called themselves at the time, even though I know that some may now use masculine pronouns or have other preferences I never thought to ask about at the time. To the best of my knowledge, all of the pregnant women and mothers I interviewed identified as hetero-normative, cis-gendered women, so I continue to call them "birthing women" and "mothers" instead of "birthing persons." Similarly, in this book, I continue to call all midwives "women" (as all of my midwife interviewees did in fact call themselves) and to use the pronoun "she" when speaking of them. Around the world, about 1% of all midwives are male. I have interviewed almost all of the male midwives in the US, as well as a few in other countries, and they all have told me that they don't mind the feminine terminology associated with the word "midwife," saying that they are happy to be included under that word, noting with humor that they wish to develop their "feminine side."

Acknowledgments

I thank Melissa Cheyney CPM, PhD, for her extremely helpful and careful review of this volume, Jeni Ogilvie at Waveland for her excellent editing, and Tom Curtin at Waveland for always believing in me and my work and his willingness—indeed eagerness—to publish this anthology.

WAYS OF KNOWING ABOUT BIRTH

PART ONE

Ritual, Paradigms, Medicine, and Mothers

1

The Technocratic, Humanistic, and Holistic Paradigms of Birth and Health Care

This chapter describes three paradigms of health care that heavily influence contemporary childbirth, most particularly in the West but increasingly around the world: the technocratic, humanistic, and holistic models of medicine. These models differ fundamentally in their definitions of the body and its relationship to the mind, and thus in the health care approaches they charter. The technocratic model stresses mind/body separation and sees the body as a machine; the humanistic model emphasizes mind–body connection and defines the body as an organism; the holistic model insists on the oneness of body, mind, and spirit and defines the body as an energy field in constant interaction with other energy fields. Of these three paradigms, the humanstic model—or humanism—stands the best chance of success in this era of the deepening penetration of technology into birth. But in order to understand

This chapter has been significantly revised and updated from its original publication in the *International Journal of Gynecology and Obstetrics*, 75, Supplement No. 1, pp. S5–S23, November 2001. Certain portions of this chapter draw heavily on *From Doctor to Healer: The Transformative Journey* (Davis-Floyd and St. John, 1998) and *Birth as an American Rite of Passage* (Davis-Floyd 2003 [1992]).

humanism in health care and obstetrics, it is essential to understand the other two approaches as well.

Based on many years of research in contemporary childbirth, most especially through interviews with physicians, midwives, nurses, and mothers, this chapter seeks to describe the 12 tenets of each paradigm as they apply to contemporary obstetrics and health care and to point out their futuristic implications. I suggest that practitioners who combine elements of all three paradigms have a unique opportunity to create the most effective obstetrical system ever known.

The 12 Tenets of the Technocratic Model of Medicine and Birth

The way a society conceives of and uses technology reflects and perpetuates the value and belief system that underlies it. Despite its pretenses to scientific rigor, the Western medical system is less grounded in science than in its wider cultural context; like all health care systems, it embodies the biases and beliefs of the society that created it (Gaines and Davis-Floyd 2003). Western society's core value system is strongly oriented toward science, high technology, economic profit, and patriarchally governed institutions (Davis-Floyd 2003 [1992]). Our medical system reflects that core value system: its successes are founded in science, effected by technology, and carried out through large institutions governed by patriarchal ideologies in a profit-driven economic context. Among these core values, in both medicine and the wider society, technology reigns supreme. As has been clear for over 50 years, most routine obstetrical procedures have little or no scientific evidence to justify them. (In fact, many common medical interventions of all kinds are not evidence-based: the *British Medical Journal*'s "Clinical Evidence" analyzed 3,000 common medical treatments and showed that a full 50% of them have unknown efficacy, while 5% were "unlikely to be beneficial" and 3% were "likely to be ineffective or harmful" [http://clinicalevidence.bmj.com/x/set/static/cms/efficacy-categorisations.html, accessed August 19, 2016].) As I hope to show throughout this book, standard obstetric procedures are routinely performed not because they make scientific sense but because they make cultural sense. As we shall see below, they exemplify certain fundamental values of technocratic life.

(1) Mind/Body Separation, and (2) The Body-as-Machine

The main value underlying the technocratic paradigm of medicine is separation. The *principle of separation* states that things are better understood outside of their context, that is, divorced from related objects or per-

sons. Technomedicine continually separates the individual into component parts, the process of reproduction into constituent elements, and experience of childbirth from the flow of life. But first and foremost, it separates the human body from the human mind.

The body presents a profound conceptual paradox to our society, for it is simultaneously a creation of nature and the focal point of culture. How can we be separate from nature when we are part of it? Descartes, Bacon, and others neatly resolved this problem in the 1600s when they established the philosophical separation of mind and body upon which the metaphor of the body-as-machine depends. This idea meant that the superior cultural essence of man, his mind—as well as the superior spiritual essence, his soul—could remain unaffected while the body, as a mere part of mechanical nature, could be taken apart, studied, and repaired.

This metaphor of the body-as-machine could have been inherently egalitarian, but the industrializing nations of the West were male-centered, patriarchal societies. Thus the male body came to be medically viewed as the prototype of the properly functioning body-machine. The female body, as it deviated from the male standard, was regarded as inherently defective and dangerously under the influence of nature, which due to its unpredictability, was itself regarded as in need of constant manipulation by man (Merchant 1983; Davis-Floyd 2003 [1992]). As a result, despite the growing acceptance of birth

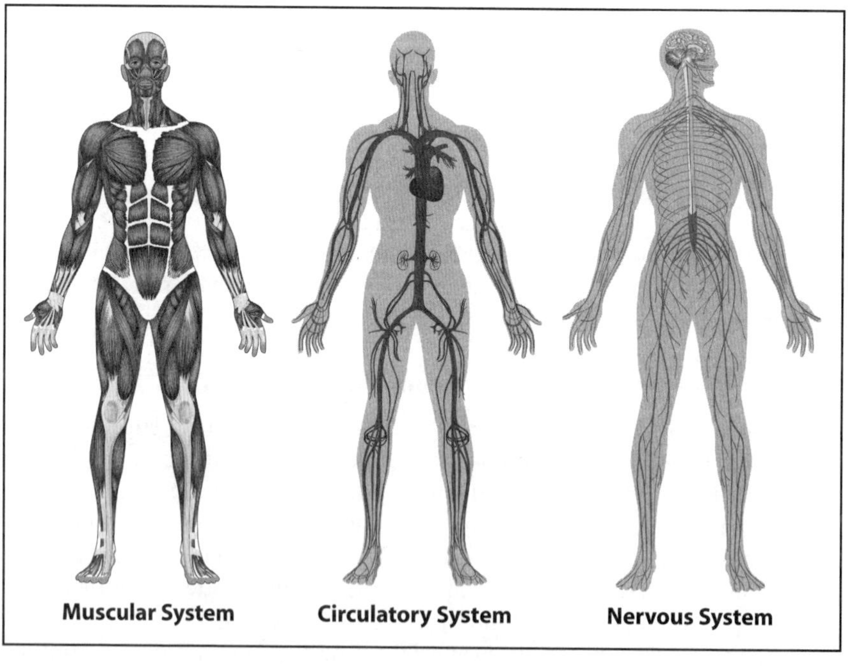

The male body as the prototype of the body-as-machine.

as mechanical like all other bodily processes, it came to be viewed as an inherently imperfect and untrustworthy mechanical process, and the metaphor of *the female body as a defective machine* eventually formed the philosophical foundation of modern obstetrics. Furthermore, as the factory production of goods became a central organizing metaphor for social life, it also became the dominant metaphor for birth: the hospital became the factory, the mother's body became the machine, and the baby became the product of an industrial manufacturing process. Obstetrics was thereby enjoined to develop tools and technologies for the manipulation and improvement of the inherently defective process of birth, and to make birth conform to the assembly-line model of factory production.

(3) The Patient as Object, and
(4) Alienation of Practitioner from Patient

Mechanizing the human body and defining the body-as-machine as the proper object of medical treatment frees technomedical practitioners from any sense of responsibility for the patient's mind or spirit. Thus practitioners often see no need to engage with the individual who inhabits that body-machine, preferring instead to think of and talk about a patient as "the c-section in 112." Jordan (1993) demonstrates how this tendency to objectify patients can extend to refusal to discuss any details of a case with the person who embodies it. This kind of alienation from their patients often becomes embedded in physicians during medical school and residency, as they are taught to protect themselves by avoiding emotional involvement. It logically follows that there is no reason to deal with the patient's emotions at all. Thus they are free to protect their own feelings from the pain of caring too much. Technocratic physicians do not value lengthy conversations with their patients, preferring to keep their visits short. Although it is well-known that touch and caring are powerful factors that can positively influence both a woman's experience of labor and the outcome of the birth, it is rare to see obstetricians touching laboring women, holding their hands, or sheltering them in an embrace.

(5) Diagnosis and Treatment from the Outside In

When most machines break down, they do not repair themselves from the inside; they must be repaired from the outside, by someone else. Thus in technomedicine, it follows that one must attempt to diagnose problems, cure disease, and repair dysfunction from the outside. The most valued information is that which comes from the many high-tech diagnostic machines now considered essential to modern health care. Such diagnostic technologies are pervasive in pregnancy and childbirth, from ultrasounds in early pregnancy to electronic fetal monitoring during labor. And treatment, too, is from the outside in—when labor slows, the amniotic sac is pierced with a hook and

pitocin is poured into a vein to speed labor up; when a baby seems stuck, it is pulled out with forceps or cut out with a scalpel.

The routine administration of IVs to women in labor is a good example of the massive overuse of this outside-in approach. There is plenty of scientific evidence (Hunt 2013; Enkin et al. 2000; Goer 1995, 1999; O'Sullivan 2009; Parsons, Bidewell, and Griffiths 2007; Rooks 1997; Singata et al 2010; Singata, Tranmer, and Gyte 2013; Vallejo et al. 2013—for just a few examples) to indicate that it's much healthier for a woman to eat and drink during labor. If a laboring woman is hungry, it generally means that birth is still a long way off; she needs to eat to keep her strength up.

A Short Side Story: Thinking Inside and Outside the Box

Many years ago, I gave a talk to the entire faculty and staff of the major maternity hospital in Texarkana, Texas, on "The Rituals of Hospital Birth" (see Chapter 2). About halfway through the lecture, I noticed that the nurses in the audience were getting restless. So I asked them why, and several of them responded that I was basically telling them that everything they were doing to laboring women was wrong. I said, "OK, what for example?" and they said, "Well, the IV for one—you're telling us it's wrong to use it. But every laboring woman in this hospital gets hooked up to an IV—100%." I asked, "Why?" and they responded, as if I were stupid, "to hydrate her." I asked, "Why?" again, and with growing impatience they responded with the same answer. I was feeling feisty that day, so I asked *why* one more time. Dead silence, until one brave nurse at the back of the auditorium stood up and said, "Because our hospital has an NPO policy"—nothing by mouth, meaning no food or drink allowed—and there was a collective gasp from the audience as just for that one moment, they stepped outside their technocratic box and realized that *laboring women could hydrate themselves* except for that hospital rule that said they couldn't. This is how paradigms work—you get stuck inside them and can't see other possibilities.

Yet the IV makes a powerful symbolic statement: it is the umbilical cord to the hospital. (Nurses often speak of their need to have a "line-in" to the laboring mother to make it easier to inject drugs later on.) Hydration via the IV with no oral intake of fluids makes it difficult to move around, and thus more likely to stay "in her place," and, at least symbolically, puts the woman in the same relationship of dependence on the institution for her life as the baby in the womb is dependent on her for its life (Davis-Floyd 2003 [1992]:95). By extension, one can see an IV as a perfect symbolic expression

of life in the technocracy: we are all umbilically linked to institutions and through them, to society. As a vein is penetrated with a needle and then with the fluid flowing through the IV line, connecting the woman to the institution, so our homes are penetrated by and thus connected to the wider world by water, sewer, telephone, electricity, and cable lines. Individuals are also connected to institutions via their drivers' licenses, credit cards, bank accounts, insurance policies, and so forth. And the technocracy wants those "lines-in" to us—so we can be counted, taxed, billed, and more and more, marketed to. The fullest symbolic extension of the IV lies in its expression and display of our ongoing fusions of ourselves with the technologies we create. A "cyborg" is a cybernetic organism, a fusion of human with machine. In the cultural arena of reproduction, we are escalating the pace of our own cyborgification (see Davis-Floyd and Dumit 1998, and the Epilogue to this anthology). Again I am speaking symbolically here; certainly nurses who put in those IVs don't think of it as umbilically linking the woman to the institution—they just want that "line-in." And yet the culturally symbolic meanings of that act are profound, indicating over and over that standard hospital procedures for birth do not make scientific sense, but they do make plenty of cultural sense.

(6) Hierarchical Organization and Standardization of Care

Like its industrial predecessor, the technocracy is a hierarchically organized society. The term *technocracy* implies use of an ideology of technological progress as a source of political power (Reynolds 1991). It thus expresses not only the technological but also the hierarchical, bureaucratic and autocratic dimensions of this culturally dominant reality model. Even as many businesses seek to make a paradigm shift by transforming themselves into "organizational networks" and "flat corporations," the medical system remains true to its role as society's microcosm, rigidly hierarchical in terms of the power of physicians as a group, the emphasis on specialty over primary care, and the subordination of individual needs to standardized institutional practices and routines.

The standardization in hospital birth is dramatically evident in most modern hospitals. Upon entering the hospital, the laboring woman is taken in a wheelchair to a "prep" or a labor and delivery room. There her clothes are removed, she is asked to put on a hospital gown, and a vaginal exam is performed. Her access to food is limited or prohibited, and an intravenous needle is inserted in her hand or arm. The external fetal monitor is attached to the woman to monitor the strength of her contractions and the baby's heartbeat. Periodic vaginal exams are performed to check the degree of the baby's descent. All of these procedures in most modern hospitals are routinely performed without scientific justification (Block 2007; Enkin et al. 2000; Goer 1995, 1999; Macones et al. 2008; Morris 2013; Romano and Lothian 2008; Rooks 1997).

As the moment of birth approaches, there is an intensification of actions performed on the woman, as she is (still in many hospitals in many countries) transferred to a delivery room, placed in the lithotomy (flat-on-the-back) position, covered with sterile sheets and doused with antiseptic, and an episiotomy is performed. (In 2017, although episiotomies are now rare in the US and other developed countries, they are still absolutely routine in most developing countries because their obstetricians are taught that "the perineum will explode" if it is not cut wider open first [see Chapter 5].) After the birth, the new mother is handed the baby for a certain amount of time, her placenta is extracted if it does not come out quickly on its own, her episiotomy is sewn up, and finally, she is cleaned up and transferred to a hospital bed. Or she may have a cesarean section; we are witnessing today a worldwide cesarean epidemic. In countries like Greece, Brazil, Iran, Turkey, Mexico, India, China, and many others, that operation has already become routine, often characterizing half or more of all births (Castro, Heimburger, and Langer 2001; Hopkins 2000; Kim 2011; Potter et al. 2001; Toan et al 2013; Victora et al 2011).

Of course, there are many variations on this theme. Some procedures that used to be standard in US hospitals in the 1940s through the 1960s such as hand strapping, the exclusion of fathers, and shaves and enemas are no longer used, although most such interventions are still common in developing countries. Other major changes since then include the father's presence and women remaining conscious during birth, usually with an epidural to keep her from feeling the pain of labor. Where there is real choice, many women opt for delivery in a birthing suite or LDR (labor-delivery-recovery room), where they can wear their own clothes, do without the IV, and walk around during labor and perhaps eat and drink. Yet in spite of these concessions to consumer demand for more humanistic birth, a basic pattern of high-technological intervention remains: most hospitals now require at least periodic electronic monitoring of all laboring women; analgesics, pitocin, and epidurals are widely administered; and cesarean section rates are increasing almost everywhere. Thus, although some medical procedures drop away, the use of the most powerful signifiers of the woman's dependence on science and technology intensifies.

(7) Authority and Responsibility Inherent in Practitioner

In line with its hierarchical structure, the technocratic model invests authority in physicians and in institutions and their personnel. Obvious cues such as titles and white coats signal the authority of physicians, who can add to their status by withholding information and using technical jargon the patient cannot understand. When the doctor is the only authority, the patient lacks responsibility. Many doctors are able to present an option as *the* answer quite easily, by simply refusing to discuss non-paradigm alternatives. In this

scenario, a patient's most comfortable role is abdication of personal preference in favor of the doctor's choice.

In childbirth, one of the most graphic demonstrations of the power of "doctor's choice" is the lithotomy position so popular with obstetricians (OBs) not because it is physiologically sound, but because it enables them to attend births standing up or sitting comfortably in front of the woman's spread legs, with a clear field for maneuvering. We know very well that this position complicates childbirth by narrowing the pelvic outlet and limiting the mother's ability to push, but the many good physiological reasons to allow women to give birth in upright positions (which include increased blood and oxygen supply to the baby, more effective pushing, and wider pelvic outlets) are far less important to most physicians than their own comfort, convenience, and status. In the West, "up" is good and "down" is bad: the person who is "on top" has the status and the power, and rarely gives it up for the good of the laboring woman and child.

Technomedicine's investment of both authority and responsibility in physicians and hospitals is a double-edged sword. Although medical personnel do have the power to give orders to patients and establish institutional policies and procedures, they can be and often are held to be accountable for deaths and outcomes that no mortal could prevent. The proliferation of lawsuits against obstetricians over the past several decades is testimony to the way citizens have turned this tenet of the technocratic model against its proponents.

(8) Supervaluation of Science and Technology

The general public tends to assume that doctors are scientists, but many medical students receive little training in research methodology and analysis. A 1978 study carried out by the Office of Technology Assessment of the United States Congress reported that "only ten to twenty percent of all procedures currently used in medical practice have been shown to be efficacious in controlled trials"; in the 1990s, it was still true that over half of the techniques physicians routinely employ have not been proven in rigorous testing and remains so today (Greenhalgh et al 2008; Grol and Grimshaw 2003; Grol and Wensing 2004). Yet the power of the technomedical paradigm is such that physicians will rapidly accept procedures and technologies in keeping with it, while rejecting those that do not. So, while science is supervalued as an ideology in this paradigm, its actual findings are often discounted or ignored.

Likewise, the technologies that predominate in medical treatment are those that support the "evolution through technology" ethos of the technocratic model, in which progress means the development of ever more sophisticated machines. When a doctor uses a "low-tech" tool like a stethoscope or fetoscope, he touches the patient, speaks to her, listens with his own ears to hers or the baby's heartbeat, interprets the sounds through his own bodily perceptions, and arrives at a diagnosis that depends in large part on his physical senses. When the same doctor uses a magnetic resonance imaging machine

(MRI) or an electronic fetal monitor (EFM), only the machine touches or interacts with the patient during the procedure. The physician's role is to interpret the mechanically mediated results, which are regarded as more objective and reliable than his perceptions.

Such new technologies are usually introduced by their marketers, who tend to describe them solely in terms of their best-case use and minimize any detrimental effects. EFM is a case in point (Kunisch 1989). Its manufacturers regularly paid physicians' trips to medical conferences; upon arrival, they found themselves walking through elaborate EFM displays to get to the meeting rooms (Wagner 1997). Now pervasive in hospital birth, the EFM has resulted not in better outcomes but in higher costs and higher cesarean rates (Alfirevic, Devane, and Gyte 2013). Nevertheless, many hospitals in the US routinely employ these machines in more than 80% of labors (Declerq et al. 2006).

Rapid diffusion and acceptance of a new technology often has more to do with its symbolic value than its actual efficacy. Machines can mesmerize:

> The amplified fetal heartbeat sounds like galloping horses . . . both the sound of the galloping and the vision of the needle traveling across the paper, making a blip with each heartbeat, are hypnotic, often giving one the illusion that the machines are keeping the baby's heart beating. (Harrison 1982:90)

So powerful is this illusion that nurses I have interviewed often become reluctant to detach the mother from the monitor because they fear that the baby's heart will stop. While they know intellectually that this is nonsense, nevertheless they are emotionally swayed by the symbolic power of these machines. Harrison's quote describes the earlier EFMs that used paper tracings; today's computerized monitors leave patients and practitioners alike staring at colorful lines on a large screen that are far more mesmerizing than the paper tracings used to be.

Once machines, like the EFM, along with CAT and positron emission tomography (PET) scanners and others, are there, they must be reckoned with, and any decision *not* to use them begins to look like substandard care—a reality that reflects both the financial and the symbolic supervaluation of technology in the American medical system. Such machines serve the powerful symbolic purpose of "upgrading" medical care in keeping with our notions of evolutionary progress; indeed, our newest cultural value is the flow of massive amounts of information through sophisticated electronic systems—just the kind of option that the EFM provides.

(9) Aggressive Intervention with Emphasis on Short-Term Results, and (10) Death as Defeat

I suggest that our culture has situated childbirth fully in risk and has normalized childbirth interventions. It is a paradox in which tremendous resources are

poured into preventing rare events rather than supporting most women to avail themselves of resources to sustain and improve their health. Fear of birth has become the foundation of childbearing in US culture. We do not usually fear things that are normal, and therefore childbirth has become culturally pathologic: it is something to be "fixed." We live in a society where women are likely to have heard only birth stories that include epidurals and cesareans. It is a culture that deifies technology and control, with no room for uncertainty of any kind and for less than perfect outcomes.

— Holly Kennedy CNM (2010)

Since the dawn of the Industrial Revolution, Western society has sought to dominate and control nature. And the more we controlled nature, including our natural bodies, the more we feared the aspects of nature we could not control. This led to the emergence of a phenomenon that anthropologist Peter C. Reynolds (1991) has labeled the "One-Two Punch" of technological intervention. Punch One: technologically alter a natural process, causing problems; Punch Two: fix those problems with more technology. For example, pollute the oceans with tons of technological trash, then try to clean up that pollution with the invention of microbes than can eat and absorb that trash. Reynolds' brilliant insight was that, while most people see Punch Two as an accidental by-product of Punch One, the deeper truth is that *Punch Two is the point*. We in the West have become convinced that altering natural processes makes them better—more predictable, more controllable, and therefore safer.

It is not hard to see how this One-Two Punch of mutilation and prosthesis applies to birth—I will say more about that in Chapter 2. For now I will simply note that Reynolds' One-Two Punch is a powerful motivating force in American society—I call it *the technological imperative*—the notion that *if it can be done with technology, it must and will be done with technology.* This impetus to improve on nature through technology has as its ultimate aim to free us altogether from the limitations of nature. The more able we become to control nature, including our natural bodies, the more fearful we become of the aspects of nature we cannot control.

Death becomes the ultimate signifier of defeat, proof that in fact we have not succeeded in transcending nature's limitations, and thus the ultimate enemy, to be battled at all costs. Lifesaving procedures for low-birthweight infants, often implemented without respect for their eventual quality of life, like high-tech intervention for the terminally ill, represent attempts at sustaining the fragile thread of life against all odds. The underlying ethos behind the routine application of so many unnecessary procedures to birth is fear of death. These procedures, which I will analyze as rituals in the following chapter, do what most rituals are designed to do: *keep fear at bay* by giving both practitioners and birthing women the illusion of control and therefore safety; they appear to minimize risk while in fact they often generate more problems than they solve.

Technomedical Hegemony: (11) A Profit-Driven System and (12) Intolerance of Other Modalities

The word "hegemony" refers to an ideology espoused by the dominant group in a given society. In a multicultural society such as that of the United States in the early 21st century, no one set of ideas about medicine, religion, economics, or anything else is shared by everyone. Nevertheless, there are ideologies that are obviously dominant: in economics, the hegemonic ideology is capitalism, and in health care, it is the technomedical/technocratic model. When an ideology is hegemonic, all other competing ideologies become "alternative" to it. Thus healing modalities such as midwifery, chiropractic, homeopathy, naturopathy, acupuncture, and so forth have been viewed as "alternative" to allopathy. While these modalities command increasing respect and usage, allopathic technomedicine still sets the standards for care. Its hegemonic status works to ensure its profitability: pharmaceutical and medical technology companies constitute by far some of the most profitable industries in the United States and the world, and childbirth management accounts for a huge amount of economic profit, most especially in the US, where a vaginal hospital birth can cost $13,000 and up (depending on what kind of insurance the mother has) and a cesarean birth can cost three times that much (May 2017; Anderson, Daviss, and Johnson forthcoming).

Any system—medical, economic, religious, or otherwise—that gains sociocultural ascendancy in extraordinarily profitable ways, and then rigidifies, shutting out new information and refusing to incorporate contradictory evidence, is in mortal danger both to itself and to the public it serves. Such hegemonic systems can benefit from frontal attacks, which can serve to keep them flexible and responsive to the changing realities of changing times. It is in that spirit that I present this analysis.

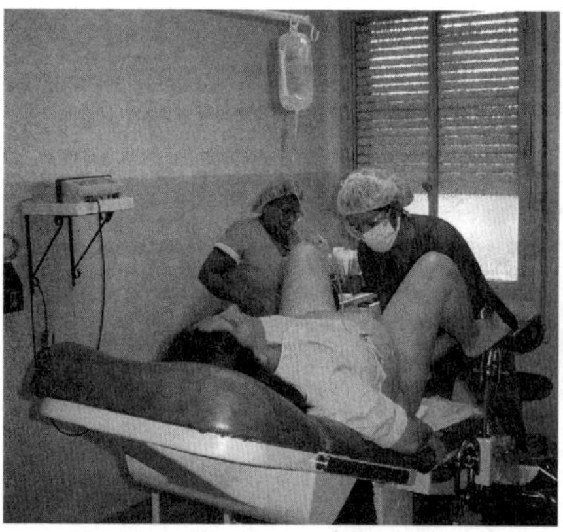

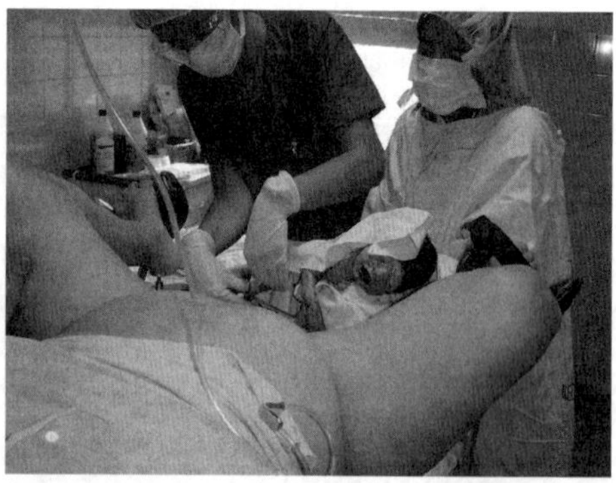

A technocratic birth in a Buenos Aires hospital.

The 12 Tenets of the Humanistic Model of Medicine and Birth

In the United States and elsewhere, the excesses of technomedicine have long been the subject of heated discussion and debate. Humanism arose in reaction to these excesses as an effort driven by nurses and physicians working within the medical system to reform it from the inside. Humanists wish simply to humanize technomedicine—that is, to make it relational, partnership-oriented, individually responsive, and compassionate. This caring, commonsensical approach is garnering wide international appreciation and support. Clearly less radical than holism, clearly more loving than technomedicine, this humanistic paradigm has the most potential to open the technocratic system, from the inside, to the possibility of widespread reform.

(1) Mind–Body Connection

The humanistic approach neither demarcates a total separation between mind and body, as does technomedicine, nor claims oneness for mind and body, as does the holistic model. Rather, it recognizes the influence of the mind on the body and advocates forms of healing that address both. Proponents of this paradigm see body and mind as being in constant communication, citing scientific research in the field of psychoneuroimmunology and elsewhere. Thus the humanistic paradigm insists that it is simplistic and narrow-minded to treat physical symptoms without addressing their psychological components. Psychoneuroimmunologist Candace Pert explained:

> Viruses use [the same receptors as the neuropeptides that carry emotions] to enter into a cell, and depending on how much of the natural juice, or the natural peptide for that receptor is around, the virus will have an easier or a harder time getting into the cell. So our emotional state will affect whether we'll get sick from the same loading dose of a virus. . . . Emotional fluctuations and emotional status directly influence the probability that the organism will get sick or be well. (1993:190)

The implications for childbirth of the notion that the mind affects what happens in the body are obvious and profound. Humanism in childbirth allows for the possibility that the laboring woman's emotions can affect the progress of her labor, and that problems in labor may be more effectively dealt with through emotional support than through technological intervention.

(2) The Body as an Organism

Although in some ways the human body is *like* a machine, it is a fact of biological life that the body is not a machine but an organism. Acceptance of this fact has powerful repercussions for treatment, as how the body is defined will shape the way it is treated by a culture's health care system. "Even medical therapies that are the most machine-like would be ineffective without the

innate healing powers of the organism," which has "properties that no machine has: those of growth, regeneration, healing, learning, and self-transcendence" (Tresolini et al. 1994:243).

Defining the body as an organism charters the development of an array of treatments that may be irrelevant to a machine but matter a great deal to an organism. Unlike machines, mammalian organisms feel pain and respond emotionally to interactions with others and to changes in their environment. Most mammals respond positively to the comfort of a loving touch and shrink from contact that is harsh or punitive. Thus a paradigm of healing based on a definition of the human body as an organism would logically stress the importance of kindness, of touch, and of caring and respectful treatment. These dimensions have special significance for the care of laboring women, from the ways they are treated during labor to the need of mother and baby to remain together after birth. The importance of this need, in addition to the successful initiation of breastfeeding, is now augmented by the growing body of literature on the "microbiome" of the baby, whose gut upon birth needs to be colonized with the bacteria of the mother's body—and not that of a practitioner—to kick start its immune system (see *Your Baby's Microbiome: The Critical Role of Vaginal Birth and Breastfeeding for Lifelong Health* by Toni Harman and Alex Wakeford 2016). The best analog for the term *humanism* in the medical literature is the term *bio-psycho-social*, which acknowledges that this model takes into account the individual's biology, psychology, and social environment.

(3) The Patient as Relational Subject

Rather than avoiding it, most humanists seek to establish a real human connection with their patients, to come to know them not just as patients but as individuals, not as "the c-section in 112" but as "the mother with twins whose sister just died." David Spiegel and his colleagues (1989) showed that women with advanced breast cancer who participated in weekly support groups not only felt better emotionally but ultimately lived an average of 18 months longer than did women with comparable breast cancer and medical care who did not attend such groups. This added survival time was, according to Spiegel et al. (1993:335), "longer than any medication or other known medical treatment could be expected to provide for women with breast cancer so far advanced." This study has been followed by a number of large-scale studies showing that more and better social support from family and friends is associated with lower odds of dying and better odds of healing at any given age (Diener and Chan 2011; Temel et al. 2010).

Starting in the 1970s, natural childbirth activists in large numbers in the US and other countries began to demand that fathers and significant others be allowed in delivery rooms, that mother and baby should not be separated after birth, and that friends and relatives be allowed to remain with the labor-

ing woman if such was her desire. The effect of the presence of caring others during childbirth does far more than simply work toward a more pleasant labor experience; it can be *central* to the positive outcome of that experience.

(4) Connection and Caring between Practitioner and Patient

Whereas the technocratic paradigm is based on the principle of separation, and the holistic model on integration, the principle underlying the humanistic approach is *connection*: the connection of the patient to the multiple aspects of herself, her family, her community and society, and her health care practitioners. Humanism requires treating the patient in a connected, relational way as any human being would want to be treated—with consideration, kindness, and respect. This paradigm insists on the deep humanity of the individuals involved and stresses the importance of the patient–practitioner relationship to the healing process. The phrase "relationship-centered care" has been suggested "to capture the importance of the interaction among people as the foundation of any therapeutic or healing activity" (Tresolini et al. 1994).

In childbirth, the strongest evidence of the power of relationship-centered care comes from the doula research. A *doula* is a female companion especially trained to give labor support. Sosa, Kennell, Klaus and their associates (1980), Kennell (1982), and Kennell et al. (1988) compared the results of laboring without and laboring with one-on-one support by a doula. They found that doula support dramatically reduced problems of fetal asphyxia and labor dystocia, shortened length of labor, and enhanced mother–infant interaction after delivery (see also Castaneda and Searcy 2015; Klaus, Kennell, and Klaus 1993; Spong et al. 2012).

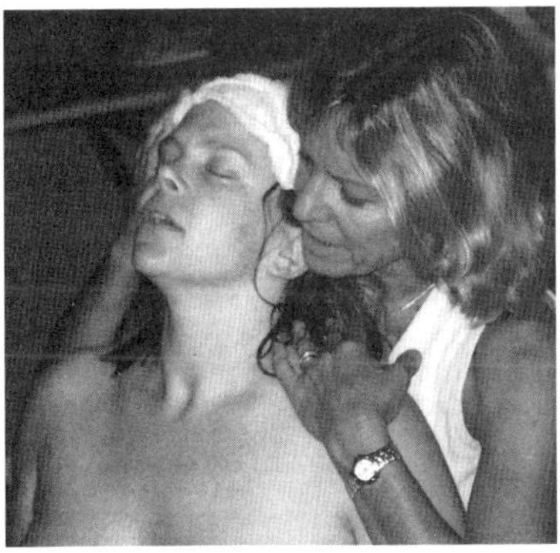

Doula Rae Davies providing labor support. Photo courtesy of Rae Davies

(5) Diagnosis and Healing from the Outside In and from the Inside Out

Where the technomedical model emphasizes diagnosis and healing from the outside in, and the holistic model from the inside out, the humanistic model calls for a moderate application of both approaches. The physician–patient communication it emphasizes allows physicians to elicit information from deep within the patient and combine it with objective findings. Accordingly, humanists find that *how to listen* is as important as knowing what to

say. Listening skills are crucial for obtaining the correct mix of data required for diagnosis.

Noting that a clinician will perform from 120,000 to 160,000 interviews during a career, Smith (1996) pointed out that the technomedical model teaches students to elicit symptoms of disease using a "doctor-centered" interviewing process. The physician elicits many bits of nonpersonal data, starting with the patient's chief complaint, then synthesizes them into a description of the patient's disease. But humanistic doctors know that the presenting complaint often masks an underlying problem. A woman complaining of fatigue, depression, and body aches may have lupus or may be despondent over a failed marriage. Practitioners must adopt an open-ended learning approach in order to create the space and time necessary to bring forth the underlying dynamic.

This open-ended learning approach forms an important part of what Smith (1996) called the "patient-centered interview." Instead of asking a series of closed, rapid-fire questions, the physician simply encourages patients to express what is most important to them, which will usually come out as a combination of data about symptoms and personal information that may turn out to highly relevant to those symptoms, even if the patient at times appears to be rambling. Allowing patients to lead keeps their ideas and concerns paramount and enhances their sense of autonomy. The patient-centered interview can form an invaluable part of the humanistic physician's ability to be both technically competent and humanistically caring (Charon 2004).

(6) Balance between the Needs of the Institution and the Individual: Superficial vs. Deep Humanism

Humanism counterbalances technomedicine with a softer approach, which can be anything from a superficial overlay to profoundly alternative methods. It is *superficially humanistic* to decorate a technocratic labor room with pretty wallpaper and bed coverings—yet nevertheless important, as pretty environments do have a calming effect. (The experience of beauty releases endorphins in our systems.) But I once heard a hospital administrator in Brazil claim that his obstetric ward was now fully "humanized" because fathers had just begun to be allowed in, and I toured another hospital in Brazil that was quite beautiful and served excellent food yet had a cesarean rate of 99%. It is better to be superficially humanistic than not humanistic at all, but the limitations of superficial humanism are clear and reveal how easily coopted the humanistic paradigm can be—for example, some hospitals in various countries install Jacuzzis and advertise via enticing pictures that they offer water birth, yet those tubs are rarely actually allowed to be used. Thus I consider it essential to contrast superficial humanism with what I term *deep humanism*; it is deeply humanistic to provide women with flexible spaces in which they have room to move around as much as they like, to actually be in water if they wish, to eat and drink and labor as they choose.

Most medical institutions are designed to support and implement technocratic principles. These institutions are so highly regulated with respect to infection control, medical/surgical and nursing procedures, security, and liability that it is often not possible for one individual to effect significant change. So sometimes humanistically inclined physicians must content them-

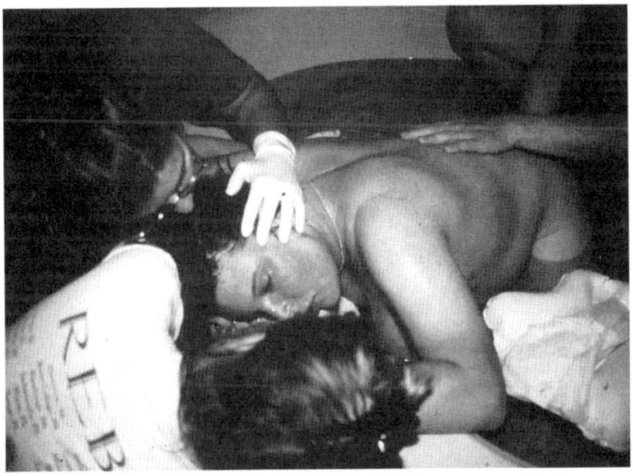

A deeply humanistic birth in a California hospital attended by nurse-midwives. This hands-and-knees position is ideal for normal birth as well as birth complications like a stuck shoulder or a breech baby, but is little used as it violates technocratic norms of appropriateness.

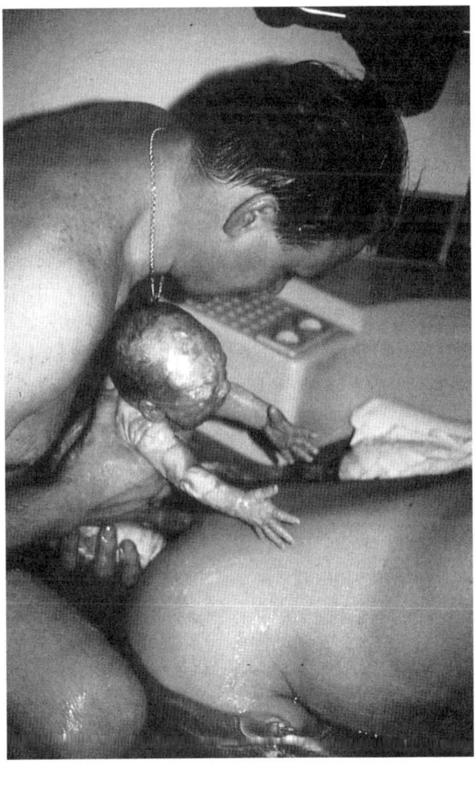

The birth outcome. The nurse-midwives stand by as the father receives the baby.

Photos by Mayri Sagady Leslie

selves with superficial improvements, but very often, committed individuals find they can do more. In the US, nurse-midwives have gained a reputation as the practitioners who try the hardest to provide deeply humanistic care within hospitals (see Davis-Floyd 2010; Rooks 1997; Wooten, Perry, and Crane 2004). Thus two humanistic changes often sought by childbirth activists include convincing hospitals to give women the right to choose midwives as their birth attendants and to have access to one-on-one doula care.

(7) Information, Decision Making, and Responsibility Shared between Patient and Practitioner

The poles between empowerment and dependence form the framework within which doctors and patients make decisions. Most health professionals are trained to bring linear information to bear in their decision making; in addition, the humanistic paradigm allows nonlinear, subjective processing to play a significant role. This is the balanced or empathic style of thinking. "Empathic" refers to the ability of one person to understand another's reality even if that reality is beyond his or her direct experience. When straightforward evidence of disease is present, doctors still have considerable latitude regarding how mutual they are willing to allow decision making to be. In the technocratic model, each situation seems to dictate a matching action. The humanistic model opens situations to multiple options.

The doctrine of informed consent and refusal establishes that patients have a right to understand their diagnosis and prognosis, their proposed treatment and its risks and benefits, and their treatment options, and to refuse some or all of them if they wish. In the technocratic model, the discussion of options outside of conventional medicine (including no treatment at all) is generally impossible due to the doctor's allegiance to technocratic approaches and ignorance of alternatives, making true informed consent impossible as patients are not given full information about the risks of the standardized procedures they may actively "choose." As Maureen May points out in *Epiduralized Birth* (2017), there can be no real choice when full information is not provided. For example, she quotes researchers Lieberman and O'Donoghue (2004:S64) as saying:

> Nulliparous women [meaning women who have not yet given birth] should be told that they are less likely to have a spontaneous vaginal delivery, that they are more likely to have an instrumental vaginal delivery, and that their labor is likely to be longer. They should also be informed of the implications of the higher rate of instrumental vaginal delivery [that accompanies the epidural], specifically the increased rate of serious perineal lacerations. . . . Women should also be informed of the higher rate of intrapartum fever [and] that if they develop a fever [because of the epidural], their infant may be more likely to . . . be treated with antibiotics for suspected sepsis.

And yet women are rarely, if ever, fully informed of such risks, which also include prolonged labor that will be augmented with pitocin, leading to a greater risk of cesarean delivery.

But in a fully humanistic approach, full and open discussion of treatment choices leads naturally to an exploration and sharing of values, and doctors are more likely to respond favorably or at least neutrally to a patient's wish to try alternative methods or to employ no treatments at all.

Arthur Kleinman (1988) expanded the notions of the patient's right to information and the "patient-centered interview" to a more dialogic approach. He suggested that the goal of the practitioner should be to enter into the experience of illness as patients perceive it by listening carefully to their narratives. To more deeply understand a patient's story, the physician can try to interpret the patient's symptoms as symbols of deeper life issues and to grasp the influence of the patient's cultural, personal, and family explanatory models. Like other humanistic and holistic physicians, Kleinman stresses the value and importance of the placebo effect, which can be activated purely through the strength of the physician–patient relationship *and thus should be tapped in every healing encounter.*

Medical sociologist Eliot Freidson (1967) asserted that the need for information is likely to result in conflict simply because a lay culture is encountering a professional culture at a moment of crisis. To balance this tension, the doctor needs to communicate trustworthiness to the patient so that the patient can accept or reject recommendations without feeling either bullied or negated. Although some physicians might fear liability with this level of information sharing, the Consensus Conference on Doctor-Patient Communication held in Toronto in 1992 found that *most lawsuits against doctors are the result of faulty communication rather than errors in medical judgment.*

(8) Science and Technology Counterbalanced with Humanism

Humanistic physicians take science as their standard and use virtually the same tools and techniques as technomedical doctors. The difference lies in timing and selection. Humanists may be more willing to wait, more apt to be conservative, more open to mind–body approaches. Humanists who are primary care doctors (family physicians, internists, pediatricians, gynecologists) may delay referring to a specialist and attempt to resolve a problem using more conservative methods, provided they have the consent of the patient to do so. Humanistic specialists will naturally be inclined to use the technology at their disposal but will emphasize caring and relationship alongside it, a combination John Naisbitt (1980) captured in the phrase "high tech, high touch."

As social scientist and midwife Maureen May (2017:244–245) points out:

> The American system of epiduralized birth will not change without a truly independent midwifery. Only independent midwifery will have the

> power and influence to carry out accurate, evidence-based informed consent . . . where women are told the unvarnished truth about the potential dangers of epidurals and pitocin, two interventions so central to our epiduralized births. This will not be easy. Modern obstetrics has convinced mothers, and themselves, that . . . totally painless childbirth through epiduralized birth is benign. Women will now be loath to hear otherwise. . . . We need to heed the call by Judith Rooks (2007) . . . that every maternity unit offer nitrous oxide for pain—a means of pain relief proven to be safe and used throughout developed countries other than the United States.

Nitrous oxide can be installed next to hospital beds and even can be used in birthing pools. It is a very effective and harmless method of pain relief, and empowering for women as they can use it when they please, on their own. As May points out, it *should* be widely available, yet is very rare in US hospitals (though quite common in Europe); American anesthesiologists don't like it because they can't control it or make any money from its use.

Poster created by Australian birth educator and activist Andrea Robertson showing the advantages of upright positions for birth, which allow gravity to help the mother push the baby out and widen the pelvic outlet and the birth canal.

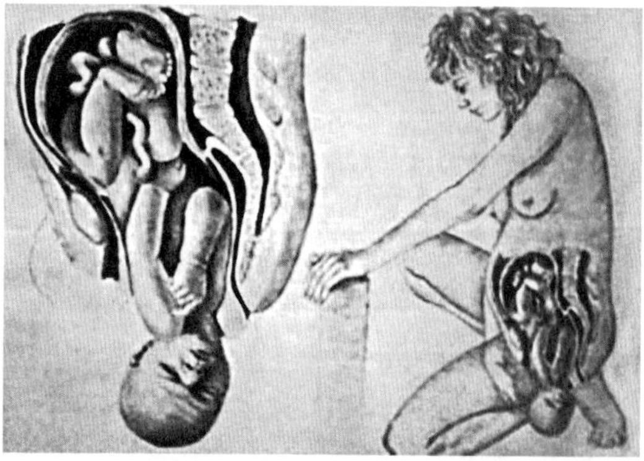

For the use of such technologies to be truly humanistic, they should be used at a patient's request or desire and their use should be soundly evidence-based. For example, epidural anesthesia can be considered a humanistic intervention because it takes away pain while allowing women to be "awake and aware." But there is nothing humanistic about forcing epidurals on women who don't want them. On the other side, how humanistic is it to allow women who arrive at the hospital demanding an epidural to have one in very early labor? A great deal of evidence now shows that if given before 6 cm dilation, epidurals can significantly slow labor because it is not yet fully established, but rather in what midwives call the "latent phase" of labor, which can take many hours or days before "active labor" (defined as beginning at 6 cm cervical dilation) is fully in progress. But when epidurals are given after 6 cm dilation, such problems are rare. Shockingly, a recent study shows that:

> In 2013, researchers published a report on 38,484 people who had their first Cesarean (primary Cesarean) in the United States during a six-year period. . . .[T]he Cesarean rate among people giving birth for the first time was 30.8%. . . . Nearly half (41.3%) of the Cesareans in first-time moms were due to Failure to Progress. This means that from 2002 to 2008, . . . (13%) of all first-time mothers in the U.S. had a Cesarean for Failure to Progress. (Boyle, Reddy et al. 2013)

> More than four in ten of the first-time mothers who had cesareans for "failure to progress" had not reached five cm dilation before they were taken to surgery (Boyle, Reddy et al. 2013). *Six cm is now considered the beginning of active labor, so this means that many of these people were still in very early labor (or maybe not truly in labor at all) when they were told that they weren't dilating fast enough.* (ACOG 2014; italics mine)

> A large number of pregnant people also have unplanned cesareans for failure to progress during medical inductions of labor. In a 2010 study that included 233,844 mothers who gave birth between 2002 and 2008, researchers found that half of all those induced who had cesareans for failure to progress had not reached six cm yet, indicating that *they were not yet in active labor when their inductions were labeled as "failed"* (Zhang et al., 2010b). (Dekker 2017; italics mine)

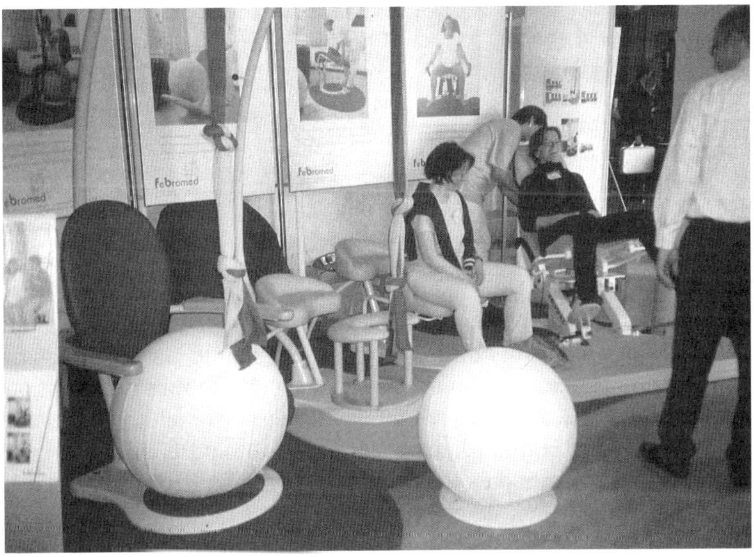

High-tech birthing stools and balls that ergonomically facilitate upright positions. A woman can even have an epidural and still utilize a ball or one of these birthing stools, as long as the tubing is long enough for her to get out of bed. The photo was taken in the Exhibit Hall at an International Confederation of Midwives conference.

Says birth activist Priya Morgenstern (personal communication), "All these women were told they were failing at something they hadn't yet been doing!!! It boggles the mind." And it follows logically that women who are not yet in active labor (6 cm) should not be admitted to the hospital, where the clock starts ticking the moment they enter. A holistic OB I interviewed some years ago noted that when he was Head of Ob/Gyn at his hospital in Louisiana, he instituted such a policy, and the cesarean rate was significantly reduced almost immediately, as there were no more cesareans performed for "failure to progress." Given that the latent stage of labor can take days, and the contractions can certainly feel like active labor, many women aware of this issue are hiring doulas, who can stay home with them to support them through the latent phase and help them to know when it is time to go in for their planned hospital birth. (Doulas are not allowed to physically check dilation, but there are many other ways by which they can tell when active labor kicks in.)

The Dekker 2017 study cited above is quite recent at this time of writing. Humanistic obstetricians and midwives work hard to evaluate these sorts of studies and to make decisions that reflect the balance between what science shows to work and the needs and desires of the women they attend.

A good example of counterbalancing science and technology with humanistic principles stems from a birth that occurred back in 1970 and described to me by midwife Faith Gibson in which an Asian woman laboring in a hospital supported by her husband and a doula rejected the delivery table

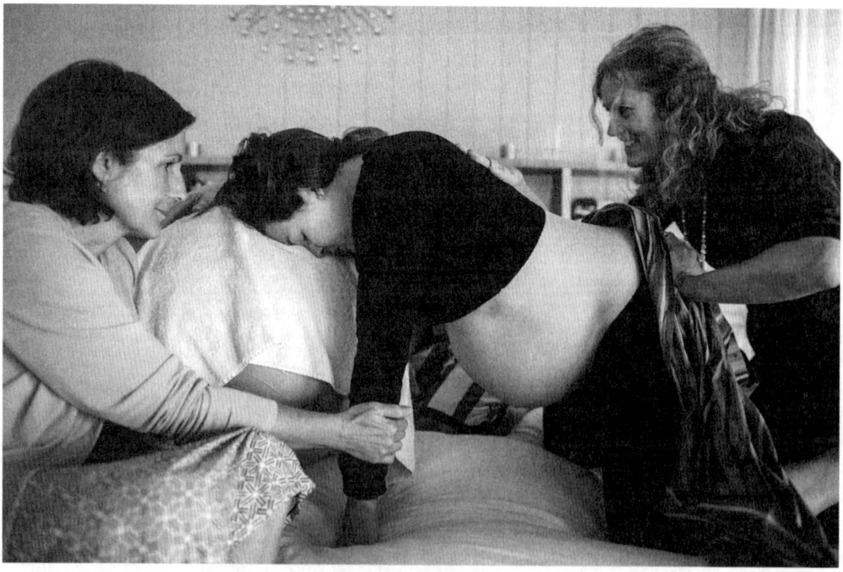

Full-on, full-bodied doula support. Photo by Monet Nicole

and asked to be allowed to give birth on the floor. The nurse-midwives attending her asked themselves what science truly demanded in that situation. The answer was that there was nothing scientific at all about giving birth flat on one's back on a delivery table; it was in fact much more evidence-based to give birth upright on the floor. What science did demand was a clean area for the delivery. So the midwives took the clean sheets off of the table and put them on the floor, and the woman, propped with pillows, cheerfully sat on top of them to give birth. In other words, ideally, humanistic care should be evidence-based care that reflects real science and not medical tradition—a reality that those CNMs figured out on their own long before upright births became more accepted in American hospitals.

(9) Focus on Disease Prevention: The Public Health Paradigm

Most proponents of humanism are also strong proponents of science-based public health initiatives that stress prevention and deal sensibly with the public environment. They point out that providing a village or a country with a clean water supply will do far more good for the health of far more people than building high-tech hospitals, as will ensuring clean air, adequate nutrition, and access to primary health care in the community. I cannot stress this point enough—*women want community-based care*; they do not wish to travel long distances, for example, for a simple prenatal exam or for birth, and so they often don't get the care they need if it is too hard and time-consuming to reach.

Prevention has been limited to the public health arena presumably because it does not turn a profit, unlike the sale of high-tech medical equipment and pharmaceuticals. No one benefits financially in any immediate sense when people stop smoking or begin drinking clean water, but a model in which compassion, not profit, is the driving force, has room for prevention and for social programs that reflect political agendas that protect the disenfranchised. Thus the *public health paradigm,* which stresses long-term, large-scale disease prevention and health promotion, corresponds closely to the humanistic paradigm, which stresses long-term biopsychosocial disease prevention and health promotion. In fact, humanists often leave private medical practice for work in the wider arena of public health. It is well worth noting here that developing countries often spend millions on building one or two high-tech hospitals that benefit only the few; whereas those millions could be spent to a much greater effect on the Number One primary health care intervention: providing a clean water supply.

The implications of this prevention-based approach in childbirth are enormous. True prevention of complications in childbirth would involve addressing the problems that lead to maternal and fetal deaths at their source. But often public health programs like the Safe Motherhood Initiative are heavily influenced by technomedical perspectives. Technomedicine identifies

hemorrhage, toxemia, anemia, and the like as the causes of maternal death, making it appear that problems inhere in individuals and should be treated on an individual basis, patient by patient, hospital by hospital. But the underlying causes of these problems, especially in low-resource countries, are the interrelated factors of poverty, poor nutrition, contaminated food and drinking water, the lower status of women, stress, and overwork. Initiatives that try to solve the problem of maternal mortality by building more hospitals and stocking them with more machines fail to address these core problems; instead, they perpetrate the agendas of technomedicine.

Both the public health paradigm and the humanistic model are compassion-driven; both focus on disease prevention, health promotion, and public education. The public health paradigm takes a broadscale, population-wide approach, while the humanistic model focuses more specifically on the individual relationships between family, patient, and provider and the effects of these relationships on illness prevention, diagnosis, and treatment.

(10) Death as an Acceptable Outcome

In childbirth, where death can arrive suddenly, the technocratic approach to the death of a baby is to whisk away the body, leaving the parents with empty arms. The humanistic way is to allow the parents all the time they need with that baby, so that the pain of death is not augmented by the pain of sudden separation. In the wider cultural arena, the humanistic approach to death is one of individual choice about the manner of dying. Individuals can sign living wills in advance, requesting that life-prolonging measures be limited. The hospice movement has brought death back into the home by supporting the dying individual and the family, not with major medical intervention but with the comfort of pain relief. This highly humanistic approach stems from a philosophy that profoundly honors a patient's individuality and freedom of choice. The process of conscious dying under both the humanistic and holistic paradigms becomes an opportunity to heal one's relationships with spouses, lovers, children, friends, oneself, and God (or a higher power). Grievances can be forgiven, old wounds mended, unmet needs and wishes fulfilled. In such cases, the death of an individual can provide tremendous opportunities for healing for families and entire communities.

(11) Compassion-Driven Care

Byron and Mary Jo Good (Good and Good 1993; Good 1995) suggested that the juxtaposed "central symbols" of *competence* and *caring* represent a cultural tension developed throughout medical education that is linked to a dualistic discourse characteristic of contemporary Western medicine. *Competence* is closely associated with the natural sciences and *caring* with the humanities. Competence is a quality of knowledge and skills, caring a quality of persons. They also note that this juxtaposition of competence and

caring, present throughout the history of Western medicine, reflects the larger struggle between science and culture, technology and humanism, which in the West are often seen as opposing forces.

It is precisely these contradictions that the humanistic approach to medicine seeks to resolve. Physicians faced with suffering are expected to process information quickly—to determine and implement a course of treatment. In technomedical circles, emotions are thought to interfere with such abilities. In both humanistic and holistic settings, feelings are accepted as part of the healing response. The driving ethos of the humanist is compassion—the ability to sense and feel the needs of others even if they are outside of one's own experience. When they sit down by a laboring woman's bed and breathe with her through a contraction, humanistic physicians are working to re-create a place in medicine for the human values of partnership, relationship, compassion, and caring. After decades of scientific research documenting the benefits of this humanistic approach, some technocratically trained physicians are allowing themselves to be human, letting go of the fear that others will think them weak and incompetent if they open themselves to their own feelings and learn skills for processing their patients' feelings without becoming emotionally overwhelmed (see Chapters 4, 5). Some find their comfort zone in *separating empathy from compassion*; too much empathy for their patients can indeed be emotionally overwhelming for the practitioner, while compassion should be a given in health care.

A different and very new approach has been adopted by Turkish obstetrician Hakkan Çoker, who has developed a model called "Birth with No Regret"; to his birth team of obstetrician and midwife/doula, he added a birth psychologist, Neşe Karabekir, who is responsible for working with the issues and emotions of the pregnant woman and her family, as well as the other members of the birth team. After every birth they attend, she helps them process their feelings about that birth; thus they are happy to empathize and engage emotionally with their patients, as they know that their own feelings will have room for expression as well. His model is gaining popularity in Turkey, which has a very high CS rate; it is spreading as fast as he and his team can teach it to others. (See his chapter in *Speaking Truth to Power: Birth Models on the Human Rights Frontier*, eds. Betty-Anne Daviss and Robbie Davis-Floyd forthcoming.)

(12) Open-Mindedness toward Other Modalities

Most humanists have no intention of learning alternative healing techniques, although in general they are open-minded and support patients who chose to use alternatives—as long as the overall treatment program includes conventional care. While many humanists adopt a sort of bemused tolerance to alternative modalities, some do advocate dietary and lifestyle changes that border on the holistic, and take a more proactive stance toward other healing

alternatives. Physicians in transition to humanism need not undergo any noticeable change in beliefs about what causes or cures disease. Simply being nicer, more caring, and more willing to touch and communicate repositions them in the humanistic model. Most will not undergo the radical shift in values that permits them to go beyond compassion to employ the healing power of that mysterious thing called "energy" in overcoming disease. This is the realm of the holistic healer.

The 12 Tenets of the Holistic Model of Medicine and Birth

The most scientific birth is often the least technological birth.
— Alice Dreger MD

If the technocratic model of medicine is the ruling hegemony, the holistic model of medicine is the ultimate heresy. Of the three paradigms I discuss, the holistic model encompasses the richest variety of approaches, ranging from nutritional therapy to traditional healing modalities such as Chinese medicine to various methods of directly affecting personal energy. Some holistic practitioners study a particular modality while others employ an eclectic approach, often of their own design. Holism often calls on individuals to be active, asking them to make major modifications in their lifestyles. It may also ask them to be passive, to simply receive prayer or a transfer of healing energy.

The term *holism* was adopted by some of the pioneers of this movement to express their inclusion of the mind, body, emotions, spirit, and environment of the patient in the healing process. The principles of connection and integration that underlie the holistic paradigm arise from the fluid, multimodal, right-brained thinking that, after centuries of devaluation in the West, has begun to regain lost ground (Eisler 1995). While the whole brain is involved in all brain functions, it is possible to say that the right hemisphere is predominantly involved in perceiving the *gestalt*, the whole. In contrast to the classifying and segmenting unimodal approach of left-brained, linear systems of thought, fluid thinkers use multimodal means of perception to apprehend the whole and to intuit the ever-shifting relationships of its parts. It is thinking of, with, and through the body and the spirit—holistic thinking, fluid thinking that transcends logical reasoning and rigid classifications in favor of what Starhawk (1989), one of its principal spokespersons, calls the "spiral dance." She means the spiral of the vortex, the tornado, the creative matrix in which things are tossed around and mixed up beyond any making sense. From the deep integrative chaos of this energy vortex arises the surprise—the unpredictable relationship, the unexpected connection, the revealing intuition—that so often constitutes a prime element of holistic healing.

(1) Oneness of Body-Mind-Spirit

Mind and body, wrought asunder by Cartesian rationalism, and reconnected in medical humanism, are re*united* in holistic medical care. The worst problem here is language: we are so used to speaking in terms of mind/body separation that even holistic healers find themselves still using the words "mind" and "body"; when they are careful, they will refer to the "bodymind" to indicate that it is all one entity. A large part of the initial impetus for the reuniting of mind and body in holistic healing was the dawning realization that the brain, the physical seat of the mind, is not located only in the head but in fact extends throughout the central nervous system. Understanding that the brain is distributed throughout the body makes it much harder to talk or think about body and mind as separate entities.

If the mind is the body, and the body is the mind, then how one responds to the treatment of even so mechanical a thing as a broken arm will have as much to do with how one thinks and feels about that broken arm, and why it got broken (was it a simple accident, or was the person unconsciously trying to harm himself to avoid taking an exam?) as about what kind of cast is put on it. In the holistic approach, addressing the psychological states and emotions of the pregnant or laboring woman is not just helpful, it is *the* essential aspect of care. Like humanists, holistic physicians are finding that they need much more engagement with the patient to get at those intangibles of mind and emotion now seen to be as much a part of the illness (or women's reactions to pregnancy and labor) as their physical manifestations.

The holistic paradigm also insists on the participation of the *spirit* in the human whole. In incorporating spirit or soul it into the healing process, holistic healers bring medicine back into the world of the spiritual and the metaphysical from which it was separated during the Industrial Revolution. The spirituality of today's holistic healers tends to be fluid and to take the form of a loose identification with Eastern, Buddhist, or New Age philosophies more often than with Judaism, Christianity, or Islam. Where the technomedical model is rigid and separatist, the holistic model recognizes no sharp divisions or distinct boundaries. This is another reason why holism is so threatening: in many people's minds, to trifle with boundaries is to invoke chaos. And indeed, chaos theory and systems theory both inform and underpin the holistic paradigm and its insistence on the oneness of body, mind, and spirit.

(2) The Body as an Energy System Interlinked with Other Energy Systems

The holistic paradigm moves far beyond the narrow view of the body-as-machine, past the humanistic view of the body as an organism, all the way to a limitless view of the body as energy. Defining the body as an energy system provides a powerful charter for the development and use of forms of medicine and treatment that work energetically—such as acupuncture, home-

"Calling the Baby"

A logical corollary of the introduction of spirit into the healing equation is the understanding that the baby is a conscious being with a spirit or soul of its own, and who can remember its own birth (Chamberlain 1998; and see the website of the Association for Pre- and Perinatal Psychology and Health). That line of reasoning leads to the conclusion that if a baby is born and doesn't immediately breathe, perhaps its soul is hesitating on the threshold, trying to decide whether to come into its body or not. Once at a conference of the American Holistic Medical Association, I was approached by a maternal-fetal medicine specialist (perinatologist) who kindly asked me, because he was worried about it, what homebirth midwives do when a baby is born and not breathing. I reassured him that all homebirth midwives are trained in neonatal resuscitation, but, wanting to give him something more, I told him that homebirth midwives also often ask the parents to "call the baby"—to invite its spirit to come through by speaking loving words and asking it to breathe—an example of what homebirth midwife Janneli Miller calls "midwives' magical speech." (1) This does no harm; (2) It gives the parents an empowering role to play in this life-or-death scenario; and (3) It just might work! He thanked me gratefully, later talking to some CNMs at the conference who assured him that they also have the parents call the baby. Some months later I received a letter from him telling me that ever since he had started to ask the parents to call the baby the second he walked into the room, by the time he was ready to resuscitate, the baby had pinked up and started breathing on its own. Again, if spirit exists, as proponents of the holistic model insist that it does, why not use it for healing in any way you can?

opathy, intuitive diagnosis, Reiki, hands-on healing, magnetic field therapy, and therapeutic touch. "Energy medicine" acknowledges the possibilities that an individual's health can be influenced by such subtleties as the vibrations of anger or hostility or the electromagnetic fields created by power plants and microwaves. Today's physicists relish documenting the vanishing frontier between matter and energy. Medical research would require complete restructuring if it accepted such conclusions from other disciplines. For example, while medicine hotly refutes the impact of the investigator on research, physics recognizes the Heisenberg Principle, which acknowledges the influence of the observer on the observed. Even the intentionality of the experimenter can profoundly affect the outcome of an experiment (Wiseman and Schlitz 1996). How can an observer separate from the observed phenomenon affect its behavior? Acceptance of this second tenet answers this question: the observer and the observed are not separate, but are energy fields in constant interaction with each other.

Many midwives I have studied in the US define themselves as holistic and consciously seek to work with what they call "birth energy" (see Gaskin 2002 [1975]). Indeed, they believe that the primary intervention a midwife can make is at the energetic level. Intervening to "redirect the energies" can ensure that no other type of intervention will be needed. If a labor stalls and a cesarean seems imminent, a midwife or doula who has a feel for the power of energy may throw open the window, put on some music, and get the mother up to dance. Or she might leave the room to allow the birthing couple some privacy, so that the loving energy of their relationship can infuse the birth experience. (Nipple and clitoral stimulation are great ways to augment labor naturally. If they bring on an orgasm, so much the better—orgasms, after all, release oxytocin ["the hormone of love"] and consist in part of strong contractions of the uterus.) The important point is that for the practitioner who works at the level of energy, these sorts of interventions will not be after-

A Short Story about Energy

A cardiologist I interviewed back in 1997 didn't believe that "energy" was anything more than what you got when you plugged something into a wall socket. Yet his oldest daughter had become an "energy healer." To finally resolve their endless arguments, he agreed to attend her energy healer group "just once." As he lay on a high table surrounded by healers laying hands on him, he had the experience of his body as pure white light. Assimilating new information requires time and effort. So he could have just rejected that experience as "brainwashing" or the like; but instead he took that time and made that effort, sitting on a park bench reliving and thus cognitively assimilating that experience as real, during which new neural networks evolved in his brain. A day or two later, while dealing with a woman's cardiac arrest, he first made sure the team was operating properly. Then he quietly stood behind the woman's head and laid his hands on her, sending her energy in the form of white light. The next day he stopped by her hospital room to see how she was doing. Upon seeing him, she exclaimed, "You're the one who saved my life!" He told her it was impossible for her to know that, as she had been unconscious the whole time he was with her. She contradicted him, saying, "No, I saw and felt you lay hands on my head and I saw the white light coming out of them. It was like I was out of my body and I could see everyone and everything in the room. You are definitely the man who saved me! I am so grateful!" Completely blown away, he joined his daughter's energy healer group and continues to practice that kind of healing today whenever possible in his work as a cardiologist.

thoughts or overlays but will be basic and primary—the first line of care. *If you intervene at the level of energy, you will most likely not need to intervene at the level of technology.*

(3) Healing the Whole Person in Whole-Life Context

This tenet of the holistic model of medicine, a logical corollary of the first two, acknowledges that no single explanation of a diagnosis, no single drug or therapeutic approach, will sufficiently address an individual's health problems; rather, such problems must be addressed in terms of the whole persons and the whole environments in which they live. It is no accident that the most commonly asked question in holistic health is "What's going on in your life?" This question expresses the holistic view that illness is a manifestation of imbalance in the bodymindspirit whole. Here holism accepts to the fullest findings from psychoneuroimmunology and other fields that the immune system, or the process of pregnancy and birth, can be impeded by exhaustion, depression, emotional stress, the loss of a loved one, toxins in the air and the water, and the stresses of technocratic life. The corollary of this view, of course, is that a healthy immune system, as well as a healthy pregnancy and birth, can be facilitated by multiple means, from dialogue to dream analysis to dance, from massage to exercise to organic food.

(4) Essential Unity of Practitioner and Client

Many holistic practitioners try to drop the word "patient" in favor of "client," as this term implies a mutually cooperative, egalitarian relationship. Where the humanistic model emphasizes the value of a mutually respectful connection between practitioner and client, still essentially separate and distinct beings, the holistic model offers the possibility that they are not separate but are fundamentally one. If the body is an energy field, then as they interact the energy fields of client and practitioner can merge, resulting in what some holistic practitioners call "intuitive diagnosis"—diagnosing the problem via shared intuition with the client (Davis-Floyd and St. John 1998). Seeking this merging of energy fields, some of the holistic physicians I have interviewed will actually ask their clients, especially those who seem overwrought, to do a breathing exercise with them for around 10 minutes to "synchronize their energies."

(5) Diagnosis and Healing from the Inside Out

While they may, if appropriate, order "outside-in" diagnostic tests, holistic practitioners will primarily diagnose and treat from the inside out—in other words, they will rely to a significant extent on the knowledge that arises from their own intuition, just as they will trust the inner knowing of their clients. Intuition is defined by the third edition of the *American Heritage Dictionary* as "the act or faculty of knowing or sensing without the use of rational processes; immediate cognition." The knowledge on the basis of which decisions are made and actions taken is defined as "authoritative knowledge" (Jordan 1993). Technomedical practitioners tend to regard textbooks, diagnostic tests, and the advice of experts as authoritative, and to dismiss the still, small voice of intuition. But holistic practitioners (like some humanists) tend to regard intuition as a primary source of authoritative knowledge, along with the books and the machines. Thus, in holistic practice, "diagnosis and healing from the inside out" can refer to the information that arises from deep inside both patient and physician—a phenomenon explained at its core by their essential unity. Midwives often consider intuition to be a primary source of knowledge about pregnancy and birth, as do all the holistic obstetricians I have interviewed (Davis-Floyd and St. John 1998; Chapters 5 and 7, this volume). Their willingness to rely on intuition comes from their deep understanding of the body as energy and their trust in right-brained, gestaltic thinking that do not rely on logic but on that sudden flash of insight from which unity and healing can arise.

(6) Individualization of Care

Holistic physicians are trained in technomedicine and have seen the damage standardized hospital policies and hierarchies can do to individuals. In general, they do their best to respond to the individuality and unique needs of each patient within the constraints imposed on them by hospital and legal regulations. For the laboring woman, individualization of care means that standardization does not apply. Her labor is uniquely her own. She eats and drinks and moves about at will. She gives birth in the place of her choice attended by the people and practitioners of her choice. And the practitioner does not respond to the variations in her labor in standardized ways. A midwife dealing with a stalled labor might invite one woman to dance, might ask another if she is afraid to give birth, and might

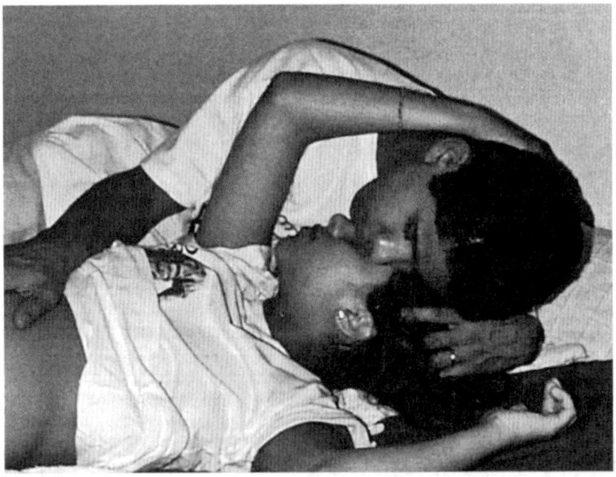

The best-kept secret: Sexual contact between the birthing woman and her partner is one of the best and most fun ways to labor. Kissing, nipple and clitoral stimulation, even to the point of bringing on orgasm, will greatly enhance the flow of hormones (oxytocin, endorphins), bring more pleasure to the experience, increase intimacy for the couple, and increase the power of the contractions to bring the baby more quickly. Photo by Ricardo Jones

suggest a long walk to a third, or a lovemaking session with her partner to get the oxytocin (again, the natural hormone generated in women's bodies during sexual intercourse, birth, and breastfeeding) flowing.

Intuition may guide the midwife to respond to individual circumstances in individual ways. The focus stays on the birthing woman. It is *her* unique needs and rhythms that will be paramount in the unfolding of her birth.

The unexpected twists that can result from holism's high value on both individualization and interconnectedness are suggested in the theory of self-organizing systems (Wheatley 1992), which states that even the smallest event, if it happens in just the right place at just the right time, can dramatically alter the whole system. Holistic healers try not to make assumptions about cause and effect. They tend to expect the unexpected and to be prepared for healing to arise in strange places and mysterious ways. A chance remark can instantly transform a woman's perception of her condition and become the foundation of a cure.

A personal example: A few days after I gave birth at home to my second child, and home alone with both children for the first time, I started feeling overwhelmed—how to generate so much love for two little beings now? I was so tired, and I felt so inadequate. A visit from my best friend, holistic healer Rima Star, solved my problem when she said, "But you don't have to generate love from inside yourself! The universe *is* love. All you have to do is open up and channel that love that is everywhere around you." I got it, opened myself, and felt the love flow through me effortlessly. A psychological issue that could have resulted in postpartum depression was resolved in an instant. Holistic healers know better than to assume they are the ones who heal the patient. They know that any one of myriad interactions over which they have no control can spark a healing process. Their genius lies in their ability to recognize that tiny flame when it is lit and help it to glow more brightly instead of extinguishing it.

(7) Authority and Responsibility Inherent in the Individual

> *Choice is an illusion in the absence of knowledge.*
> — Maureen May

A basic tenet of holistic healing is that ultimately, individuals must take responsibility for their own health and well-being. No one can really heal anyone else; individuals must decide for themselves if they want to be healed, and if so, they must take action to achieve that goal—give up smoking, exercise, eat right, maybe even let go of a lucrative job that makes them unhappy or a relationship that is harmful to their health. Holistic practitioners in general tend to see themselves as part of a healing team, of which the patient is a full-fledged, indeed the most significant, member. Many of my holistic interviewees repeatedly expressed their frustration with patients who refused to take responsibility for their own health. They may greet the new client prepared to offer her empowerment, full participation in decision making, informed choices, and so on, yet the patient may want only to be handed a prescription and told how many pills to take, or to schedule her cesarean between conference calls (Davis-Floyd and St. John 1998; Chapter 3). Although some interviewees refuse to revert to the hierarchical mode and may refer such patients to another MD, most accept and work with the patient's desire to place the physician in charge, or try to re-educate clients to take back the authority and responsibility they have surrendered.

(8) Science and Technology Placed at the Service of the Individual

If the technocratic model of medicine can be snappily characterized as "high-tech/low-touch," and the humanistic model as "high-tech/high-touch," then it would seem to follow logically that the holistic model of medicine would be "low-tech/high-touch." Sometimes this is true, as in the case of hands-on energy work, nutritional medicine, and herbal therapies—healing modalities for which few technological artifacts are used.

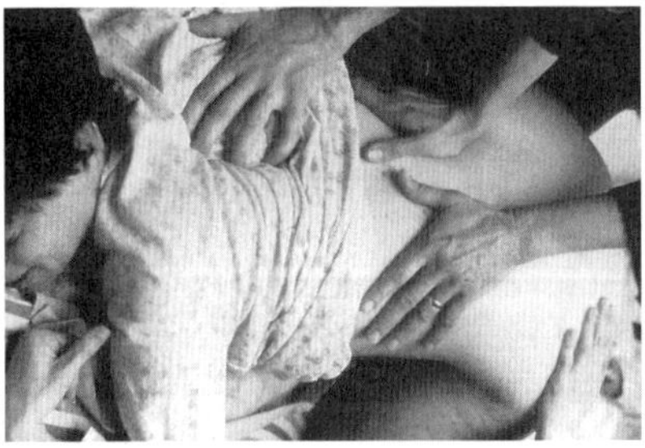

Low-tech, high-touch hands-on labor support. Photo by Mary Kroeger

Yet holistic healing can and often does incorporate high technology, from biofeedback machines to lab tests and diagnostic computers. Holistic healers in general do not reject technology; rather, they place it at the service of their clients, instead of allowing the technologies of health care to dominate, intimidate, and lay the ground rules for treatment. Usually these technologies are not invasive, nor do they produce the toxic effects of many of the technologies of conventional medicine. In childbirth, they range from administering oxygen to a laboring woman in need of extra energy, to birth balls that facilitate changes in position, to Jacuzzis with overhead ropes to pull on as the woman bears down. Such technologies do not dominate and control; rather, they work with physiology to empower the woman to give birth.

And what of science? As we have seen, physicians are reluctant to change many commonly used procedures even when evidence reveals them to be inappropriate. French physician Michel Odent, a world leader in holistic childbirth, often notes that "science will save us." He is referring to the trend in Western obstetrics toward evidence-based care. If obstetric care in most hospitals were to become truly evidence-based, then most standard interventions, including routine IVs, routine use of pitocin, and the lithotomy position would have to be eliminated; women would eat, drink, and move about freely during

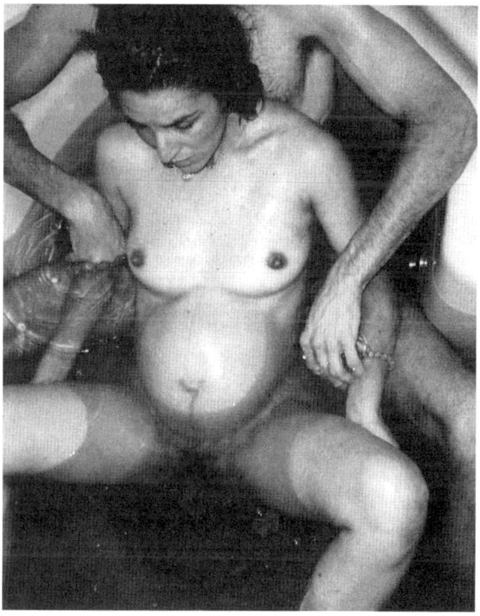

Science and technology combining to facilitate a holistic water birth in a Brazilian hospital. Upright positions are evidence-based, and high technologies (such as pipes and electricity) have allowed the tub to fill with hot water. But the technologies merely support, not dominate, the birth process. Photo by Brazilian obstetrician Adailton Salvatore

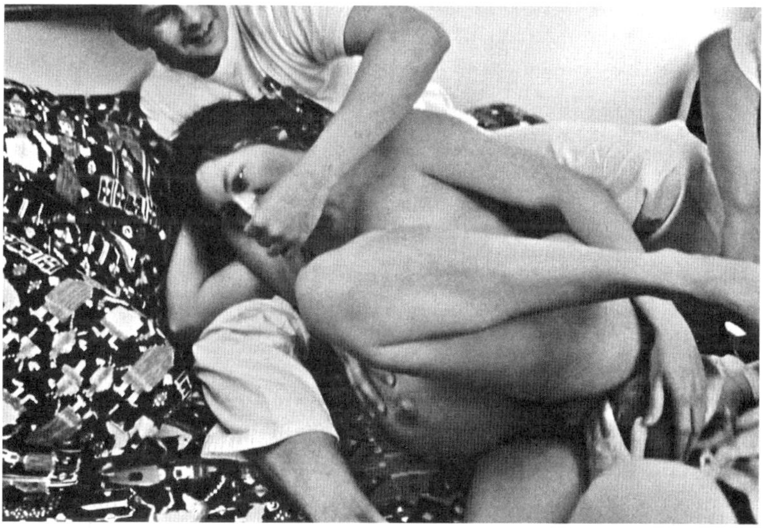

Side-lying during my holistic homebirth in Austin, Texas, 1984. I was exhausted from a long labor so the midwives asked my husband Robert to hold the oxygen mask for me to give me more energy during pushing. I found this to be an extremely empowering use of technology that facilitated my ability to give birth vaginally to a 10-pound baby after a previous cesarean. Note that both I and my midwife have our hands on the baby's head—the midwife had said, "Reach your hand down—you can welcome your baby!" I can still vividly recall the sensation of my baby's head in my hand—it gave me the strength I needed for that final push. Photo by Peter Gonzalez labor; and they would give birth in side-lying, or upright sitting or squatting positions (Bryers, MacKenzie, and Van Teijlingen 2010; Enkin et al. 2000; Goer 1995, 1999; Rooks 1997; Walsh 2007).

(9) A Long-Term Focus on Creating and Maintaining Health and Well-Being

Technocratic physicians often express extreme frustration over the patient's failure to follow doctor's orders. In contrast, holistic physicians most frequently voice frustration over patients who make no long-term commitment to improving their health but want the doctor to provide them with a quick fix and let them get on with their lives as before. Quick fixes are poor substitutes for long-term lifestyle changes that can maintain good health. Holistic practitioners want their clients to make long-term changes in their diets and lifestyles that will not simply prevent illness but will actively generate good health. Giving up sugar, caffeine, and processed foods and taking vitamin supplements, eating nutrient-rich organic vegetables, exercising regularly, and dealing with stress through meditation are examples of the kinds of long-term changes that are often necessary to the creation of wellness. Holistic obstetric practitioners know that pregnancy is an important time to be making such changes, not only for the health of the baby but also to ensure the long-term health of the mother. The problem is of course that many people are resistant to such long-term lifestyle alterations. Holistic practitioners must engage in a great deal of client education, and must maintain a great deal of patience, in order to support people in making this kind of change.

(10) Death as a Step in a Process

Beyond the humanistic view of death as "the final stage of growth" lies the holistic paradigm's redefinition of death not as any kind of final end but as an essential step in the process of living. This view stems from holists' definition of the body as an energy field, and from their deep-seated understanding of the transmutable nature of energy. Because of their integrated views on the essential oneness of body, mind, and spirit, it is only at the moment of death that holists grant these a conceptual separation. At death, in this view, the energy of the body decays and returns to earth, while the energy of the spirit or the individual consciousness continues on. Most holists seem to accept some version of Eastern philosophies of reincarnation, a processual view that allows the interpretation of death as an opportunity for continued growth into a new kind of life in spirit and then again in flesh. While this positive view of death does not lead holists to rush to embrace death, it does tend to give them a strong sense of trust in the essential safety of the universe and in the wisdom and worth of its ways.

Abortion as Death or New Life: A Side Story

Some years ago I conducted a brief study of the differences in abortion views held by New-Age mothers and fundamentalist Christian ministers (Davis-Floyd 2000). The ministers saw abortion as baby-killing and thought it immoral and wrong. The New-Agers believed that only the body died—the spirit of the child simply went back through the gateway to be reborn to someone else at some future time. When I explained this view to the curious ministers, who had asked me to do so, they were astonished; one exclaimed, "Well, that is a legitimate religious belief—I am going to have to rethink this whole issue to try to see it from their point of view."

(11) Healing as the Focus

To say that the holistic model focuses on healing instead of on profit is not to dismiss the role of money and the practitioner's need to make a livelihood within the system. Holistic practitioners have strong views about money—both for themselves and as part of their professional identity. While they are conscious of the need to earn a living, that need *follows* their personal commitment to work rather than drives it. Few of the holistic physicians I have interviewed practiced within the framework of managed care, for example, where medicine and money are strongly affiliated. Only a few were on staffs of hospitals, where major health expenses are incurred, and virtually none were members of organized medicine (as exemplified by the American Medical Association and its regional counterparts). Many belonged instead to the American Holistic Medical Association (AHMA).

Recognizing that healing occurs not in response to their actions but in the support and stimulation of the vital force, in the exchange of energy between individuals, or in the long, slow progress toward health that often rewards major lifestyle changes, holistic doctors are keenly aware of their partnership with patients. Money is part of this exchange. Unlike doctors who practice technomedicine and are apt to live stressful and harried lives wherein they are unable to care for themselves adequately, holistic doctors tend to find that their own healing often accompanies that of their patients, as it is practically impossible to espouse a holistic philosophy without applying it to oneself. In the mutual appreciation that often arises between holistic doctor and patient, a deep experience of *value* replaces the physician's focus on money (Davis-Floyd and St. John 1998; Chapter 5). Thus holistic MDs tend to make less money than their more technocratic colleagues, yet count themselves happier for the healing rewards they and their patients' experience.

(12) Embracing Multiple Healing Modalities

As we have seen, the holistic paradigm's definition of the body as an energy field in constant interaction with other energy fields makes possible its embrace of multiple modalities that remain unacceptable to proponents of the technomedical paradigm. The ultimate holistic vision entails a profound revolution in health care. Were this paradigm to gain cultural ascendance, the dominance of the technocratic model would be replaced with the cultural valuation of a multiplicity of approaches. Midwifery, homeopathy, naturopathy, acupuncture, and other approaches to well-being would take their places as respected and legitimate disciplines, as indeed they have increasingly been doing. Practitioners of each modality would know enough about the others for appropriate referral. Above all, the public would be educated in the techniques of self-care, a healthy lifestyle, and the appropriate use of a variety of approaches to healing.

Holistic medicine's embrace of multiple healing modalities is gaining growing public attention and acceptance. The clearest evidence for this statement comes from a study that determined that one-third of Americans sought the services of a non-MD practitioner in a one-year time period—and paid out of pocket for three-quarters of the cost of these services (Eisenberg at al 1993; Eisenberg et al. 1998; see also Barnes, Bloom, and Nahin 2008; Harris et al. 2012; Hunt et al. 2010). Another finding of this survey was that 72% of the maverick patients did not tell their doctors about their use of alternative medicine. Perhaps the center stage given to this study reflects the financial impact on medicine it uncovered, as well as the finding that the users of non-conventional therapies were well educated, middle-income whites, 25–49 years of age—a prime market set for orthodox medicine.

Stratified Holism and the Limitations of a Focus on the Individual

The notion that authority and responsibility for health inheres in the individual is useful for thinking about the health care of the middle and upper classes. But the poor often do not have the luxury of choosing their diet, their job, or their lifestyle. Nor can they afford the many options presented by holistic healers, as these are usually not covered by private or government insurance systems. A huge limitation of holistic healing has been its confinement to the wealthier segments of society and its almost total unavailability to the poor—a sort of "stratified holism"—a term I am coining to index the embeddedness of holistic practices within the structural context of the middle- and upper-classes (just as the widely-known term "stratified reproduction" [Ginsburg and Rapp 1995] indexes the availability of many reproductive

The Technocratic, Humanistic, and Holistic Models of Medicine

The Technocratic Model of Medicine	The Humanistic (Biopsychosocial) Model of Medicine	The Holistic Model of Medicine
1. Mind/body separation	1. Mind-body connection	1. Oneness of bodymindspirit
2. The body as machine	2. The body as an organism	2. The body as an energy system interlinked with other energy systems
3. The patient as object	3. The patient as relational subject	3. Healing the whole person in whole-life context
4. Alienation of practitioner from patient	4. Connection and caring between practitioner and patient	4. Essential unity of practitioner and client
5. Diagnosis and treatment from the outside in (curing disease, repairing dysfunction)	5. Diagnosis and healing from the outside in and from the inside out	5. Diagnosis and healing from the inside out
6. Hierarchical organization and standardization of care	6. Balance between the needs of the institution and the individual	6. Lateral, networking organizational structure that facilitates individualization of care
7. Authority and responsibility inherent in practitioner, not patient	7. Information, decision making, and responsibility shared between patient and practitioner	7. Authority and responsibility inherent in each individual
8. Supervaluation of science and technology	8. Science and technology counterbalanced with humanism	8. Science and technology placed at the service of the individual
9. Aggressive intervention with emphasis on short-term results	9. A long-term focus on disease prevention	9. A long-term focus on creating and maintaining health and wellbeing
10. Death as defeat	10. Death as an acceptable outcome	10. Death as a step in a process
11. A profit-driven system	11. Compassion-driven care	11. Healing as the focus
12. Intolerance of other modalities	12. Open-mindedness toward other modalities	12. Embrace of multiple healing modalities
Basic underlying principle: separation	Basic underlying principles: balance and connection	Basic underlying principles: Connection and integration
Type of thinking: unimodal, left-brained, linear	Type of thinking: bimodal	Type of thinking: Fluid, multimodal, right-brained

options to the wealthy and very few to the poor). Perhaps the greatest challenge confronting proponents of holism is to make their services more financially accessible: it will take a global paradigm shift of epic proportions in order for governmental and private insurance systems in all countries to cover multiple forms of care. But this is the ultimate holistic vision: that allopathic hegemony would be replaced with systems in which all modalities would be equally accessible to all people.

It is of course worth pointing out that biomedicine is heavily stratified as well, in socioeconomic, racial, ethnic, and gendered terms, and that its positive effects would be greatly enhanced by wider accessibility to all. From a cross-cultural point of view, both the technocratic and the holistic paradigms are limited by their focus on the care of the individual. In contrast, social science research in countries with the highest maternal mortality rates (e.g., sub-Saharan Africa) highlights the general poor health of women, who in many patriarchal societies suffer from overwork, exhaustion, anemia, malnutrition, and a variety of diseases resulting from polluted water, showing that, as noted above, the most important interventions required for improving women's health and for increasing safety in birth are clean water, adequate nutrition, and improved educational and economic opportunities for women. Such issues *are* addressed within the humanistic paradigm, which is closely related to the public health approach, which encompasses an emphasis on the socio-structural issues that generate illness and on wide-scale disease prevention and cure.

Functional Medicine: A Brief Note

In recent years many practitioners, aware of the cultural views of "holistic" or "integrative" or "energy" medicine as "New-Agey" or "airy-fairy," have switched to using the term "functional medicine" instead. As explained on the website of the Institute for Functional Medicine:

> Functional medicine addresses the underlying causes of disease, using a systems-oriented approach and engaging both patient and practitioner in a therapeutic partnership. It is an evolution in the practice of medicine that better addresses the healthcare needs of the 21st century. By shifting the traditional disease-centered focus of medical practice to a more patient-centered approach, functional medicine addresses the whole person, not just an isolated set of symptoms. Functional medicine practitioners spend time with their patients, listening to their histories and looking at the interactions among genetic, environmental, and lifestyle factors that can influence long-term health and complex, chronic disease. In this way, functional medicine supports the unique expression of health and vitality for each individual. (https://www.functionalmedicine.org/about/whatisfm/)

In my terms, functional medicine combines elements of both the humanistic and holistic models and may in the future replace these terms as the number of its practitioners continues to grow. In fact, a number of my physician interviewees who formerly called themselves holistic practitioners now use the "functional medicine" label instead, presenting widely on that topic at conferences and fine-tuning the model in their daily practices.

The Importance of Ideology: Why Paradigms Matter

The importance of ideology was definitively demonstrated by a systematic review of 137 reports on factors influencing women's evaluations of their childbirth experiences carried out in 2002 by Ellen Hodnett. Her objective was to summarize what is known about satisfaction with childbirth, with particular attention to the roles of pain and pain relief. The reports in Hodnett's review included descriptive studies, randomized controlled trials, and reviews of intrapartum interventions. The results were as follows:

> Four factors—personal expectations, the amount of support from caregivers, the quality of the caregiver-patient relationship, and involvement in decision making—appear to be so important that they override the influences of age, socioeconomic status, ethnicity, childbirth preparation, the physical birth environment, pain, immobility, medical interventions, and continuity of care, when women evaluate their childbirth experiences. (Hodnett 2002a:S171)

The review's conclusion was: "*The influences of pain, pain relief, and intrapartum medical interventions on subsequent satisfaction are neither as obvious, as direct, nor as powerful as the influences of the attitudes and behaviors of the caregivers*" (italics mine). Attitudes and behaviors stem from particular philosophies/paradigms that form the template for the caregiver's beliefs about birth. In other words, it's the model behind the model of practice that most determines the kind of care a practitioner will provide.

As a society's medical system mirrors its core values in microcosm, so the evolution of medicine can influence the evolution of the wider culture. We must ask, Who do we want to make ourselves become through the kinds of health care we create? Contemporary obstetric practitioners have a unique opportunity to weave together elements of each paradigm, including the wide-scale public health emphasis of the humanistic model, to create the most effective system of care ever designed on this planet. Information is available about indigenous childbirth practices from many cultures, some of which (such as massage, certain hand maneuvers, and upright positions for birth) are highly beneficial and should be incorporated. More information than ever is available from scientific studies that tell us much of what we need to know about the physiology of birth and the kinds of care that truly support women

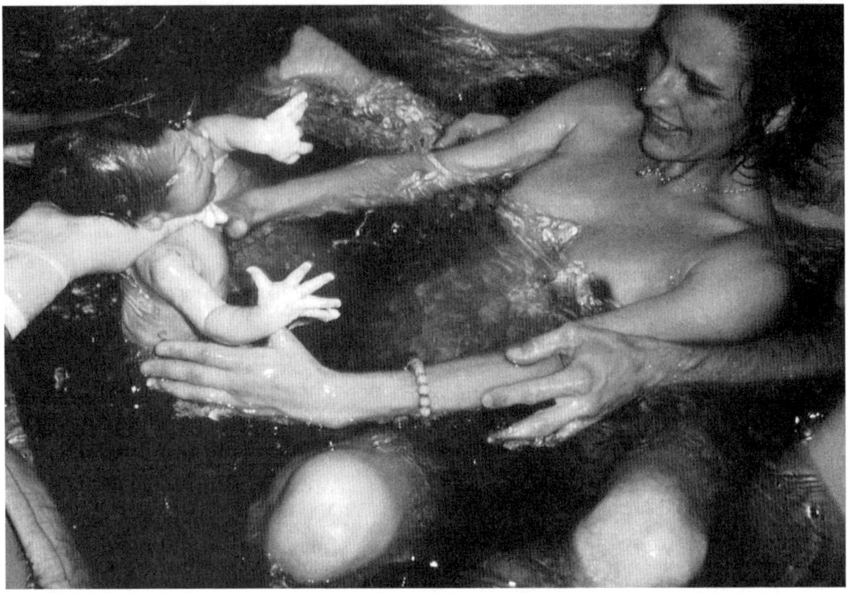

The paradigm-combining outcome of the previously shown water labor in a Brazilian hospital, as science (which supports water birth), technology (the tub), and holism work in sync to facilitate this birth. Photo by Adailton Salvatore

to give birth. And technologies exist to support every kind of labor choice. If we could apply appropriate technologies, in combination with what science shows us actually works, the values of humanism, the wide-seeing vision of the public health paradigm, and the spontaneous openness to individuality and energy chartered by holism, we could in fact create the best maternity care system the world has ever known. This is the challenge I offer![1]

Questions for Thought and Discussion

1. How is the body defined in the three paradigms described in this chapter?
2. What are the implications for treatment of these bodily definitions?
3. What is the difference between superficial and deep humanism in the treatment of labor and birth and why does it matter?

[1] And indeed some practitioners around the world have done just that. We describe their outstanding, evidence-based, and functional models in *Birth Models That Work* (Davis-Floyd et al. 2009), *Speaking Truth to Power: Birth Models on the Human Rights Frontier* (Daviss and Davis-Floyd forthcoming), and *Sustainable Birth* (Gutshow, Daviss, and Davis-Floyd forthcoming); see also Chapter 5, this volume. And we hope to see the development of many more such models in future years.

Recommended Films

Born in the USA: produced by Marcia Jarmel and Ken Schneider, 2000. This film shows a technocratic hospital birth, a humanistic birth in a birth center, and a holistic homebirth, so is a perfect complement to this chapter. www.patchworkfilms.net; https://www.fandor.com/films/born_in_the_usa; https://www.youtube.com/watch?v=krnoLMz1a18; http://www.imdb.com/title/tt3670708/. Students can be asked to identify which elements of each paradigm are identifiable in this film, as well as in the other films recommended for subsequent chapters.

Laboring Under an Illusion: Mass Media Childbirth vs. The Real Thing: produced by Vicki Elson, 2009. A documentary showing over 100 video clips of "media-generated myths about childbirth," illustrating how culture affects our birth experiences. www.birth-media.com

Why Not Home? The Surprising Birth Choices of Doctors and Nurses: producer/director Jessica Moore. This film focuses on hospital birth providers who choose homebirth with the goal of moving toward improvements to maternity care in hospitals and at home. A list of screenings is available at http://www.whynothome.com/

Microbirth: a 60-minute documentary exploring the latest scientific research into the microscopic events that occur during childbirth and strongly affect the baby's "microbiome"—the bacteria that colonize its gut and body as it travels through the birth canal and that can have life-long consequences for the baby's health and potentially impact the future of mankind. Winner of the Grand Prix award at the Life Sciences Film Festival in 2014, the film features leading world experts including Martin Blazer and Maria Gloria Dominguez Bello. Available at https://vimeo.com/ondemand/microbirthfilm

2

The Rituals of Hospital Birth

Enacting and Transmitting the Technocratic Model

The overwhelming use of epidurals for pain relief, and the inevitable augmentation of labor with pitocin that accompanies it, has cemented a mechanized and routinized system of childbirth that is now conceived of as normal.
— Maureen May, *Epiduralized Birth and Nurse-Midwifery*

Why is childbirth, which is a unique and individual experience for every woman, treated in such a highly standardized way in the United States (and around the world)? No matter how long or short, how easy or hard their labors, the vast majority of American women are hooked up to an electronic fetal monitor and an IV, are encouraged to use pain-relieving drugs, most often an epidural, and give birth flat on their backs in the lithotomy position.[1] Approximately one-third of them also receive doses of the synthetic hormone

[1] Semi-sitting positions are increasingly common in American birth, though not in developing countries—a welcome humanistic improvement, yet still with the disadvantage that most of the mother's body weight is on her pelvis, which does not allow for maximum pelvic opening. Yet that does not matter too much if the mother has been moving around a lot during labor, and not stuck in just one position.

The full results of this study appear in Robbie Davis-Floyd. 2003 [orig. pub. 1992]. *Birth as an American Rite of Passage*. Berkeley: University of California Press. This chapter is derived from that book in its updated form.

pitocin to speed their labors, and one-third of American babies are delivered by cesarean section.

Many Americans, including most of the doctors and nurses who attend birth, view these procedures as medical necessities. Yet mothers in many low-technology cultures give birth sitting, squatting, semi-reclining, or on hands and knees—all positions far more physiologically efficacious—and are nurtured through the pain of labor by experienced midwives and supportive female (and sometimes male) relatives. What then might explain the standardization and technical elaboration of the American—and now the global—birthing process?

One answer emerges from the field of symbolic anthropology. Decades ago Arnold van Gennep (1966) noticed that in many societies around the world, major life transitions are ritualized. These cultural rites of passage make it appear that society itself effects the transformation of the individual. Could this explain the standardization of American birth? I believe the answer is yes.

I came to this conclusion as a result of my study of American birth between 1983 and 1991 (Davis-Floyd 2003 [1992]). I interviewed more than 100 mothers and many of the obstetricians, nurses, childbirth educators, and midwives who attended them. I realized that American society's deepest beliefs center around science, technology, patriarchy, and the institutions that control and disseminate them and that there could be no better transmitter of these core values and beliefs than the hospital procedures so salient in American birth.

Rites of Passage

A *ritual* is a patterned, repetitive, and symbolic enactment of a cultural belief or value; its primary purpose is alignment of the belief system of the individual with that of society (Davis-Floyd and Laughlin 2016). A *rite of passage* is a series of rituals that move individuals from one social state or status to another.

Rites of passage generally consist of three stages, originally outlined by van Gennep: (1) separation of the individuals from their preceding social state; (2) a period of transition in which they are neither one thing nor the other; and (3) an integration phase, in which, through various rites of incorporation, they are absorbed into their new social state.

In the year-long pregnancy/childbirth rite of passage in American society, the separation phase begins with the woman's first awareness of pregnancy; the transition stage lasts until several days after the birth; and the integration phase ends gradually in the newborn's first few months of life. By making the naturally transformative process of birth into a cultural rite of

How Rituals Enact Paradigms: A Comparative Example

In *The Power of Ritual* (from which this section is adapted), Davis-Floyd and Laughlin (2016:94–96) explain how the hegemonic technocratic paradigm of medicine is daily enacted through numerous ritualized procedures that are usually viewed not as rituals, but as "necessary" procedures of traditional medical care. Before we get to the rituals of hospital birth, I illustrate my point about how rituals enact paradigms in this section through one small but revealing example. Imagine a woman going into a doctor's office for a pelvic exam. In a technocratic practice, she is ushered into a usually cold room, told to take off her clothes and put on a paper gown (a symbol of her status as a patient), and asked to lie down on a high table with her bare feet up in cold metal stirrups. The doctor enters, accompanied by the nurse, walks to the end of the table, and greets her while looking down at her genitals. With few words of preparation or explanation, he inserts his gloved hand into her vagina to examine her. If she tightens up in alarm or fear, he orders her to relax and if she doesn't, he forces his way in until he obtains the information he seeks.

In a humanistic practice, the doctor either first meets the woman in his office or enters the room to chat with her while she is still in her street clothes (a symbol of her status as an individual, not a patient). He/she asks the patient about her concerns around this visit and anything else that may be on her mind. After this conversation, he asks her to undress as he leaves the room. The cold metal stirrups are covered with socks or pads. During the exam the doctor explains what he is doing and checks with the woman to make sure she is feeling OK. If she tightens her muscles in alarm, he immediately withdraws his hand and talks to her about what is causing her to close up. If she is truly distressed, he helps her sit up, speaks reassuring words, and promises not to continue with the exam until she is ready. He talks with her about her past—was she sexually abused at some point?—and will recommend counseling or perhaps a support group.

In the first scenario, the doctor is enacting the beliefs and values of the technocratic paradigm of medicine—the body is a machine, time is of the essence, information is important, his status is higher than hers, the coldness of the metal on her feet is irrelevant, as are her experience of the exam and their relationship. In the second scenario, the doctor is enacting the values of humanism: status is not relevant, relationship is; body and mind are connected; if her muscles tense in fear, there is a good reason, possibly having to do with past sexual abuse, or simple, momentary fear that can easily be addressed. Obtaining needed information from a pelvic exam is not as immediately important as addressing the woman's emotional state and not repeating or adding to

(continued)

past abuses. In each case, the procedures are ritualistic: they are patterned and repetitive (being ushered into the examining room, being told to put on the gown, lying down on the table with legs spread, etc.). They are also symbolic: in the technocratic case, the white coat of the doctor contrasts with the naked genitals of the patient, and he is "up" and she is "down," both literally and interactionally. In the humanistic case, the white coat of the doctor is paralleled to some degree by the clothing of the patient during their first conversation, which takes place eye to eye, on a much more equal level. The pad over the stirrup sends the symbolic message that her experience matters, a message that is heavily reinforced if the doctor stops the exam to accommodate the woman's needs.

The technocratic practitioner may not think much about what he is doing—he may simply be enacting the beliefs and values he was taught in medical school and residency, without awareness of the paradigm underlying them. The humanistic practitioner, in contrast, will very likely be aware that he is "doing it differently"—his choice to enact the values of humanism in his medical practice will usually be a very conscious one because it is alternative to the norm. In both cases, it is through ritual that each practitioner enacts and displays—and thus reinforces—the values that he or she holds.

In contrast, in a fully holistic practice, a homebirth midwife (see Cheyney 2011) would be performing any necessary vaginal exams in the mother's home, both dressed in regular clothes, on the mother's own bed or sofa. The mother and the midwife would likely spend an hour or so talking about any concerns the mother has, reinforcing their preexisting relationship. The midwife, who sees the mother's body as sacred, would proceed with the exam ever-so-gently and immediately share with the mother any information she is obtaining as she is feeling it with her fingers. The midwife would be sensitive to the mother's energy and to the energy field established between them, and would be quick to address the mother's reactions and feelings, as the mother would also be sensitive to the midwife and trust in both her expertise and their relationship. She would also encourage the mother to be sensitive to her baby's energy, to talk to her baby, touch her belly a lot, and send love to that baby all during pregnancy and during the labor and birth process. In this situation, we find less actual ritual and more actual, interactive communication between client and practitioner, because (in contrast to the technocratic model, which is *implicitly* transmitted in ritual, as we shall see more clearly below), *the humanistic and holistic ideologies are explicitly spelled out* in many books, articles, blogs, and websites and frequently enacted in explicit conversations between practitioner and mother.

passage, a society can ensure that its basic values will be transmitted to the three new members born out of the birth process: the new baby, the woman reborn into the new social role of mother, and the man reborn as father.

The Characteristics of Ritual and Obstetric "Routines": Hospital Birth as a Technocratic Rite of Passage

The following primary characteristics of ritual are particularly relevant to understanding how the initiatory process of cognitive restructuring is accomplished in hospital birth.

Symbolism

Rituals transmit their meaning through symbols. A symbol is an object, idea, or action that is loaded with cultural meaning. Instead of being analyzed intellectually, a symbol's message will be *felt* through the body and the emotions. Thus, even though recipients may be unaware of incorporating the symbol's message, its ultimate effect may be extremely powerful.

Routine obstetric procedures are highly symbolic. For example, to be seated in a wheelchair upon entering the hospital, as many laboring women are, is to receive through their bodies the symbolic message that they are disabled; to then be put to bed is to receive the symbolic message that they are sick. One woman told me:

> I can remember just almost being in tears by the way they would wheel you in. I would come into the hospital, on top of this, breathing, you know, all in control. And they slap you in a wheelchair! It made me suddenly feel like maybe I wasn't in control any more.

As I explained in great depth in Chapter 1 (pp. 7–8), the intravenous drips commonly attached to the hands or arms of birthing women to "hydrate" them and administer drugs via what nurses call a "line-in" make a powerful symbolic statement: as I detailed in Chapter 1, they are umbilical cords to the hospital. By making her dependent on the institution for her life, the IV conveys to her one of the most profound messages of her initiation experience: in the contemporary American technocracy, we are all dependent on institutions for our lives, "umbilically" linked to them through the water and sewer pipes, electrical wires and cables, wireless systems, and TVs that pervade our homes, through our banking and insurance accounts and credit cards, and increasingly through our laptops, smartphones, iPads, and the like. The rituals of hospital birth are not accidental—they are profound symbolic and metaphoric expressions of technocratic life.

A Cognitive Matrix

A matrix (from the Latin *mater*, or mother), like a womb, is something from within which something else comes. Rituals are not arbitrary; they come from within the belief system of a group. Their primary purpose is to enact and thereby transmit that belief system into the emotions, minds, and bodies of their participants. Thus analysis of a culture's rituals can lead to a profound understanding of its belief system.

A *technocracy* as I define it is a society organized around an ideology of progress through the development and increasing utilization of high technology and the global flow of information. Analysis of the rituals of hospital birth reveals their cognitive matrix to be the technocratic model of reality that forms the philosophical basis of both Western biomedicine and American society.

As described in Chapter 1, the technocratic model's early forms were developed in the 1600s by Descartes, Bacon, and Hobbes, among others. This model assumes that the universe is mechanistic, following predictable laws that the enlightened can discover through science and manipulate through technology, in order to decrease their dependence on nature. In this model, the human body is viewed as a machine that can be taken apart and put back together to ensure proper functioning. In the 17th century, the practical utility of this body-as-machine metaphor lay in its separation of body, mind, and soul. The soul could be left to religion, the mind to the philosophers, and the body could be opened up to scientific investigation.

The metaphor of the body-as-machine was central in the development of modern obstetrics. Wide cultural acceptance of this metaphor accompanied the demise of the midwife and the rise of the male-attended, mechanically manipulated birth. As society industrialized, the rising field of obstetrics adopted the assembly-line model of production of goods as its template for hospital birth. Accordingly, a woman's reproductive tract came to be treated like a birthing machine by skilled technicians working under relatively inflexible timetables to meet production and quality-control demands to produce "the perfect baby." As one resident explained: "There is a set, established routine for doing things, usually for the convenience of the doctors and the nurses, and the laboring woman is someone you work around, rather than with." The most desirable end product of the birth process is the new social member, the baby; the new mother is a secondary by-product.

Repetition and Redundancy

Ritual is marked by repetition and redundancy. For maximum effectiveness, rituals concentrate on sending one basic set of messages, repeating it over and over again in different forms. In hospital birthing, the message is repeatedly conveyed that the laboring woman is dependent on the institution. She is also reminded in myriad ways of the potential defectiveness of her birthing machine. These include periodic and sometimes continuous electronic monitoring of that machine, frequent manual examinations of her cervix to make sure that it is dilating on schedule, and, if it isn't, administration of the synthetic hormone pitocin to speed up labor so that birth can take place within the standard 12–24 hours. These procedures repeatedly convey the messages that time is important, you must produce on time, and you cannot do that without technological assistance because your machine is defective.

Cognitive Stabilization

When humans are subjected to extremes of stress and pain, they may become unreasonable and out of touch with reality. Ritual assuages this condition by giving people a conceptual handle to keep them from "falling apart" or "losing it." Labor subjects most women to extremes of pain, which are often intensified by the alien and frequently unsupportive hospital environment. They look to hospital rituals to relieve the distress resulting from their pain and fear. One woman expressed it this way:

> I was terrified when my daughter was born. I just knew I was going to split open and bleed to death right there on the table, but she was coming so fast, they didn't have any time to do anything to me. . . I like cesarean sections, because you don't have to be afraid.

When you come from within a belief system, its rituals will comfort and calm you.

Order, Formality, and a Sense of Inevitability: The "Cascade of Interventions"

Its exaggerated and precise order and formality set ritual apart from other modes of social interaction, enabling it to establish an atmosphere that feels both inevitable and inviolate. In tandem with this sense of inevitability, a "cascade of intervention" often occurs when one obstetric procedure alters the natural birthing process, causing complications and inexorably "necessitating" the next procedure, and the next. Many of the women in my study experienced such a "cascade" when they received some form of pain relief, such as an epidural early on, which slowed their labor. Then pitocin was administered to speed up the labor, but it suddenly induced longer and stronger contractions. Unprepared for the additional pain, the woman asked for more pain relief, which ultimately necessitated more pitocin. Pitocin-induced contractions, together with the fact that the mother is usually lying down with electronic monitor belts strapped around her stomach, often caused the supply of blood and oxygen to the fetus to drop, affecting the fetal heart rate. In response to the "distress" registered on the fetal monitor, an "emergency" cesarean was performed. Countless mothers have found themselves thanking the obstetrician for saving their baby, when the danger to the baby came in fact from the interventions the doctor ordered. As May (2017:69) describes it.

> If the mother has an epidural, she *will* automatically have an IV catheter. She *will* have IV fluids. She *will* have augmentation of labor with pitocin. She *will* have a urinary catheter. . . . This unitary set of interventions is held together by the epidural. . . . The epidural is central to the uniformity of what is now the norm in America's system of birth. Under these conditions, the labor and delivery unit runs like a well-oiled machine. (Italics in original)

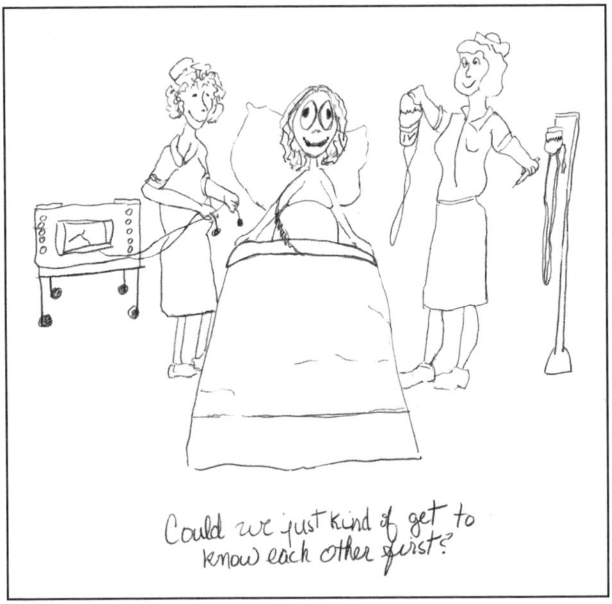

"Could we just kind of get to know each other first?" A woman asking for a less ritualistic/technocratic, more humanistic approach to birth care. Drawing by Sharon Gill, from my description of a "Cathy" cartoon I once saw

Cognitive Transformation

The goal of most initiatory rites of passage is cognitive transformation: the symbolic messages of ritual fuse with individual emotion and belief. Routine obstetric procedures map the technocratic model of birth onto the birthing woman's perceptions of her labor experience, aligning her belief system with that of society. Take the way many mothers come to think about the electronic fetal monitor, for example. The monitor is a machine that uses ultrasound to measure the rate of the baby's heartbeat through electrodes belted onto the mother's abdomen. Observers and participants alike report that the monitor, once attached, becomes the focal point of the labor. One woman described her experience this way:

> As soon as I got hooked up to the monitor, all everyone did was stare at it. The nurses didn't even look at me anymore when they came into the

room—they went straight to the monitor. I got the weirdest feeling that *it* was having the baby, not me.

This statement illustrates the successful conceptual fusion between the woman's perceptions of her birth experience and the technocratic model. So thoroughly was this model mapped onto her psyche that she began to feel that the machine was having the baby, that she was a mere onlooker. Soon after the monitor was in place, she requested a cesarean, declaring that there was "no more point in trying."

And it's not only laboring women who are emotionally affected by the EFM; a nurse I interviewed stated, in some confusion, "I know it's irrational, but after a mother is on the monitor for a while, *I get afraid to take her off because I get the feeling that the machine is keeping the baby's heart beating.*" This high emotional affect generated by the EFM is partially responsible for its continued routine use during even normal labors—it makes

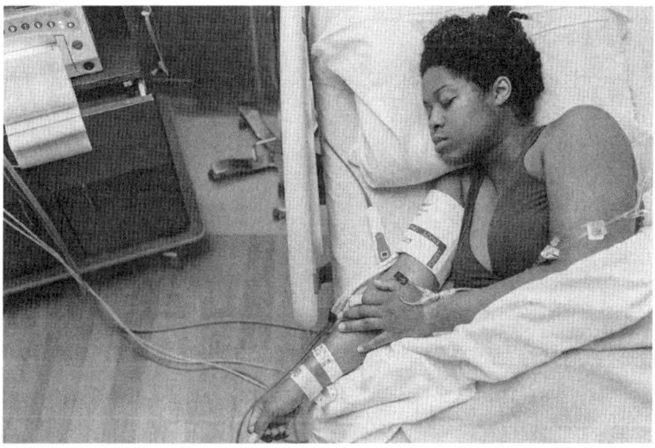

A laboring mother hooked up to a fetal monitor. Photo from austinbirthphotos.com

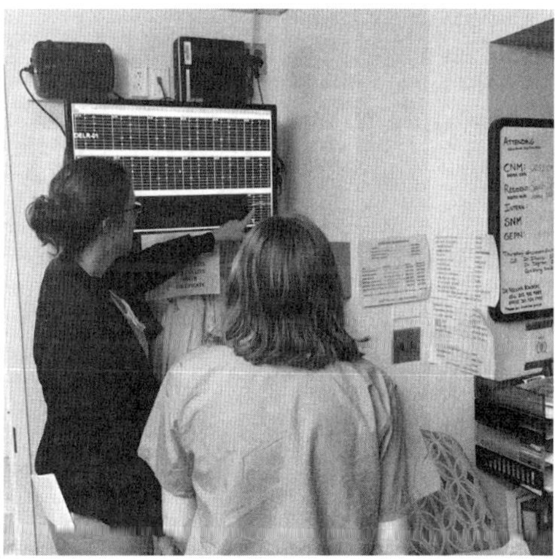

A senior nurse-midwife (CNM) teaches a student nurse-midwife (SNM) how to monitor the monitor. In many hospitals, practitioners trying to be with the laboring woman have to constantly go out of the labor room to enter information into computers, which really ought to be in the labor rooms themselves, given their constant use. Many former homebirth midwives who become CNMs note that the hardest part of the transition is learning how to use the machines and cope with the insistent focus on the machine instead of the mother. Photo by Richard Jennings CNM hospital staff, and some mothers, feel safer, and insurance companies as well. I have spoken with several heads of obstetrics who have tried to eliminate the routine use of the monitor in their departments, only to discover that insurance will not cover births that occur when, during labor, mothers are not hooked up to an EFM. And lawyers tell doctors they are more vulnerable to lawsuits when they do not use it. Thus these different sectors of society com-

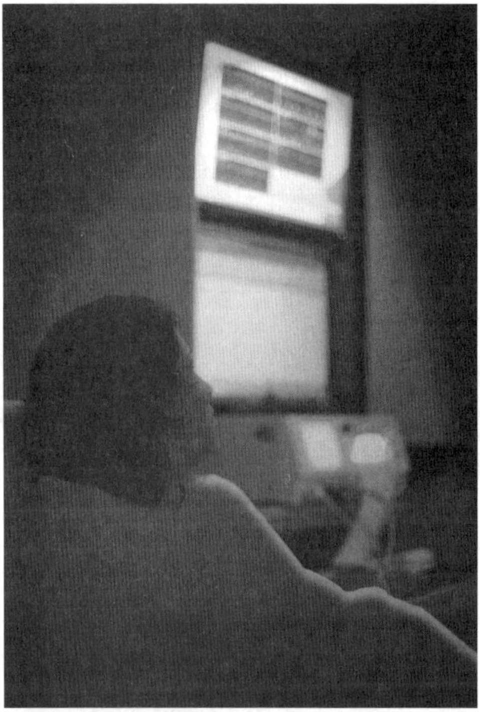

The laboring woman's visual field in the hospital. Note that both of these women are lying down without movement, despite the fact that movement is the essence of normal birth physiology; walking, standing, sitting, and moving are essential aids in the effectiveness of uterine contractions and fetal descent. Top photo by Leif Osmundson

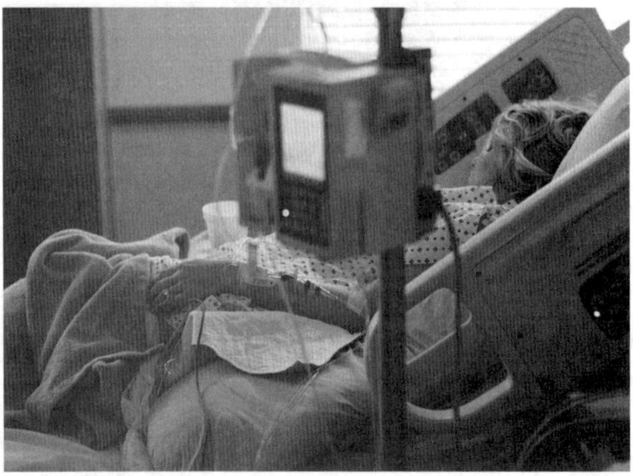

bine to ensure that high technology remains primary in hospital birth. We must never underestimate the power of high-technology symbols like the EFM—our technocratic cultural faith in such symbols utterly ignores and transcends the huge body of scientific evidence against their routine use.

If we stop a moment now to consider the visual and kinesthetic images that a laboring woman will be experiencing—herself in bed, in a hospital gown, staring up at an IV pole, bag, and cord on one side and a big whirring machine on the other and down at a steel bed and at a huge belt encircling her waist—we can see that her entire visual field conveys one overwhelming perceptual message about our culture's deepest values and beliefs: Technology is supreme; you are utterly dependent upon it.

Affectivity and Intensification

Rituals tend to intensify toward a climax. The order and stylization of ritual, combined with its rhythmic repetitiveness and the intensification of its messages, methodically create the sort of highly charged emotional atmosphere that works to ensure long-term learning. As the moment of birth approaches, the number of ritual procedures performed upon the woman will intensify toward the climax of birth, whether or not her condition warrants such intervention. For example, once the woman's cervix reaches full dilation (10 cm), the nursing staff immediately begins to exhort the woman to push with each contraction, whether or not she actually feels the urge to push. Yet if the obstetrician has not arrived by the time the head starts to crown, the laboring woman is then exhorted, with equal vigor, *not* to push. Such commands constitute a complete denial of the natural rhythms of the woman's body. They signal that her labor is a mechanical event and that she is subordinate to the institution's expectations and schedule. Similar high drama may pervade the rest of her birthing experience.

Preservation of the Status Quo

A major function of ritual is cultural preservation. Through explicit enactment of a culture's belief system, ritual works both to preserve and to transmit the culture. Preserving the culture includes perpetuating its power structure, so it is usually the case that those in positions of power will have unique control over ritual performance.

In spite of tremendous advances in equality for women, the United States is still a patriarchy. Nowhere is this reality more visible than in the lithotomy (supine) birthing position for birth. Despite decades of effort on the part of childbirth activists, including many obstetricians, the majority of American women still labor and give birth lying flat on their backs. This position is physiologically dysfunctional. It compresses major blood vessels, lowering the mother's circulation and thus the baby's oxygen supply. It increases the need for forceps or cesarean because it both narrows the pelvic

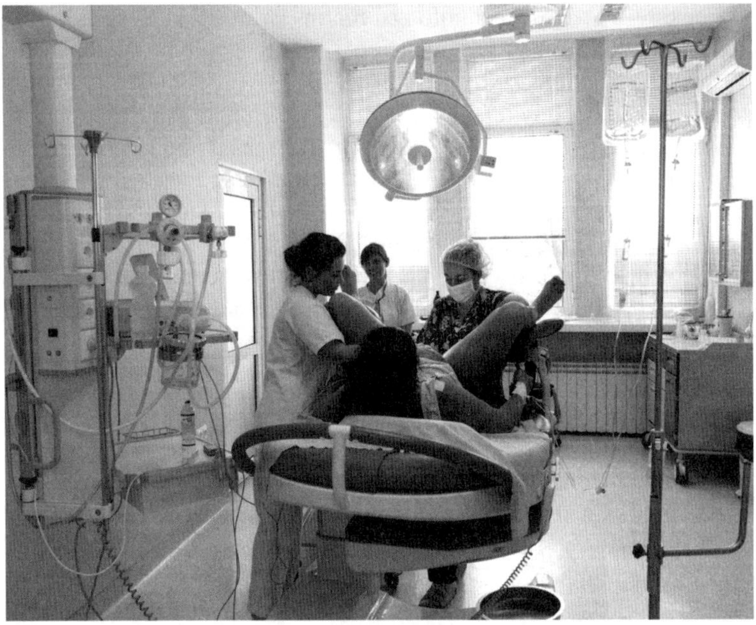

Lithotomy position for birth. Note that the mother has nothing to hold on to to help her push, and completely lacks any kind of labor support. Her inability to push effectively in this dysfunctional position led to the use of forceps to get the baby out. Photo by Suzanne Arms

outlet and ensures that the baby, who must follow the curve of the birth canal, quite literally will be born heading upward, against gravity.

This lithotomy position completes the process of symbolic inversion that has been in motion ever since the woman was put into the hospital gown. Her normal bodily patterns are turned, quite literally, upside-down—her legs are in the air, her vagina totally exposed. The doctor—society's official representative—stands in control not at the mother's head nor at her side, but at her bottom, where the baby's head is beginning to emerge. Interactionally, the obstetrician is "up" and the birthing woman is "down," an inversion that speaks eloquently to her of her powerlessness and of the power of society at the supreme moment of her own individual transformation.

The episiotomy sometimes performed by the obstetrician just before birth also powerfully enacts the status quo in American society. This procedure, which used to be performed on over 90% of first-time US mothers (those who did not have a cesarean) as they gave birth, expresses the value and importance of one of our technocratic society's most fundamental markers—the straight line. Through episiotomies, physicians can speed up the birth in accordance with our cultural value on time, and can also symbolically deconstruct the

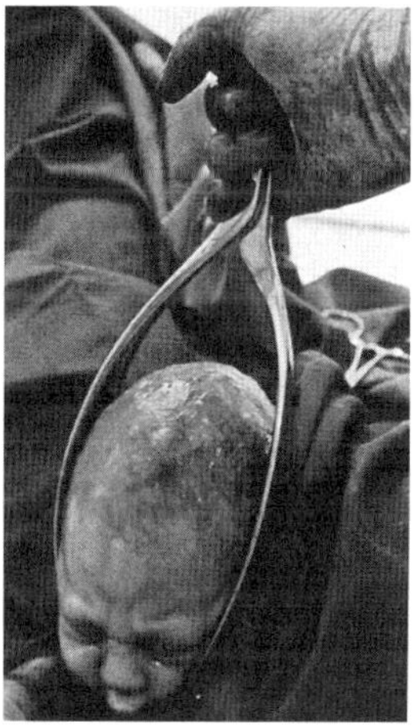

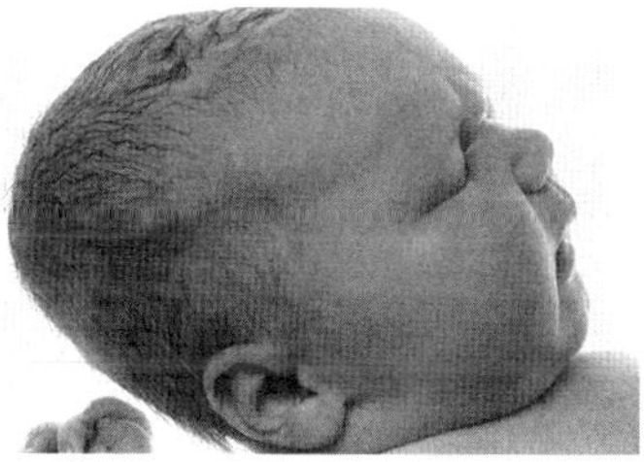

Forceps delivery in photo on left, and the consequences to the baby in photo on right. Photos by Mary Kroeger CNM

vagina (stretchy, flexible, part-circular and part-formless, feminine, creative, sexual, nonlinear), then reconstruct it in accordance with our cultural belief and value system. Doctors used to be taught (incorrectly) that straight cuts heal faster than the small jagged tears that sometimes occur during birth—but in fact, episiotomies often cause severe tearing that would not otherwise occur. These teachings dramatize our technocratic belief in the superiority of culture over nature. Because it virtually does not exist in nature, the line is most useful in aiding us in our constant conceptual efforts to separate ourselves from nature.

So much scientific evidence has accumulated over the past 40 years about the detriments of episiotomy that its use in the US has dramatically decreased to under 10% of births, showing that change *can* occur when the evidence to support it is overwhelming, and that US doctors do sometimes pay attention to the evidence. Yet episiotomies are still used in over 90% of vaginal births in most Latin American countries and in many others around the world where the practice is so ingrained that the evidence, if known, is simply ignored. As one Brazilian obstetrician exclaimed to me, "I was taught that if I did not perform an episiotomy, the baby could not possibly come out!" (See Chapter 5.) In Romania, where close to 100% of birthing women have episiotomies for this very reason, I met a mother who was allergic to the materials in the thread used to sew up episiotomies. She told her doctor this and he promised not to cut her; but so deep were his beliefs that the baby can't come out or the perineum will rip if an episiotomy is not performed, during the birth he did it anyway, and she ended up in the hospital for three weeks for the major infection she got from her allergy to the thread.

Effecting Social and Individual Change

Paradoxically, ritual, with all of its insistence on continuity and order, can be an important factor not only in individual transformation but also in social change. New belief and value systems are most effectively spread through new rituals designed to enact and transmit them; entrenched belief and value systems are most effectively altered through alterations in the rituals that enact them.

Fifty-two percent of my 100 interviewees did experience cognitive fusion with the technocratic model during labor and birth, 42 of them with ease because they both expected and accepted the need for high technology during birth and did not mind its deployment, and nine with distress, because they had striven for a normal, unmedicated vaginal delivery and had not achieved that goal. Fifteen percent entered the hospital intent on a natural childbirth and did succeed in reaching that goal, thereby avoiding conceptual fusion with the technocratic model. These women were personally empowered by their birth experiences. They tended to view technology as a resource that they could choose to use or ignore, and they often consciously subverted their socialization process by replacing technocratic symbols with self-empowering alternatives. For example, they wore their own clothes, drank fluids, and ate their own food, rejecting the hospital gown and hydration via the IV. They walked the halls instead of going to bed. They chose perineal massage instead of episiotomy and gave birth sitting up, squatting, or on their hands and knees. Most importantly, they waited until labor was well advanced before heading to the hospital, usually supported at home by a doula who could tell them when they were in truly active labor (6 cm); from that point, labor usually proceeds fairly rapidly and unnecessary interventions can be avoided.

One woman, confronted with the wheelchair, said, "I don't need this," and used it for a luggage cart. This rejection of customary ritual elements is

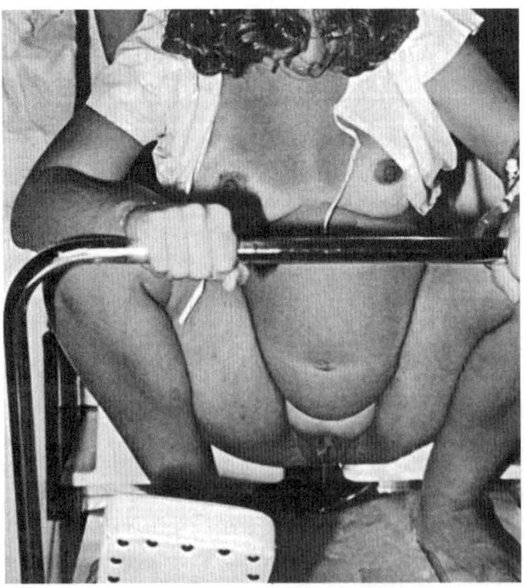

A physiologic squatting birth.
Photo by Ricardo Jones

an exceptionally powerful way to induce change, as it takes advantage of an already charged and dramatic situation.

During the 1970s and early 1980s, the conceptual hegemony of the technocratic model in the hospital was seriously challenged by the natural childbirth movement. Birth activists succeeded in getting hospitals to allow fathers into labor and delivery rooms, mothers to birth consciously (without being put to sleep), and mothers and babies to room together after birth. They fought for women to have the right to birth without drugs or interventions, to eat and drink at will, to walk around or even be in water during labor. Prospects for change away from the technocratic model of birth by the 1990s seemed bright.

Changing a society's belief and value system by changing the rituals that enact it is possible, but not easy. To counter attempts at change, members of a society may intensify the rituals that support the status quo. Thus a response to the threat posed by the natural childbirth movement was to intensify the use of high technology in hospital births. During the 1990s, although the routine use of episiotomy declined significantly and has continued to do so, the epidural rate shot up to 60% and remains there today.

And starting in 1970, periodic or continuous electronic monitoring of nearly all women was introduced and became standard procedure during that decade, resulting in a dramatic rise in the cesarean section (CS) rate, from 6% in 1970 to 23% in 1979. Why does routine EFM use raise CS rates? Because the machine provides *too much information*—when you see every fetal heart rate deceleration, even though such fluctuations can be normal, you are more likely to rush the mother to the OR for a cesarean only to find once the baby is delivered that it was not, in fact, in distress. By 2012, the US cesarean rate had reached 32%.

Yet, fascinatingly, the American cesarean rate still remains at 32% today, in 2017. Back in 2012, all indicators were that it would continue its steep rise, yet it appears in my view that five decades of birth activism have had a profound effect. American obstetricians are quite aware that cesarean rates in countries like Brazil, Turkey, and Greece, and in Chinese cities have reached epidemic proportions—50% or higher in these and other countries. And they seem to be trying to prevent that sort of excess from occurring here. Today, possibly because of the influence of birth activists and the increasing presence of nurse-midwives and doulas in American hospitals, obstetricians are doing a very good job of keeping the CS rate stable—a result that to my mind goes in tandem with other humanistic changes that are quite common here now. The enema, the separation of the mother from her husband or partner, the rushing of the mother from labor to delivery room for birth, the routine separation of mother and baby after birth—all these are still absolutely routine in hospitals in low-resource countries yet have, in the US, the UK, and other high-resource countries been eliminated in favor of labor-delivery-recovery rooms where women can stay the whole time, with partners and friends allowed to be present. "Rooming-in" (where the baby stays in the room with the mother) is quite common in the US and UK, as is skin-to-skin contact immediately after birth and the encouragement of immediate breastfeeding. These humanistic (see Chapter 1) changes offer hope for a more evidence-based future for the American treatment of birth.

Ritual Change: Induction Only at or after 39 Weeks

Some years ago, a Florida pediatrician in charge of her hospital's NICU noticed that it was constantly full because so many babies were born prematurely because of scheduled inductions of labor and scheduled cesareans. "Due dates" are only estimates, and they are often wrong. So women who think their babies are nearly due might seek labor induction simply because they are "sick of being pregnant," and doctors usually complied. The result was that NICUs across the US were full of babies born prematurely who should not have been. This Florida pediatrician got angry, and demanded that her hospital establish a policy of *no inductions or scheduled CS before 39 weeks* (full-term is 40–42 weeks, but at least that was an improvement over delivering babies at 32–38 weeks, whose lungs are not yet fully developed, so they have to be intubated and on oxygen to survive). Once that policy was implemented, the NICU emptied out and word spread. Eventually ACOG (2013) itself came out with an official policy of no induction or scheduled CS till 39 weeks or later, thereby saving many thousands of babies from prematurity (Osterman and Martin 2014). This change in the rituals of induction and scheduled cesareans resulted from both incontrovertible evidence and the righteous indignation of one Florida doctor at the dysfunctionality of allowing women and doctors to decide, for convenience's sake, to get that baby out whenever they felt like it. (As Maureen May [2017] points out, it is a fact of life that "convenience" is not always a self-indulgent choice: many women, especially the poor, have tremendous logistical challenges in preparing for birth, including arranging care for the children they already have and transportation to the often-far away hospital. Yet they too are compelled by the risks to their baby to follow this new policy and wait.)

Ritual Change: Waiting to Cut the Umbilical Cord

Cutting the cord immediately after birth has long been a ritual practice symbolic of removing the baby from the worlds of the womb and nature and initiating it into the realms of technology and culture. There has never been any scientific evidence justifying this ritual, and by now there is plenty of evidence to its contrary. Immediate cord-cutting deprives the newborn of its blood and oxygen supply, which will keep coming into the baby until the cord stops pulsating. The pure logic of leaving the cord intact until then, now backed up by multiple studies, has finally resulted in the establishment of an international policy endorsed by the International Confederation of Midwives (ICM), WHO, FIGO (the International Federation of Gynecology and Obstetrics—the acronym is for its name in French), and many other organizations to stop immediate cord-cutting and wait patiently for the pulsating to stop. This new practice enables the baby to take its time to establish effective breathing, and stands as another example of how scientific evidence can sometimes create ritual change.

Ritual Change: The Woman-Centered Cesarean

Science and technology can be counterbalanced with humanism in the performance of cesarean sections—a growing trend. A woman-centered cesarean, first and foremost, results from a consensual decision made by the woman and her practitioner(s) that a CS is a necessary one in her case (unless there is an extreme emergency that allows no time for discussion), or also in the case that the woman has chosen to schedule a cesarean rather than go through labor at all. In either case, the woman is the protagonist, is fully informed of her rights and the reasons for the CS, and gives full informed consent. She will have an epidural or a spinal (unless she chooses general anesthesia, which hardly ever happens). Her hands will not be strapped down so that she can be free to hold her partner's hand during the procedure and to hold the baby immediately after birth. (This is outdated information in the US, where hand-strapping during CS has not been routinely done for decades, yet is still a very common practice in developing countries.) Also if she wishes, soft music will be played, and possibly the lights in the room may be dimmed, except for the light above the OBs performing the operation. The conversation, if there is one, will focus on the mother and not on the latest sports event (unless she prefers ordinary chit-chat), and, again if she chooses, the mother's partner, doula, and/or midwife will be with her, holding her hand or massaging her head gently. Most hospitals only allow one companion during a cesarean, but it is increasingly common to allow more. One of them may even sing for her, as a midwife friend of mine recently did for my goddaughter's very necessary CS here in Austin a few years ago (she had planned a homebirth at my house, but the baby was well and truly stuck).

Many women report feeling disconnected from their babies if they cannot see them born, so to remedy this problem, the sheets delineating the sterile field around the abdominal incisions can be put *behind* the mother's head so that her face is inside the field and she can see the birth. (The mother can wear a mask as the practitioners do—this is possible but rare, as it requires a huge shift in thinking about the ritualized boundaries of the sterile field.) Another option is to demarcate the field with clear plastic sheets so that the mother can see through them—a creative solution invented by my colleague and friend William Camann, who is the head of obstetric anesthesiology at the Harvard-associated Brigham and Women's Hospital in Boston. He told me several years ago that the clear plastic sheets are now quite common there and women love them as they can watch their babies appear. His preferred terms for these types of cesareans are "gentle cesarean" or "family centered cesarean."[2] In a recent article, "Mother- Baby- and Family-Centered Cesarean: It Is Possible" (Camann and Barbieri 2013),[3] which describes in detail how to perform this type of CS, the authors say:

> In most obstetric units, babies born by cesarean delivery are brought to a newborn resuscitation unit, examined, cleaned, banded, administered medications, weighed, and swaddled before being introduced to the mother. In cesarean deliveries early skin to skin (STS) contact and early initiation of breastfeeding are not common. . . . Research indicates that the traditional surgical rituals [Davis-Floyd 2003 (1992)] and processes of cesarean delivery prevent mothers from connecting to important physical and emotional aspects of the birth process. Practices that prevent early maternal-infant bonding and slow the initiation of breastfeeding may result in lower breastfeeding rates at 6 months of life and impact maternal behaviors. A new approach to cesarean delivery is the mother- and baby-centered cesarean delivery, also known as the "natural cesarean" delivery. In this approach, there is a reduced emphasis on traditional surgical rituals and an increased emphasis on facilitating the early interaction of the mother and family with their baby. The mother- and baby-centered cesarean celebrates the momentous birth event and encourages early mother–infant bonding.[4]

In a very few hospitals around the world, women are allowed to wear gloves with long sleeves and to reach down and pull up their babies themselves if they wish—this is a huge change in CS rituals, as doctors often commented during our interviews that delivering a baby by cesarean "makes you feel like God"—an adrenaline rush that some find hard to give up. Much evidence suggests benefits if the baby's body colonizes with the mother's bacteria, which it does as it moves through the birth canal and when held by the mother for immediate skin-to-skin contact. Skin-to-skin has multiple benefits, including helping to colonize newborns with beneficial bacteria and greatly aiding in the establishment of breastfeeding, as well as regulating the baby's body temperature, heartbeat, and respiration. As always, the attitude of the caregivers during the operation will have the greatest effect on how the woman experiences her birth; in a woman-centered cesarean they will treat her and any who accompany her with dignity, respect, compassion, and kindness. Such changes in the rituals surrounding the performance of cesareans, while still rare, are becoming more common, and constitute a clear example of how a new global awareness of the rights of the woman during birth and a humanistic orientation can result in changing the rituals surrounding birth—a

[2] See http://commonhealth.legacy.wbur.org/2013/01/whats-a-natural-cesarean-and-how-natural-is-it-really and http://www.cnn.com/videos/tv/2015/01/28/the-gentle-c.cnn.

[3] http://www.mdedge.com/obgmanagement/article/65052/obstetrics/mother-baby-and-family-centered-cesarean-delivery-it-possible

[4] See the video "The Natural Caesarean: A Woman-Centred Technique" by the Jentle Childbirth Foundation (www.youtube.com /watch?v=m5RIcaK98Yg).

These transparent plastic sheets are now commonly used at Brigham and Women's Hospital in Boston during cesareans.

All photos by William Camann MD, who originated the idea.

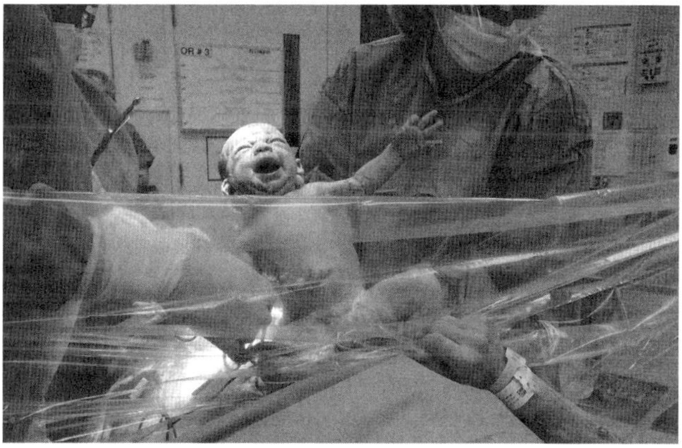

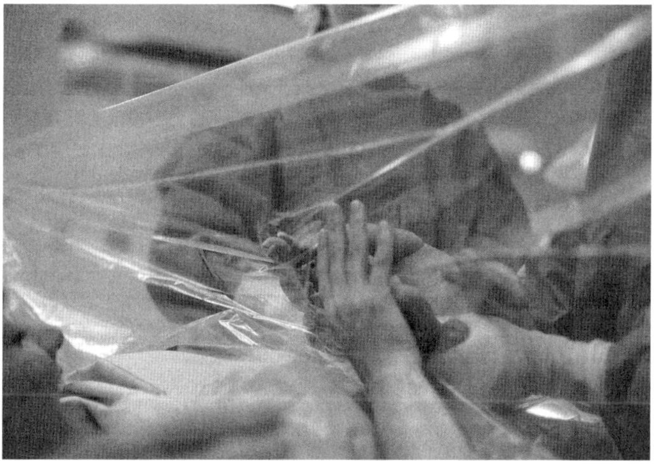

The mother is handed the baby immediately after birth.

Immediately after the cesarean birth shown above, the mother pulls the baby to her chest.

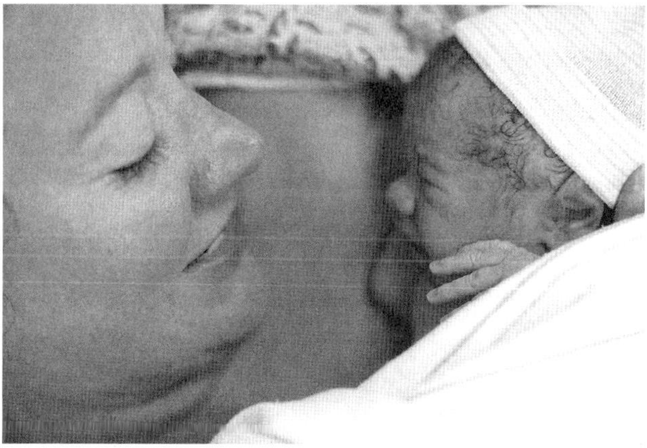

clear example of how culture change can result in ritual change, and vice-versa. (I am not recommending routine CS here, just noting that when truly necessary or the woman's own choice, cesareans can be transformed in highly humanistic ways.)

The Rituals of Homebirth

Six of my 100 interviewees completely rejected the technocratic model altogether and chose to give birth at home under an alternative paradigm, the holistic model. This model stresses the organicity and trustworthiness of the female body, the natural rhythmicity of labor, the integrity of the family, and self-responsibility. Although homebirthers constitute only 1.36% of the American birthing population, their conceptual importance is tremendous, as through the alternative rituals of giving birth at home, they enact—and thus guarantee the existence of—a paradigm of pregnancy and birth based on the value of connection, just as the technocratic model is based on the principle of separation. In her article "Reinscribing the Birthing Body: Homebirth as Ritual Performance" (2011:519), Melissa Cheyney describes homebirth rituals as "not simply evidence-based care strategies" but also as "intentionally manipulated rituals of technocratic subversion designed to . . . peel away the fictions of medicalized birthing care." She gives many examples of homebirth rituals in that article, which I strongly encourage any of my readers interested in homebirth to explore. Here below I will provide some examples from my own homebirth experiences.

During my second birth in 1984, I was anxious and nervous for the first 26 hours of labor, because that's how long I had labored in the hospital before having an unnecessary cesarean for my first birth for the much-abused reasons "failure to progress" (see Chapter 1, p. 22) and "cephalo-pelvic disproportion" (CPD), meaning my pelvis was supposedly too small for the baby to pass through. (My daughter only weighed 7 pounds and 14 ounces, whereas my son, whom you see in the picture below, weighed a full 10 pounds, and so it appears that my pelvis was big enough after all.) The contractions during that 26-hour period sure felt real, but my midwives kept telling me, whenever I asked them to check my dilation, that I was only at 4 cm and thus still in the latent phase of labor, which, they assured me, could take days. And indeed it was only on the morning of the third day that I reached six cm and active labor kicked in—that was enlightening, as the contractions of active labor were indeed qualitatively different—much stronger, much more powerful. I was mightily relieved after the first 26 hours passed—now I could know for sure that my mind and my fears would not map the pattern of my first birth onto this second one. My midwives and doula helped by making a circle of tall, lit candles around me, letting me talk and cry out my fears, and then (symbolically) throw them into the candles to be consumed by the flames as we chanted prayers and empowerment songs, such as:

Circle round for freedom, circle round for peace
For all of us in prison, circle for release
Circle for the planet, circle for each soul
For the children of our children, keep the circle whole

And after the birth, we spontaneously performed the ritual you see in the second photo below.

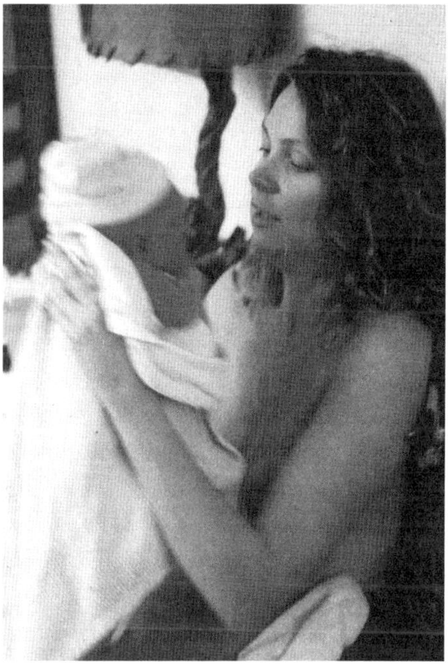

A silent, intuitive moment with Baby Jason about 20 minutes after the birth. After multiple attempts to breastfeed him—he was not hungry so kept refusing the breast and crying—I couldn't figure out what to do because the midwives and everyone else kept talking and giving me advice and there was just too much noise in the room. I sent everyone out except my wonderful photographer (the only one staying silent) so I could get in touch with my baby and ask him why he kept fussing and what he needed me to do. Once it was just the two of us, I could hear his silent answer clearly. Photo by Peter Gonzalez

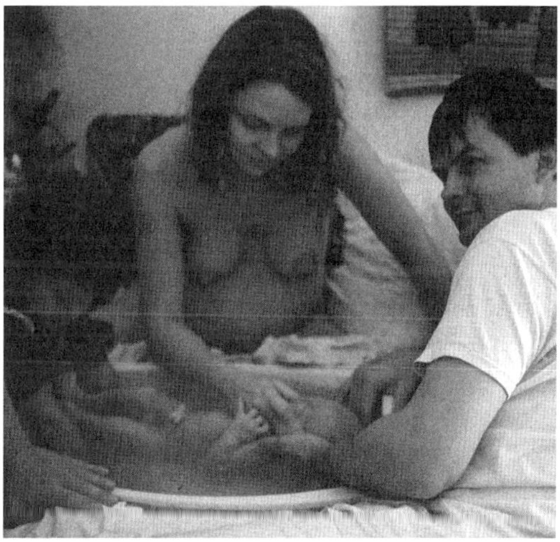

[bottom] A spontaneous homebirth ritual: The answer I received from Baby Jason was that he wanted to be in water. So my photographer Peter filled up the tub with warm water and laid it on the bed. Once Jason had wiggled his head around to get my finger in his mouth, he completely relaxed. As he opened his eyes and began to look around with interest, everyone who had been present at the birth came over to encircle him, including his 4-year-old sister Peyton. One by one, as he gazed at each in turn, they spoke ritualistic words welcoming him to the world. And so we enacted our own personal values and beliefs in community, family, individuality, and love, as well as our mutual belief that babies are conscious beings and need to be treated as such. Photo by Peter Gonzalez

As I will discuss in depth in Chapter 3, I suggest that the existence of homebirth as a model for the ideal, woman-centered birth has heavily influenced practitioners' efforts in many countries to increasingly humanize hospital birth.

Mutilation and Prosthesis: The One-Two Punch of Technocratic Birth

Industrialized childbirth causes disturbed labor, thus impeding the secretion of maternal oxytocin. It then attempts to solve the very problem it has brought about through the infusion of pitocin (artificial oxytocin) to promote labor. The addition of the epidural to the mix of medical interventions solves the problem of the increased pain that often accompanies the administration of pitocin. This occurs with no research as to the safety of the concomitant use of these two very potent medications.
— Maureen May, *Epiduralized Birth*

In the vast body of literature on birth, what has been missing is a work that describes American childbirth from an ethnographic standpoint, utilizing the rich, insightful data that can only be derived from real-life observations. A new ethnography, *Epiduralized Birth and Nurse-Midwifery: Childbirth in the United States* by Maureen May CNM, PhD (2017), helps to meet that need. Based on a year of on-site observation and interviews at one midwifery service in a community hospital, the book describes "epiduralized birth"—a process of managing labor and birth that is antithetical to what May terms "ecological birth." The book shows how nurse-midwifery care involves a "normality paradox" among midwives who must negotiate highly technocratized care that often runs contrary to their professional and personal values. May demonstrates that "epiduralized birth is an assembly-line process where all interventions are integrated, inseparable, and interdependent elements of a single process—a process that has the epidural at its core." In this new work, May has managed to capture via ethnography much of what I have long been saying about the rituals of hospital birth and their systemic, integrated nature.[5]

To recap from Chapter 1, In *Stealing Fire: The Mythology of the Technocracy* (1991), Peter Reynolds describes the fundamental act of ritual transformation in technocratic culture as the "One-Two Punch." Take a highly successful natural process (e.g., salmon swimming upstream to spawn). Punch One: render it dysfunctional with technology (dam the stream, pre-

[5] Although I have toured many hospitals around the world, and spent considerable time in some, I have never carried out long-term hospital ethnography; most of my data comes from interviews with mothers and practitioners.

venting the salmon from reaching their spawning grounds). Punch Two: fix it with technology (take the salmon out of the water with machines, make them spawn artificially and grow the eggs in trays, then release the baby salmon downstream near the ocean). Reynolds identifies this One-Two Punch—destroy a natural process, then rebuild it as a cultural process—what he calls "mutilation and prosthesis"—as an integral result of technocratic society's supervaluation of science and technology over nature (1991:3–5).

Prosthesis is a term used in medicine for artifacts that replace lost bodily functions and parts, but in technocratic rituals, the culture first produces the mutilation of nature that the prosthesis is designed to replace. For example:

> In a recent article on what the authors refer to as "the top 10 coming attractions" in biotechnology, among the innovations listed are genetically engineered crops that contain genes for making pesticides—mutilation and prosthesis folded into one; and genetically engineered bacteria that will clean up oil spills and chemical dumps by eating the pollutants—a man-made fix for man-made mutilation. In some cases, both phases of the One-Two Punch are implemented by the same organization. In an advertisement for the DuPont Corporation, one of the major purveyors of munitions in the Vietnam War, a Vietnam veteran plays basketball on artificial legs manufactured by DuPont. Industrial society is a master of the One-Two Punch: send nature reeling with a hard Right, then finish it off with the Left. Industrial society destroys natural cycles with one hand while building fabrications of them with the other, but the integrated operation of these two disparate processes is almost invisible to people. (Reynolds 1991:5)

Reynolds shows that when the One-Two Punch of mutilation and prosthesis *is* culturally recognized, as in the building of the salmon hatcheries, it is usually dismissed as an accidental by-product of industrialization or embraced as a compromise solution to unfortunately competing demands. But taking off from Ellul (1964), who pointed out that "technological society" is not defined by its tools and techniques at all, for these are always changing, but by its underlying system of values, Reynolds demonstrates that "the dominant value of contemporary industrial society is in fact the One-Two Punch itself" (p. 7)—the creation of dysfunctions in nature through technical intervention and their replacement by fabricated analogs of natural processes. I suggest that the cultural management of American birth is a perfect example of the One-Two Punch and that, as such, it is a complete cultural and ritual expression of our technocratic core value system.

As we have seen, technomedicine mutilates the natural rhythms of birth by multiple interventions in every phase (drugs to speed labor and eradicate pain, frequent cervical checks, rupturing the membranes), then prosthetizes the skewed results via electronic fetal monitoring and the often-resultant delivery by cesarean section. In the process, and in the name of progress, this mutilation can harm women and fetuses: iatrogenic damage to mother or baby is all too common in hospital birth. In other words, the dangers of this mutilation and prosthesis in birth are real and their resultant dysfunctions are multiple; they range from the current global epidemic of unnecessary cesareans to the overpopulation of the NICUs around the world with babies born prematurely from labors that should never have been artificially induced.

To be sure, normal physiologic birth carries its own set of risks. In societies in which women are malnourished and overworked, rates of both infant and maternal mortality are high. But when women are healthy, well nourished, and receive adequate social support, the percentage of complications in childbirth is very low—under 15%. And the majority of complications that occur can be screened for in advance. The problem is that far too often, technomedical interventions are not reserved for the small percentage of births that actually need them; rather, they are performed on the majority of laboring women. By interfering with the normal process of labor, such ritualized interventions often generate the very complications they are designed to prevent. (See www.childbirthconnection.org.)

Yet many women demand their own technocratization and that of their unborn and newborn children because its rituals speak to them compellingly of controllability and predictability, which contrast favorably in their minds with the out-of-control nature of "natural childbirth." To recap again from Chapter 1, the transcendent message of technocratic birth—that technology is better than nature—aligns with their own experience of order imposed on chaos by the dishwasher, the smartphone, and the computer. The transcendent message of the One-Two Punch is that *Punch Two is the point*: we truly and deeply believe that to technologically re-create a natural process is to make it better. Damming a river seems better than letting it flood, and hooking a woman up to an EFM seems better than letting her labor on her own, because both processes allow us to control, or appear to control, nature with technology. Decades ago, *Life* magazine declared:

> If we think of the human body as a kind of machine, doctors of the future will be like mechanics, simply replacing those parts that can't be fixed. . . . Succeeding generations of artificial devices will perform as well as their natural counterparts and may prove more reliable. For instance, gains in microelectronics will lead to a bionic heart with an internal power pack. . . . The circuits controlling man-made limbs and hands will be packed with more computing power, making the prosthetics increasingly dexterous. . . . Tiny TV cameras mounted on eyeglass frames will transmit electronic images directly to the visual cortex of the brain, bringing limited vision to the sightless. (1989:57)

Although humanistically redesigned hospitals tout a smorgasbord of options for birth, from Jacuzzis to home-like birthing suites, in fact the vast majority of birthing women are constrained by the basic processes of the technocracy to the same realities faced by the dammed-up rivers and those thousands of salmon trying to swim home. The question arises, if this One-Two Punch of technocratic de- and reconstruction is in fact so integral to American society that it must be enacted a thousand times a day in the ritual production of new social members, to what extent does it define women's own perceptions of the proper cultural treatment of their pregnant bodies? Women's own conceptualizations of those bodies? In other words, how do the women to whose bodies these technologies are applied think about the relationships between their bodies and these technologies? And given that as conscious human agents they may have more choices than the salmon and the rivers, what do they choose? I have sought to provide answers to these questions in the following chapter, via a study that contrasts the ideologies and body images of women who choose highly technocratic birth and women who choose completely natural childbirth at home.

Conclusion: Ritual Socialization

I have seen the wide variations of normal birth as a midwife. The utter sameness of the births I witnessed at Community Hospital continued to unnerve me throughout my year of fieldwork.

— Maureen May, *Epiduralized Birth and Nurse-Midwifery*

Every society in the world has felt the need to thoroughly socialize its citizens into conformity with its norms, and citizens derive many benefits from such socialization. Cultures often find ways to socialize their members from the inside, by making them *want* to conform to society's norms. Ritual is one major way through which such socialization can be achieved. Obstetric procedures can be understood as rituals that facilitate the internalization of cultural values at the same time as they mutilate and prosthetize the physiologic process of birth, deconstructing its natural flow and reconstructing it as a mechanistic process of production. These procedures are patterned, repetitive, and profoundly symbolic, communicating messages concerning our culture's deepest beliefs about the necessity for cultural control of natural processes. Obstetric interventions also attempt to contain and control the physiological process of birth and to transform the birthing woman into a mother who has internalized the core values of technocratic society. From society's perspective, the birth process will not be successful unless the woman and child are properly socialized during the experience, transformed as much by the rituals as by the physiology of birth.

Questions for Thought and Discussion

1. How does Davis-Floyd define ritual?
2. Why does the author insist that standard obstetric procedures for birth are rituals? Do you agree with her analysis? Why or why not?
3. What cultural purpose do the rituals of hospital birth perform?
4. How do women tend to respond to hospital birth rituals? How would you respond?

Recommended Films

The Business of Being Born: produced by Ricki Lake and Abby Epstein. http://www.thebusinessofbeingborn.com/. This film provides a clear demonstration of the rituals of hospital birth and contrasts them with depictions of birth at home.

Trial of Labor: A Documentary about Childbirth from a Mother's Perspective: produced by Robert Humphreys and Elliot Berlin, 2016. This documentary follows four women on their quest to have a vaginal birth after cesarean (VBAC). The women came from all walks of life, but all had one thing in common—the determination not to be forced into unnecessary surgery. Each woman in the film chose her own path to natural birth: some chose a formal hospital setting—one chose to labor at home with a doula—and another chose a homebirth with a midwife. Irrespective of outcome, they all found healing in truly informing themselves, making their own decisions, and fighting for "a trial of labor." http://www.trialoflabor.com/

Birth produced by Suzanne Arms, 2017. This soon to be released film examines routine modern hospital-based interventions in the physiologic process of labor and birth and compares the midwifery model with the medical-hospital-intervention model. suzannebirthing@gmail.com

The Natural Caesarean: A Woman-Centred Technique by the Jentle Childbirth Foundation (www.youtube.com /watch?v=m5RIcaK98Yg). 12 minutes.

The Gentle C. http://www.cnn.com/videos/tv/2015/01/28/the-gentle-c.cnn. 5 minutes.

Acknowledgments

This chapter/article in its original version has been reprinted 17 times in various books and journals and translated into several languages; I would like to thank all those who found it so useful. I also thank Peter Gonzalez for his wonderful photos of my and Jason's homebirth, and Sarah Culver, who searched the Internet for me and found some of the photos used in this chapter.

3

The Technocratic Body and the Organic Body

Hegemony and Heresy in Women's Birth Choices

Women's Agency in Birth: Body Image as Microcosmic Mirror of Worldview

All orthodoxies need heresies, all political regimes need dissenters, not only to jail or burn them, but also to co-opt them. For as marginal figures, they hold the secret of creative transformations. If anomalies can be plowed back into the system—composted, as Mary Douglas puts it—the system becomes stronger.
— Morris Berman

This chapter addresses women's agency in childbirth. It describes the technocratic ideology that women's culturally mediated desires and choices helped to hegemonize since the mid-20th century *from mothers' points of view,* and contrasts that hegemonic ideology with the heretical holistic model

This chapter is part revised, adapted, and updated from the following two sources: Davis-Floyd, Robbie. 1992 "The Technocratic Body and the Organic Body: Cultural Models for Women's Birth Choices." In *The Anthropology of Science and Technology*, eds. David J. Hess and Linda L. Layne, a special issue of *Knowledge and Society*, Volume 9. Hartford, CT: JAI Press. And Davis-Floyd, Robbie. 1994. "The Technocratic Body: American Childbirth as Cultural Expression," *Social Science and Medicine* 38(8):1125–1140.

of birth and the organic view of the body it charters, also from the mothers' points of view. In *Coming to Our Senses: Body and Spirit in the Hidden History of the West*, historian Morris Berman (1989) points out that dominant hegemonies, religious or secular, need heretical movements to oppose them so that the hegemonies can co-opt them and steal their heretical energy. When the natural childbirth movement first came to American popular attention in the 1950s and 1960s via the works of European authors Grantly Dick-Read, Ferdinand Lamaze, and Frederic Leboyer, *it* was the heretical model, as it sought to empower women to educate themselves about pregnancy and birth, to reject total domination by physicians, to give birth consciously, awake and aware, with their husbands present. All these were radical ideas at the time. Yet currently, as we have seen in the first two chapters, the heretical energy of the natural childbirth campaign has been redirected into making technocratic birth more humanistic, more appealing, more palatable to the women who are choosing it. As May (2017:11–15) points out, "The vast majority of mothers choose to avail themselves of highly technical births, demanding inductions and epidurals. . . . An analysis of epiduralized birth that emphasizes patriarchy camouflages the extent to which mothers are involved in decision-making within today's labor and delivery units."

Why do so many women choose to have their labors induced and give birth under epidural anesthesia? Why do they elect to be monitored, when they could reject the imprisoning and uncomfortable monitor and walk during labor—a more physiologically sound option? Why do we find a 32% cesarean rate culturally and medically acceptable? This chapter derives from a study I undertook after finishing the research for my dissertation/first book. It addressed these and similar questions by focusing on the correlations between US women's self- and body images and worldviews. My fundamental assumption was that *body image is a microcosmic mirror of worldview.* I examined that assumption through the widely divergent body images and worldviews of two specific groups of women: I interviewed 32 professional, career-oriented women who chose to give birth in the hospital, and eight women (four professionals, four stay-at-home mothers) who chose to give birth at home. During our in-depth interviews, I tried to get at their body images especially as they dealt with the physical changes of pregnancy and the symbolic aspects of motherhood in relation to their conceptions of self.[1] Later, as I sought to make sense of the pile of transcriptions before me (scholars didn't have sophisticated coding programs back then—we simply printed out our transcriptions and coded them by hand), I began to see that certain fundamental notions about the nature of reality were mirrored in the words these women used to describe their thoughts and feelings about their physiological experiences of pregnancy and motherhood.

[1] These interviews were conducted between 1988 and 1991. Nevertheless, I have kept this chapter mostly in what is termed the "ethnographic present"—writing in the present tense to create more engaging reading. All names used are pseudonyms.

In classic works, Emily Martin (1987, 1990) focused her anthropological lens on revealing differences in the images of body and birth held by middle- and working-class American women—differences that center around the issue of control. In their efforts to wrest control of birth away from the medical establishment, the middle-class women in Martin's study strove not only for control of their birth settings and attendants but also, and most fundamentally, for control of themselves as they labored and gave birth. Meanwhile, their working-class sisters rejected this middle-class emphasis on self-control during birth, saying, "They were talking about breathing and panting and—what are you talking about? It hurts!"

The differences between the two groups in my study are equally compelling. The women in both groups were all relatively affluent members of the white middle-class between the ages of 28 and 42: the fact that they held so many other things in common makes all the more noteworthy the dramatic contrasts in their images of body and birth, and in the worldviews I could glimpse through their expressions of those images. I chose to study white middle-class women because they carry a great deal of what anthropologists call "cultural capital" (which implies certain degrees of status and power) that would seem to grant them the highest levels of choice, unconstrained by socioeconomic, ethnic, or racial barriers to full freedom of choice. Since their choices varied so widely, I was interested in the ideological differences behind those choices. Just as Martin sought not only to present the differences between middle- and working-class women's ideologies of the body and birth but also to discover the meanings of those differences, so I sought both to delineate the ideological differences between these two groups of white middle-class home- and hospital birthers, and to discover what these differences reveal about American culture and its engendered and embodied—or disengendered and disembodied—future.

Women's Body Models: Technocratic and Holistic

Birth. *This is the complete expulsion or extraction from the mother of a fetus irrespective of whether the umbilical cord has been cut or the placenta is attached.*
— Cunningham, MacDonald, and Gant, *Williams Obstetrics*, 17th edition

We value the oneness of the pregnant mother and her unborn child, an inseparable and interdependent whole.
— Excerpt from the Midwives Alliance of North America "Statement of Values and Ethics"

When I first began research on American birth in 1981, most of the 100 women I interviewed over the years of my dissertation research (which later became my first book, *Birth as an American Rite of Passage*) said they wanted some form of "natural childbirth in the hospital," in resistance to the consciousness obliterations their mothers experienced as they gave birth from the 1930s to the 1960s via the widely used drugs scopolamine and general anesthesia. Given this desire for natural childbirth, I expected to find, as Martin had, that most women would resent and resist the increasing number of impersonal intrusions of technology into birth, and what I and others (Arms 1981 [1975]; Haire 1972; Hazzell 1976 [1969]; Romalis 1981; Rothman 1982; Shaw 1974) perceived as women's concomitant loss of their power as birthgivers. But when my initial study was completed several years later (Davis-Floyd 2003 [1992]; Chapter 2, this volume), I instead found that 70% of my 100 interviewees, if not exactly thrilled, were at least rather comfortable with their highly technologized obstetrical experiences and were not much interested in resistance.

Of these 70 women, nine seemed especially to have actively sought and been personally empowered by the technological interventions in their births. (They stood in sharp contrast to nine other women in my sample who had sought natural childbirth but were in the end utterly devastated by their hospital experiences, and who expressed long-lasting feelings of disempowerment, alienation, and rage.) Although this earlier study did not specifically focus on occupation, I noticed that these nine women were all high-powered professionals in positions of prestige, power, and authority. When they hired an obstetrician, they were hiring another professional to perform a service. From him or her they expected the same sort of professionalism and competence in matters of the body as they expected from themselves in their own areas of expertise. They seemed to see technology as integral and central to all areas of American life and fully expected that the very best of modern technology would be brought to bear on their pregnant bodies and the babies within to ensure that their births were competently managed and controlled, and therefore safe.

I was both surprised and intrigued by the attitudes and desires these professional women expressed, and by their ability to manipulate medical ideology and procedures to their advantage. On the other hand, I was equally intrigued by the nearly total resistance to such ideology of the women I came across who had chosen to give birth at home. I was fascinated to see that the women in both these categories actively defined themselves, in myriad ways, as future-shapers. It seemed to me that these two groups represented fruitful ground for further study.

In the book in which I describe that earlier study, *Birth as an American Rite of Passage* (2003 [1992]), I utilized medical texts, childbirth literature, the analyses of other social scientists, and my own data obtained from interviews with women and practitioners to formulate descriptions of two fundamentally opposed models of birth that define the ends of a spectrum of beliefs about birth in the US. I labeled these the "technocratic" and "holistic" models (see Chapter 1, this volume). In that book, since I had not yet become aware of what I later came to call the humanistic model of birth (see Chapter 1), I described the middle range of this spectrum as defined by various "natural childbirth" models; these were given considerable attention in the book, but will not be discussed in this chapter, nor will the humanistic paradigm, as my focus here is on the conceptual extremes, which provide baselines for understanding the experiences and attitudes of the two groups of women in this study.

To briefly recap, the technocratic extreme is dominant in most American hospitals and hegemonically defines the American way of birth. This technocratic paradigm metaphorizes the female body as a defective machine unable to produce a healthy baby without technological assistance. In contrast, the holistic paradigm interprets the female body as an organic system, and birth as an ecological process that can be significantly harmed by dissection and intervention. This chapter investigates the interplay between these paradigms and women's lived experiences of body and self. The basic tenets of these two opposing paradigms will be presented in italics throughout the chapter as they emerge from the words and experiences of these two groups of white middle-class women, and then will be summarized in a chart near the end.

The Technocratic Body and the Professional Woman: A Cultural Hegemony

> *When it came time for Susan Blume to deliver her baby, she was blessedly calm. No sweat soaked her brow, no pain lined her face. She uttered not a sound. As the baby squeezed down the birth canal, Blume [anesthetized by an epidural] lay placidly on her side, reading People magazine and robbing the gods of one more woman bringing forth children in sorrow.*
>
> — Elaine Herscher, *San Francisco Chronicle*

> *Orthodoxy, in other words, opts for the map instead of the territory, the travelogue instead of the trip.*
>
> — Morris Berman, *Coming to Our Senses*

The 32 professionals in my study who chose hospital birth held a wide range of occupations: four were mid-level managers for banks, two for insurance companies; two were fund-raising managers for political campaigns, one was a museum curator; two were realtors, two physicians, three college professors, two regional sales managers, six managers or directors of large government agencies, one accountant, one high-level manager for a major airline; and five owned their own companies. Most of them made as much or more money than their husbands.

The Professional/Personal Split

During the interviews, it quickly became apparent that these women live their lives in terms of a fundamental and clear cut distinction between the personal and professional realms. How they primarily define themselves in relation to society at any given moment is usually a function of what realm they are in. In the professional realm they *are* their role: professor, division manager, CEO. Secure in their professional identities, in the personal realm many of these women seemed to actually be amused to define themselves as "John's wife," or "Suzie's mother," almost as if being John's wife or Suzie's mother was a sort of game they played sometimes. Some perspective on this security of identity was provided by an older woman I spoke with, who had been Mrs. James Bowen since she was 20. She said, "I have always been defined by who my husband was. Now that he is dead, I am forced to confront the fact that I am 65 years old and have no identity of my own." In dramatic contrast stands Lina's description of why she defines herself so strongly in terms of her career, while many of her friends do not:

> I find that some of my friends that I was in college or graduate school with have given up too much. . . . They have compromised their careers in really significant fashion. Either they don't work or they will work part-time, and they just haven't really made a go of it professionally but . . . have put their energies into the relationship and into the family. [That] is very dangerous.
>
> Q. Why?
>
> Men leave. . . . They are relying on their husbands to such a degree that if they leave they are really in trouble. They have totally compromised their careers. They have great potential and they let it go. . . . They in essence capitulated to the family.

Presence in either the personal or professional realm is expressed through bodily adornment: suits and tailored dresses at work, shorts or jogging suits at home. Leah explained:

> I see [the body] as a way to have people respond to you. The way you present yourself draws an equal reaction from the bodies that respond to you. . . . I definitely see that in the professional environment. The way I dress reflects the level of professionalism that I have and the type of response I get from other people. I don't dress in flounces and frills, I dress very tailored and that is reflected even in the glasses I wear. They are pretty much straightforward and businesslike. . . . I like to give a straightforward presentation so that people can deal with me straight.

I found it noteworthy that when I interviewed these women in their homes, they almost invariably would glance down at their casual sweats and tennis shoes and laughingly comment, "You are seeing my other self, my home self"; but when I went to their offices, they never said, "You are seeing my professional self." For most, the professional self was the primary self.

In general, any overlap between the personal and professional realms went one way: personal aspects, like children, relationships, emotional display, did not belong at work, while professional aspects, like paperwork, computer work, and phone calling, often were taken home. (The specific and notable exceptions to this rule will be discussed later on.) Enforcing the boundaries of this one-way street did not present much of a problem for most of these women at first; even those who dated and/or married male colleagues were usually able to keep these relationships separate from their everyday professional activities.

Pregnancy as a Violation of the Professional/Personal Split

Pregnancy perforce entails a violation of the conceptual boundary separating these personal and professional realms of life. Sexuality and children are plainly part of the personal domain; they do not belong at work. But pregnant women visibly and obviously take their children not only into the workplace but also to even the most important meetings! Predictably, many of these women worried about how this boundary violation would affect their work relationships with their colleagues and superiors:

> Q. Were you worried about how your colleagues might react to your pregnancy?
>
> Yes, that's an unqualified yes. . . . They look at me as the President, and I . . . was worried that they might start thinking about me not as much as a professional, but as a woman, and that shouldn't necessarily be bad, but I was worried that it might affect the respect level. . . . It's kind of more obvious that you're a woman, I think, if you're pregnant, I mean it's just constantly reminding people of that rather than just thinking of you as a professional. It gave them another thing to think about, and it wasn't something I wanted them to think about, because I wanted them to think about me as a business kind of guy. [Kay]

However, very few of these women found their fears to be justified. Only three reported that they suffered any sort of job discrimination as a result of their pregnancy, while most others reported the joyful discovery of unexpected benefits from their physical blurring of the personal/professional distinction:

> When I was pregnant for the first time, I was working in a large corporation, and always it was to dress for success, and you were very much on guard as a woman. And as soon as I revealed I was pregnant, people who were not friends of mine, executives many levels up on the corporate ladder, just opened up their personal lives. They identified so strongly with being a father or having a wife who was pregnant. I mean, they would go into 10 or 15 minute conversations. I was stunned at how open and personal everything became when they were around a woman who was bearing a child. [Joanne]

As it evolved for most of these women, the conflict between work and pregnancy was not between their pregnant bodies and their male colleagues, as most had expected, but between their own expectations for their work performance and the biological realities of those pregnant bodies. Catherine said:

> I hated it that people were always wanting to have personal conversations with me about how I was feeling. I was not interested in that at all, and so I made it very plain right at the start that I didn't want to deal with any of that stuff. When I'm at work I am strictly business. I think the reason I didn't have any problems with how I was treated when I was pregnant was that I made it so clear that there was no difference.
>
> Q. Did pregnancy pose any problems at all for you at work?
>
> I would sometimes get so tired that I would tell my secretary to hold my calls, and put my head down on my desk and just sleep for an hour. But I never let anyone know about it, and I made sure that I always got just as much work done anyway, even if that meant I had to stay there longer.

The Centrality of Control

This tension between the professional and personal domains is often heightened by the woman's own perception of herself in relation to her body. Just as with the middle-class women in Martin's study (1990), an overriding concern of these professional women is *control*. They hold the strong belief that *life is controllable*, and that *to be strong and powerful in the world, one must be in control*. As long as these women feel in control, they are "happy," "everything is fine." They achieve control over their *lives* through careful planning and organization of their time and activities. (I asked all of them what they thought about the notion of applying corporate management techniques to family life, such as scheduling family summit meetings, etc. A few thought the notion detracted from the unstructured flow that they saw as the essence of the personal, as opposed to the professional domain, but most heartily approved of the idea.) They achieve control over their *bodies* through regularly scheduled exercise (most were very athletic in school) and over their own *destinies* through reaching positions of independence and importance in the wider society. Interestingly, those who admitted to wanting and enjoying power insisted that it was not power over others that appealed to them, but power to make things happen in the world. Lina said:

> I didn't want to be like my mother . . . I didn't want to be picked on by my husband all the time, and be powerless. You know, she was powerless.
>
> Q. What did you do to be powerful?
>
> I got a PhD and a job.

The Self/Body Split: Pregnancy and Birth as Out-of-Control

These professional women seem to judge every situation by the degree of control they feel they can maintain over it. Even their pregnancies are usually carefully controlled, planned to occur at just the chosen time in their careers.

But once those processes were set into motion, they became uncontrollable, and thus presented these women with a division within their most treasured notions of self: between the cultural, professional parts within their control, and the personal, biological processes outside of it. Lina experienced this division so intensely that she could hardly believe it when she became pregnant:

> Deep down inside of me I believed that I had desexed myself by being the successful professional and I would have to pay for that. I thought I would have a hard time getting pregnant because I thought I would have to pay for what I had gotten away with. . . . I have succeeded at a man's game. . . . A couple of my male faculty colleagues, when they would see me on the campus with the baby, would constantly say, "I can't believe you are a mother, I can't believe you are such a good mother—you are like my mother. I can't believe it." What they were really saying to me is, "I thought you were a guy."

This separation of self from biology is clearly reflected in the body concepts held by many of these women. I asked each one, "How do you think about your body? What is your body?" I was interested to notice that most, instead of giving me a definition, immediately began to talk about how they judged their bodies—as too fat, not in good enough shape, or healthy, in good shape. Such statements reflect their shared belief that *the body is imperfect*:

> I think it's pretty functional [but] . . . it's fat around the middle, and my boobs are too small. [Lou]

> I used to always hate my body. I always had this joke that I got my mother's eyes and my father's chest. I used to think I was flat, you know, I wanted new boobs and liposuction. In the last five or six years, I like it better. It's mine. That's a really loaded question, because you know—women, unless we've had it greatly enhanced by plastic surgery, I don't think we like it. I don't know anybody who *likes* their body. But I've gotten OK about it, and my husband thinks it's the cutest thing he's ever seen. [Louise]

The words of most of those who did provide definitions expressed the additional and equally fundamental belief that *the body is separate from the self*:

> You know, I think there is me and then there is what I'm like physically which can be changed or modified—clothes, makeup, exercise, hairstyles, food. [Georgia]

> My body is mine. It's only mine. I think it was something that was given to me for a reason, you know, to get around in this particular life, because I think it's a place for my soul to be. [Lou]

> A vehicle. Something that moves me from place to place. A repository for thought, for creation, for beliefs, philosophies. [Leah]

> My body is a vehicle that allows me to move around, a tool for my success in the world. [Joanne]

> My body is the recipient of the abuse from the lifestyle that I choose. . . . It's my weakest link—it's like you have to pay the price somewhere—I'm out of shape, overweight, and not eating right—my body to me is what has paid the price for this career.
>
> Q. Can you describe your relationship with your body?
>
> Abusive. [Beth]

Predictably, then, the physical state of pregnancy was problematic at best for some of these women. For intrinsic to the notion of the *body as a vehicle*, a *tool for the self*, are the corollary ideas that *the body is worth less than the self it houses, which, being worth more, should control the body*, should be "in charge." Concomitantly, most of these hospital birthers experienced the bodily condition of *pregnancy as unpleasant because it is beyond the control of the self*, or, as they put it, "out of control." Here is how they expressed that feeling. Linda said:

> I think there are a lot of women who love being pregnant and they would say that. My sister, the Earth Mother, did. Especially before I got pregnant, I thought, "Maybe I'll get into it." But I didn't get into it. I felt bad and large and awkward and nauseated. And oh, I love having the baby, but I wish there were an easier way.

To the question, "How did you feel about your body while you were pregnant?" Lina responded:

> I didn't like it. It just overwhelmed me, the kinds and the variety of sensations, and the things that happen to your body because of the pregnancy. I didn't like it at all. I felt totally alienated from my body.

Even Leah's positive experience of pregnancy is expressed in terms of separation and a feeling of lack of control:

> I really did feel very healthy. It was different being so focused in my body. That's what was so curious. I was watching all this happening. It was something taking control all over me and it was all good. To a certain extent I try to live outside my body so it doesn't control me. Only in this case it was very much controlling me. And that's ok—it was guiding me.

Joanne added:

> I was real apprehensive about going into labor. It kind of terrified me, mostly because I like to be in control . . . and you don't have any control when that happens. I used to have nightmares about standing in front of the president and making a presentation and having my water break.

And here is how Beth experienced birth:

> I mean, it's like a demon to me. There's another being in your body that has to get out and it's looking for a way to get out. And all of a sudden,

> it's like my center of control left my brain and went to this, this thing in my body. And I had no control. I'm very much an in-control person. I like to think that I'm in control of what's going on here, that I can control whatever happens. It was like the control center moved from me to this other being. And you know, all I was doing was lying there—I had to do whatever this other being said was going to happen. And it was *my* body that it was happening to. That was the thing I liked the least.

As they viewed the body as a vehicle for the mind or soul, so these women tended to see the pregnant body as a vessel, a container for the fetus (who is a being separate from the mother) and to interpret its growth and birth as occurring through a mechanical process in which the mother is not actively involved. (Sarah flatly stated, "You're just a vessel. That's all you are, just this vessel.") These beliefs were behaviorally expressed in myriad ways during pregnancy. For example, the evidence these women relied on for proof of the baby's health and growth was objective, coming primarily from ultrasound photographs and electronic amplification of the fetal heart rate. They understood the importance of nutrition and knew that they had to eat well so the baby would be well nourished. But, unlike the homebirthers, they saw this in terms of a simple, mechanical cause-effect relationship. If they ingested good foods, the necessary nourishment would travel to the baby through the placenta, enhancing overall development and especially brain growth. Excessive ingestion of alcohol or junk food, however, might result in a child with less-than-optimal brain capacity. Thus, eating well was a mother's duty to her unborn child to ensure optimal growth conditions. And all of these women had both regular ultrasound scans and underwent amniocentesis in efforts to ensure that they would have perfect babies. Although most of these women experienced giving up alcohol and junk food as something of a burden, to them it was also a logical necessity, something they did as a matter of course. But it did not, conceptually speaking, entail their active participation in growing the child. It merely made them into the best possible "vessels."

In keeping with these attitudes, most of these women did not view the processes of labor and birth as intrinsic to their feminine natures. Said Linda, "If my husband could do it the next time instead of me, that would be just fine." Added Joanne:

> Even though I'm a woman, I'm unsuited for delivering . . . and I couldn't nurse. . . . I've told my mother—I just look like a woman, but none of the other parts function like a mother. I don't have the need or the desire to be biological. . . . I've never really been able to understand women who want to watch the birthing process in a mirror—just you know, I'm not, that's not—I'd rather see the finished product than the manufacturing process.

The Mind/Body Split: Mind over Biology

Emergent in Joanne's words we see the technocratic notions that birth is a mechanical process and that there is no intrinsic value in giving birth "naturally," because technology is better than nature anyway. Thus we can understand when Joanne says that she enjoyed her cesarean birth because her anesthesiologist explained what was happening step by step, and because, since she felt no pain, she was able to be so intellectually attentive to the birth that she could watch the time to see which of her many friends who had placed bets on the time of the birth would win the $18 in the pot. She stated:

> [I liked that because] I didn't feel like I had dropped into a biological being. . . . I'm not real fond of things that remind me I'm a biological creature—I prefer to think and be an intellectual emotional person. So you know, it was sort of my giving in to biology to go through all this.

Here Joanne expresses a view held by most of the women in this group: *The ideal, whole woman is intellectual and emotional, but not necessarily biological.* (Some behavioral ramifications of this notion will be discussed later on.)

Like Joanne, Katie preferred the sense of control provided by a cesarean, and in no way saw this as a disempowering loss, but only as an empowering gain because it was something *she* had caused to happen. When her baby was two weeks overdue and labor had not begun, she told her doctor, who was urging restraint, "I am really getting sick of this. Please schedule [the cesarean]." In response to the question, "How did you feel about yourself after the birth?" she responded, "I felt pretty special. Proud. . . . I felt as if I had accomplished quite a bit."

Kathy, who also described her cesarean as personally empowering, said:

> I don't feel like I missed out on anything. With my first two I was put to sleep. With my third, Bryan, I was given an epidural. Heaven! I would never do it any other way. A cesarean with an epidural. I was awake, everything. Ah, it was just wonderful. . . . I would have to say, hey, I participated in it. I was awake and I felt the pulling and the tugging. I did not push or anything. But I was definitely a part of what was going on.

Elaine summarized:

> Well they induced labor and I wasn't very good at my relaxation techniques and my breathing and after about four hours of labor I decided I would prefer to have a cesarean and so that's what we did. . . . I know some women get all uptight about that, that it wasn't a normal delivery, but I didn't feel the least bit cheated and I feel my birth experience was just as happy as it would have been. I was very happy when I heard them cry, and it was a very pleasant experience.

In their words we hear again the belief these women strongly hold, that the mind is more important than the body, that as long as their minds are aware, they are active participants in the birth process. We hear this expressed even in Clara's recounting of her rapid and unmedicated vaginal delivery:

> Travis came in a little over an hour and that was just not enough time to get mentally prepared. I felt . . . my body was pushing me into having this baby. My mind was not there to work with it. I needed more time to be able to get on top of it and be there.

As a corollary of the idea that technology is better than nature, most of the hospital birthers in this study felt rather strongly that *labor is naturally painful, that pain is bad, and that not to have to feel pain during labor is good and is their intrinsic right as modern women*. To the question, "What did you want out of the birth experience?" Joanne responded, "Out of the birth experience itself I wanted no pain. I wanted it to be as simple and easy and uncomplicated as most everything else has been for me." Said Leah, "I made the decision: I had two hits of Demerol in the IV. I controlled the pain through that." Beth, who "had planned for but did not end up with natural childbirth," was nevertheless very pleased to feel that she also was in control of the decisions that were made. She had expected a long labor with little pain. When the pain became severe, she asked for relief, "and you know, even though I hadn't planned on an epidural, they were very responsive when I said I wanted one." The next time around, Beth planned for an epidural: "When I got there, I was probably about five centimeters, and they said, 'Uh, I'm not sure we have time,' and I said, 'I want the epidural. We must go ahead and do it right now!' So, we had an epidural." And Elaine stressed: "Ultimately the decision to have a cesarean while I was in labor was mine. I told my doctor I'd had enough of this labor business and I'd like to have a cesarean and get it over with. So he whisked me off to the delivery room and we did it."

In keeping with this *high value on making their own decisions* (fully exemplified in the "we" part of "we did it"), the major discontents these women expressed with the medical handling of their labors and deliveries resulted not from the administration of anesthesia, but from its withholding. Kay reported:

> I [asked] for an epidural at one point, but they said they didn't have time to do it.
>
> Q. Was that okay with you?
>
> Not really! I was awfully uncomfortable and I had remembered how wonderful it was [with my first birth] and that I had instantly felt terrific. . . . I was mad that I was in so much pain, and then they would tell me something like "we don't have time," you know—that just drove me wild. I didn't like that at all—I wanted to have it when *I* wanted to have it.

Another woman expressed outrage that a friend of hers in advanced labor had been denied anesthesia for the same reason as Kay, saying earnestly, "No one has the right to tell you that you have to go through that kind of pain." Although a good bit of evidence exists on the depressive effects of analgesia and anesthesia on the baby during labor and birth (see May 2017 for an excellent summary), most of these women felt very strongly that they had an absolute right to the mind/body separation offered by such drugs, especially the epidural. Lina spoke for the majority:

> I read all this stuff that told me I would be a complete asshole to have an epidural and I revolted. [The books said that] I would be able to see that it's much better for the baby and it's a natural experience, and there's just all this pressure. . . . I quit smoking, ate meat, drank milk for months and months—I had been such a good girl. A couple of hours of whatever an epidural was going to do to me, tough. You can put up with it, kid.

Later on Lina insisted that her physician would be the one to know if the drugs used in labor posed any dangers. She and many others stated firmly that they did not believe that their doctors would let any harm come to their babies. In this belief is illustrated yet another technocratic precept: *medical knowledge is authoritative* (Jordan 1997). In contrast to the homebirthers, as we shall see in a moment, none of the 32 hospital birthers reported much respect for or reliance on their own intuition or "inner knowing."

Mediation and Integration through Nurturance—at Home and in the Workplace

Hand in hand with their intense desire for control, for not dropping down into biology, goes, at least for some of these women, a lack of interest in breastfeeding for any extended length of time. To breastfeed is to be out of control—the milk comes unbidden and runs down your blouse; you must drop what you are doing and attend to the child's hunger, a job that cannot be delegated. Bottle-feeding, on the other hand, enables someone else to do that for you, and frees you from enslavement to biology as surely as does an epidural. I recall reading about a woman in a 1930s novel telling her daughter, "The bottle was the battle cry of my generation!" That cry was echoed by my interviewees:

> I really thought I wanted to breastfeed, but I didn't. I wanted my body back. [Lina]

> Yes, it's good for the baby, but if you're uncomfortable with it, for any reason, don't do it. It just isn't worth the trauma. This time I'm not going to do it at all, uh-uh. Part of it goes back to not having the need or the desire to be biological. The other is the confinement of nursing. You know, I wanted to be able to get up and go, and let somebody else feed the baby, and the idea of expressing just nauseated me. [Joanne]

Linda did want to nurse, but ran right up against the boundary between the personal and professional realms:

> I don't have my own office, so I've been trying to think where I'm going to pump when I'm at the hospital. The best I've come up with is the examining room, you know, because that has a lock on the door and I hope it'll work out, because it's not optimal, it's not optimal at all.

Yet, in spite of the difficulties, she was willing to find a way because, as she expresses it,

> a lot of my friends who have worked and have nursed say they feel a little better about working if they're nursing. You know, you still have that connection. I was talking to one of my friends yesterday and she said, "That's one thing the babysitter can't do, you know. That's mine." And I sort of feel that way too. That makes it a little better, a little easier about going back to work. Plus the immunological aspect about putting him in day care—I feel a little better about that, giving him a little better chance of fighting all the germs out there.

Nursing for Linda, as well as for several others, provided a much-valued mediation–integration of the personal and professional realms. Another seeker of integration was Kay, president of her own company, who nursed and kept both her babies in her office until they were a year old. (When I went in to interview her, her two-month-old was sleeping on a chair.) Joanne expressed her difficulties with the personal/professional dichotomy:

> I think there is that split, and that's one of the toughest transitions that professional women have to deal with, and that is: I want to be the soft mommy, and then I have to strip my gears and get back into being the tough businesswoman. And I think that's a tough transition to make.

She goes on to describe two women who serve as role models for her who are "very tough businesswomen," yet will bring their children to the office and will even get down on the floor in full corporate attire in the middle of a busy day to play with someone else's children. She continues:

> It's very encouraging to see people break out of the corporate mold because the corporate personality is so hard and cold and really kind of distasteful . . . I think having families makes people kinder. . . . If people would just step back from corporate greed and get back into relating to people in terms of their interdependence and their affection for each other, it would be a better world.

Louise, when asked what she thought about applying corporate strategies to family life, replied that for her, it was more a question of applying family strategies to the business world: "I treat my clients as if they were as important to me as my family, and it pays off. They really respond, and I have turned this business around from losing to making money in less than a year because of it." As is evident in Louise's statement, these women place *high value on their emotional and nurturing abilities*, abilities they feel spill over from the personal to the benefit of the professional realm. For example, when Janis was head of the electric customer service office, she often worked intensively one-on-one with delinquent bill payers to help them develop an overall economic plan that would work for them. She said, "And I still get visits from people who tell me that I turned their lives around for good, because instead of being their adversary, I nurtured them, and I'm proud of that. I think being a mommy makes me a better professional." Likewise, Kay specifically designs her presidential style to be "participative, democratic, understanding, and kind." Thus caring for her children in her office can be viewed as an extension of her presidential self rather than a contradiction to it; their presence simply represents further integration of the personal and professional spheres that she as president has tried to bring together from the beginning of her company.

These women in general, even as they devalued feminine biological processes, consistently placed high value on what they saw as the feminine qualities of nurturance and emotionality, and sought to bring these qualities into the workplace in a very conscious effort to "humanize" the office environment. Their efforts toward such integration included both more personalized relationships with clients and employees (such as implementing client education programs, flextime, etc.), and creating friendlier environments. Wherever these women had enough control, they redecorated sterile office buildings with softer colors, warmer lighting, conversational areas, artwork, and potted plants, finding that such efforts repeatedly paid off in enhanced intraoffice relationships and increased productivity.

Such integration of the personal and professional realms, however, is usually minimal compared to the degree of separation between these realms. For example, about leaving her six-week-old baby at a day care center, Linda the pediatrician had this to say:

> Q. Do you feel that it would be better for your baby to be with you?
>
> Possibly. On the other hand, I also feel like I probably wouldn't be very happy. I'd probably start climbing the walls, and in a way that would be a bad thing to do to him, to say well alright, I'm going to throw away 20 years of education to stay home with you so that you can be the perfect child.

Thus we arrive at a central question for most of these women: where are they going to put their bodies, carriers of their selves, in relation to their children, the products of those bodies? The answer in general is that as the children were thought of as separate in the womb, so this separation achieves nearly immediate geographical reality after birth. The majority of these women work ten-hour days, and so they see their children only for a maximum of one-and-a-half to two hours per day. I suggest that this situation is a logical extension of their own body images. To rationalize the time/attention differential between work and parenting, most of these women hung their hats on the popular notion of "quality time." (Please note that I am not preaching here, just analyzing—my own family life pretty well reflected this model when I was raising my own children.)

The Dichotomies of Technocratic Life

The similarities in the desires, experiences, and perceptions of pregnancy and birth of these professional women raise many questions. For example, what happens when you can't control everything? Janis had fibroids in her uterus that made her pregnancy very difficult and dangerous. Carolyn, after not exercising for one very busy year, woke up one morning with such a severe pre-arthritic condition in her legs that she could not walk for days. Susan experienced a hormone shift toward the end of her pregnancy that resulted in intense and long-lasting anxiety attacks from which she did not recover until an effective medication was found five years later. Bewildered and angered by their out-of-control bodies, rather than surrendering, these women intensified their commitments to control: Janis was determined to keep working until time for birth, and she did; Carla embarked on a rigorous exercise program and is doing much better; and Susan fought her nearly paralyzing anxiety so successfully that no one at work ever knew of her problem.

When the body works right, it is a vehicle for success. When it does not, it is an impediment to be overcome. As professional and personal are separate domains, so are mind and body, so are mother and baby (even when contained in one body), and so are parents and child:

- professional/personal
- self/body
- mind/body
- mother/baby
- parent/child

These dichotomies seem to encapsulate and express the separations and divisions of technocratic life as most of these women experience it. To some degree, they appear to be mediated by the emotional and nurturant qualities through which these women see themselves as enriching both the workplace and the home.

Homebirthers and the Organic Body: A Cultural Heresy

The contractions kept coming. Each one of them pushed. . . . I tried joining in, very carefully. I pushed with my stomach muscles, just a little . . . but whoa, my uterus grabbed me and drove me along with itself. I couldn't push just a little. It had to be a lot. . . . It was so powerful and uncontrollable. I might push myself inside out if I went too far. But who cares? I didn't try to hold back anymore. I pushed hard. I grabbed onto Vic, onto the folds of his clothes. I held my breath and pushed as hard as I could and it felt good. It felt better. The contractions didn't hurt as much anymore. It was exciting. I'm pushing!

— Janet Isaacs Ashford, "Doing It Myself"

Natural birth is difficult, but a woman's body is designed for this function. When a woman births without drugs, anesthesia, or medical intervention, she learns that she is strong and powerful. She learns self-confidence. She learns to trust herself, even in the face of powerful authority figures. Once she realizes her own strength and power, she will have a different attitude, for the rest of her life, about pain, illness, disease, fatigue, and difficult situations.

— Paulina (Polly) Perez, RN, doula and coauthor of *Special Women*

We will turn now to consideration of the body images and worldviews of the eight homebirthers in my study. Four of these—Kristin, Ryla, Karen, and Liza—were the most extreme proponents of what I have called the holistic model of birth. These four, like Linda's sister, were the sort of women that Linda would call "Earth Mothers." They did not have professional careers in the business or academic worlds; they worked out of their houses as "New Age" counselors and rebirthers, and devoted a large proportion of their waking hours to motherhood. The other four—Tara, Susan, Elizabeth, and Sandra—are professionals of the same ilk as the hospital birthers (Tara and Susan run political campaigns, Elizabeth teaches at a university, and Sandra manages a store).

Self–Body Integration

Interesting differences emerge between the body images of these two subsets of homebirthers. The women in the first group (the home-workers) place no distance between self and body, saying "I *am* my body," or "My body is the physical expression of me." In so saying, they are expressing a basic tenet of the holistic model (which emphasizes union instead of separation)—the very un-Cartesian notion that *self and body are One*.

Differing in many ways from these "Earth Mothers," the four professionals who gave birth at home share much with the hospital birthers in this study, most notably including their desire to be in control and their feelings that body and self are separate. Yet somehow they sense that these notions are inconsistent with their choice of birthplace and the philosophy that accompanies it, as well as with their lived experiences of pregnancy and birth. You can hear them struggling with this inconsistency in the way they discuss their relationships with their bodies. Tara gets herself halfway toward wholeness:

> It has a lot to do with who I am and how I feel about myself. . . . I think that probably 50% of who I am is my body, just in terms of the way I interpret my physical being and try to project that to my family and to the people around me.

And Susan shows us how her lived experience of pregnancy contradicted and changed her former notions. She stated:

> I used to see my body as the vehicle in which I can run around and project myself to the world. . . . I never thought about my body as being me until I did get pregnant. And then you feel very much in tune because you can feel everything that is going on . . . and now I am so much more comfortable with my body, and more and more I see it as part of my Self.

These homebirthers, like Martin's working-class women, tended to reject medical definitions and value judgments in favor of their own lived experience. Experiencing the body as the self, or as part of the self, they came to stress in belief and behavior the body's *organic interconnectedness*, as opposed to its mechanicity, and to view *the female body as normal, attractive, and healthy.* Susan said.

> Before, I was very uncomfortable with my body—the way I looked, the way I felt, just everything. Since I gave birth, it's just not a problem. I'm not all that modest any more. We went to Canada, stripped off all our clothes, and jumped in the ocean, and it didn't bother me that somebody might look at me and say "she could lose ten pounds." . . . I kind of like the way I look.

These homebirthers felt deeply and strongly that female physiological processes, including birth, are healthy and safe:

> Well this one customer—I guess she's maybe 28—she said, "Sandra, are you still thinking about having this baby at home?" She said, "I'm not going to say anything but I think you're absolutely insane. What if something happened?" I said, "Are you not going to drive your car because you could have a wreck? You've got a higher risk doing that than having a baby at home." My friends think I'm crazy. But I think they are. I mean really, *they* are—they're the ones that have missed the whole birth experience, not me.

Letting Go of Control

In dramatic contrast to the high value placed on control by the hospital birthers, the four nonprofessional, spiritually oriented Earth Mothers in my study felt that *giving up control was far more valuable in birth and in life than trying to maintain it*—a philosophical position again arrived at through lived experience. Said Liza:

> I was brought up in the mainstream, and I used to knock myself out trying to control everything. Then I got sick, and I realized that I actually can't control anything or anyone. As soon as I let go of trying, and just began to surrender to what is, everything in my life started to work. I got well, I got married, I had a baby. And if the lesson needed reinforcing, labor did it. That is a force beyond control, a powerful wave that will drown you if you fight it. Better then to dive into it, to relax, let it carry you. Whenever I tried to control my labor or myself during labor, I was in agony. But when I let go and surrendered to the waves, they carried me.
>
> And honestly, contractions only last around 45 seconds, and then you get a break. I think anyone can handle 45 seconds of pain, especially if you stay focused in the moment, on relaxing into this contraction, and then the next, without constantly asking, "How much longer do I have to go?" Because if the answer is hours and hours, you can get really discouraged. But if you just dive into one contraction at a time, and just stay right there in that moment, again, the waves will carry you. (Originally quoted in Davis-Floyd 1994:1133)

Again, we see Tara and Susan moving in that philosophical direction through their lived experience. To the question, "How important is it to you to be in control?" Susan responded, "You know the answer to that! It's more important than it should be. Because I get very carried away with it sometimes, and [I need to learn to let it go sometimes]. I've been a lot happier since I started practicing that." Tara put it this way:

> I always had in my mind that morning sickness was psychological and that basically I could control all these things. If I did things right, ate the right things, and treated my body the right way, then I wouldn't have to worry about kinds of morning sickness that people have, and I could have a quick and easy labor. I exercised a lot, you know, I paid attention to my diet and everything, and I realized, finally, after nine months and a birth, that there are a lot of things you just don't have control over. But it took me that long to admit it.

Tara's kinship with the professional women discussed in the prior section is reflected in her early desire for control over the birth process, and her belief that she could achieve such control by doing all the "right" things in preparation for the birth. Her holistic view of birth kept her from wishing to utilize the technocratic forms of control so important to her professional sisters. Unlike them, she was willing to give up her desire for control to the experience that such control was not and had never been hers.

Pregnancy as Integration

As we might expect, Tara and Susan, like Linda's "Earth Mother" sister, enjoyed pregnancy's constant changes, and came to value their lack of control over these changes. Tara declared, "I loved being pregnant. I just loved all of it. I liked looking at my body in the mirror. I couldn't wait to see what would happen next." Susan said, "I was in awe. . . . Being pregnant was fascinating. . . . It isn't when you're barfing in the toilet bowl every morning, but when that part is over, you feel good. You feel better than you ever had in your life."

To the direct question, "Other women I have interviewed experienced their body changes during pregnancy as being out of control, meaning that they didn't have control. Why didn't you?" Susan responded:

> Whenever anything like that happened to me, I had already read up or talked to midwives and I knew it was coming. I knew that that was going to happen next and it was all part of this wonderful experience of getting pregnant. It felt like it was natural. It was what your body was supposed to do. One step closer to having that baby there.

This response and others like it show that these homebirth women place just as much importance on their minds as do the hospital birthers in this study, but in a rather more integrated way that sees the body and its changes as equally important and holds body and mind to be equally important parts of the whole.

According to the holistic model espoused by these homebirthers, *like self and body, mother and baby are essentially One*—that is, they form part of an integrated system that can only be harmed by dissection into its individual parts. Much more than a passive host, or "vessel," the mother sees herself as *actively growing the baby.* Susan said: "Especially when you're actually actively doing all the exercises you're supposed to be doing and you're actively eating and drinking what you're supposed to be eating and drinking, then you really feel like you are feeding and nourishing and growing the baby." For Kristin, this feeling of active involvement in pregnancy combined in an unusual way with psychic experiences that generated in her sensations of, and then belief in, the reality of active communication, unity, and partnership with her unborn baby:

> When I was about two months pregnant I was lying on my waterbed one night in the dark, not sleeping, but also not really thinking, just drifting along, when suddenly, from somewhere inside of the front of my head I heard these words, "I'm here, I'm a girl, and my name is Joy Elizabeth." . . . One night [much later on], I had a Braxton Hicks contraction and I heard a voice inside say "I'm scared." I told her I was scared, too, and that everything would be okay because we were partners and we would do this thing together.

Elizabeth experienced this sort of active communication and sense of partnership with her unborn in a rather dramatic way:

> Two weeks before he was born, he was still breech. My midwives felt confident about a breech delivery, but I . . . very much wanted him to turn. I went to a therapist who, several people had told me, was really good at visualization, and asked her to help me get in touch with him. I imagined myself in the warm waters of my uterus until I could see him. I told him I loved him, and couldn't wait to hold him in my arms, and then I asked him please to turn. I told him it was really important to me. He looked right at me and I suddenly felt that if I would show him what to do, he would do it. So I started swimming down, towards my cervix, motioning for him to follow me. . . . By the time I woke up the next morning, he had completely turned, and he stayed that way until he was born!

Mind–Body Integration: Active Agency and Inner Knowing during Birth

For these homebirthers (as, in their very different way, for the hospital birthers) this active, agentic role was key. Near the beginning of her first pregnancy, during her very first interview with an obstetrician, Susan became angry because his response to her questions was, "You don't need to worry about that. I'll take care of that." She said, "He thought he knew more about it than I did!" When I asked her, "Why didn't you assume that he did know more than you?" she replied:

> Well, I didn't consider having a baby something I wasn't supposed to take part in. That I was just there to grow this baby and he was going to take it out of me, but I couldn't do that on my own. I knew better than that. I knew enough about the way a body functions and the way people have babies to know that it was me 100% that was going to get this baby through the birth canal and out into the world. And once it's out there, you know, you do need people to take care and make sure the baby is OK and to make sure that I'm OK and that everything went well, but as far as bringing that baby through, that was my job. And I needed to know something about it. I needed to know exactly how that was going to work and I wanted somebody who would work with me to do the best job I could.

Just as these homebirthers see themselves as actively growing their babies, so they also see *labor and birth as hard work that a woman does*. This holistic view that does not separate the woman from the process of labor accepts *pain as an integral part of that process*. To eliminate that one part would interfere with the systemic whole, and would begin a cycle of interference that might have unforeseen results. When I asked, "Did it mean anything to you that you went through the pain?" Tara responded:

> Oh yes. It's part of the whole experience. In this society, we try not to experience pain. We take lots of drugs, I mean legal things. And I feel that's why a lot of people get into other forms of drug abuse. . . . Even though during labor I remember feeling it was almost unbearable, it never entered my mind to wish I had "something for the pain." . . . I wanted the pain to stop, but not because somebody gave me something. I guess part of it is . . . the wonderful physical and emotional stuff that is going on at the same time as the pain. If you took drugs for the pain, you would change all the rest of it, too.

Susan Irwin and Brigitte Jordan define authoritative knowledge as "legitimate, consequential, official, worthy of discussion, and useful for justifying actions by people engaged in accomplishing a certain task or objective" (1989:13). Under the technocratic model, only technologically obtained medical knowledge is said to be authoritative. But homebirthers operating under the holistic model often regard *a woman's intuition or "inner knowing" more highly than the objectively obtained information of tests* (see Chapter 7).

For example, Elizabeth's midwife became concerned during labor because the baby's heart tones were dropping, and muttered under her breath about possibly going to the hospital. Elizabeth heard her, and was "flooded with the total certainty that her baby was fine." She leaned forward between pushing contractions and whispered this inner knowing to the midwife, who immediately and visibly relaxed. Later Elizabeth asked the midwife about her response. The midwife replied, "Over the course of my years of doing homebirth, if I have learned anything it is to trust what mothers know."

On the subject of whose knowledge to trust, homebirth professional Susan expressed herself very strongly. She said:

> I went to an OB when I found out I was pregnant. And I told him, son of a bitch, that I was pregnant, and he said, "Let's test you and see." And I said, "No, I am pregnant and I'm trying to pick an OB." And he said, "Let's pee in the little cup and let me see." And that infuriated me. . . . He sent me home with this little pink book about how you had to act differently now that you are pregnant, and at the back of this book, it said . . . to be sure to take a frilly sexy nightgown to the hospital for after the birth and little notes and a pen so that you'll have something to do. . . . And I just called him up and said, "Cancel my appointment." It was a throwback from the fifties. It was ridiculous. And then I was really upset because I didn't know what to do, [and someone I ran into suggested that I call a midwife named Nikki], and we just hit it off like that. Instantly I knew that this was what you were supposed to do. This was the way to have a baby.

In technocratic reality, not only are mother and baby viewed as separate, but the best interests of each are often perceived as conflicting. In such circumstances, the mother's emotional needs and desires are almost always subordinated to the medical interpretation of the best interests of the baby as the all-important product of this "manufacturing process." Thus individuals operating under this paradigm often criticize homebirthers as "selfish" and "irresponsible" for putting their own desires above their baby's needs. But under the holistic paradigm held by these homebirthers, just as mother and baby form part of one integral and indivisible unit until birth, so *the safety of the baby and the emotional needs of the mother are also One. The safest birth for the baby will be the one that provides the most nurturing environment for the mother.* Said Tara: "The bottom line was that I felt safer [at home] and I think that's what it boils down to for most people. . . . It seemed strange to me that people feel safer with drugs and that type of thing." Elizabeth confirmed, "My safest place is my bed. That's where I feel the most protected and the most nurtured. And so I knew that was where I had to give birth." And Ryla added, "I got criticized for choosing a homebirth, for not considering the safety of the baby. But that's exactly what I *was* considering! How could it possibly serve my baby for me to give birth in a place that causes my whole body to tense up in anxiety as soon as I walk in the door?"

According to the technocratic model, the uterus is an involuntary muscle, and labor proceeds mechanically in response to hormonal signals. Both Susan and Tara were attended at home by midwives who see *the uterus as a responsive part of the whole*, and who therefore believe that *the best labor care will involve attention to the mother's emotional and spiritual desires, as well as her physical needs*. The difference between these two approaches is clearly illustrated by the responses of a physician and a lay midwife to the stopped labor of a client. The physician said, "It was obvious that she needed some pitocin, so I ordered it," and the midwife said, "It was obvious that she needed some rest, so she went to sleep, and we went home for awhile, until active labor kicked in." Here is Susan's story:

> Nikki [the midwife] kind of got worried about it towards the afternoon. Because it just kept going on and nothing was changing. And she took me to the shower and said, "Just stay in there till the hot water goes away." And Ira went with me to massage me and try to get everything relaxed. And then Nikki asked my friend Diane, "What's the deal with Susan? . . . Is she stressed out about work?" And Diane said, "Well, yeah, I think she's afraid to have the baby. She's afraid that once she's had the baby . . . she's not going to be able to go back to her job and all that." So when I came back out and laid back down, Nikki started in on me about it. She said, "Right now your job is not important. What you have to do right now is have this baby. This baby is important." And I just burst into tears and was screaming at her and started crying, and I could feel everything when I started crying just relax. It all went out of me and then my water broke and we had a baby in 30 minutes. Just like that.

A powerful and revealing example of the mind–body integration so profoundly believed in by homebirthers comes from Lynn Richards' book on *The Vaginal Birth after Cesarean Experience* (1987:159–160). A woman called Linda and her midwife recount their experience of Linda's severe postpartum hemorrhage after a homebirth:

> Linda: I felt the sweetness of my baby's body sliding out from within me. I opened my eyes and saw her—my big, beautiful, wide-eyed, alert and vibrant sweet girl. My need for her exploded within me and I asked for her. I held her on my abdomen and named her. How I loved her! . . . and then the blood . . . began to flow.
>
> Midwife: Blood was gushing down from Linda's uterus, and no amount of uterine stimulation, either naturally or medically, would stop it. I reached inside her vagina, following the cord up to the top of her uterus where the placenta still partially clung to her uterus. I looked at her and said, "You can stop this bleeding any time you want to." She replied, in amazement, "I can?" "You can. Let go of your pregnancy, let go of your placenta."
>
> Linda: The midwife's voice brought me back to contact and responsibility. Her face gave me peace and power once again. I welcomed the peace, and took the responsibility and power. The peace flowed through my entire body and the power hit the top of my uterus. Out came the placenta.
>
> Midwife: And the bleeding stopped.

> Linda: At last I accepted . . . the truth of my healthy body and my right to give birth, love with it, live with it. . . . Shanna and I were both born that night.

Such dramatic experiences of the reality and viability of the mind–body connection are common in the narratives of homebirthers. For example, Kristin said:

> Somewhere during this time I remembered my birth during a rebirthing session. . . . I didn't want to come out of my mother, and finally the obstetrician had to deliver me with forceps. I remembered being inside trying not to come out . . . setting it up so that someone else did it for me and forced me to be born. I have had to deal with issues of helplessness and force my whole life. I had a powerful emotional release and cried for a very long time. Steven held me and provided safety to experience the tremendous trauma that surrounded that incident.
>
> [Well into labor] my screams clued the midwives that transition had completed and it was time to push. This was the point where having remembered my own birth was invaluable. I was thinking how much I wanted to just forget this whole thing and go do something else, that I didn't know what to do, I didn't know how to push, that I couldn't do it, that I should give up, that no one could make me do it—all the helplessness and force issues I had glimpsed in the rebirthing. . . . I remember telling myself I would do whatever I had to do. . . . The next time I felt a contraction coming on I pushed with all my might and yelled at the same time. It was a yell from deep in my throat, and definitely not from pain, but from putting every aspect of my being into that push. I did that for about 35 minutes, whenever a contraction would come . . . and the baby's head came out. One more push and her shoulders were delivered. Then the midwives invited me to reach down and pull her out, which I did. . . . The midwives had slit the sac because she was still inside it, and I pulled her out and laid her on my chest. . . . She coughed gently once, and then she lay there very peacefully. Someone put a blanket over her and we lay there like that for probably thirty minutes. I have no idea of the time. I was completely transfixed.

Later, Kristin added:

> Pregnancy and birth changed my whole view of myself. I discovered that I had never valued myself as a woman. I valued the masculine aspects of my personality, but I considered my womanly traits weak and counter-productive. [Birth was] an incredible discovery of the power of my intuition, and of the value of trusting myself.

Living the Paradigm at Home, in the Workplace, and in the World

Just as the principle of separation governs so many domains of life for the hospital birthers in this study, so the principles of integration and interconnectedness that these homebirthers internalize through pregnancy and birth spill over into many other areas of their lives. For example, Susan reports that she is learning to put the principle of giving up control to use in the office and is finding that the results include lowered stress levels and improved relationships with subordinates, who feel freer to innovate and take on more responsibility as she becomes less controlling. Elizabeth began experimenting with the same principle in her teaching and finds that when she gives up trying to control her students by making them see things her way, potentially tense confrontations and disagreements transform into mutually productive discussions. Likewise, when her children become ill, Elizabeth rarely takes them to a doctor:

> Since I learned so much about mind–body integration from giving birth, I know that most of the time, they can heal themselves, if I can just listen well enough to help them figure out what's really wrong emotionally. Once we handle that, usually their bodies can quickly take care of the rest.

Susan uses her experience of birth to conceptualize more concretely her link to all of life:

> I think birth is going to become much more technological, more geared toward more testing, early intervention, genetic selection. But I would prefer that birth remain as natural as possible. There's something emotional, psychological, involved. If we lose that, we will regret it in the future, because we're missing out on something that links us to life in a very fundamental way. Birth is what ties us to other forms of life, creates a bond between human women that goes back hundreds of generations, and bonds us to other species as well. The more technological birth becomes, the more it differentiates us, and the more unlike other species—and other members of our own species—we become.

Some Commonalities: Active Agency and Control

A caveat: In my efforts to make clear the profound differences in body image and worldview between these two groups of women, I have no doubt overemphasized the polarities, which, although evident and real, can obscure some important commonalities that need to be acknowledged. Most important, I think, and most reflective of recent events in American society is the fact that all these women are far from resembling the passive victims of technocracy that many of their mothers may have been. All were active agents in their birthgiving, although in radically different ways, as we have seen. For both groups, curiously enough, that agency took the form of control. We have seen the importance of control to the hospital birthers; we should also note its importance to the homebirthers. For although they gave up trying to control their bodies, they very actively sought to retain control of other sorts of things, most particularly of their birth space. "Nosy neighbors," "nervous parents," and "medical types" were to be kept out; besides partners and children, only carefully selected midwives, relatives, and/or friends were allowed in. As Elizabeth put it, "I had to control my birth environment, so that nobody would control my birth."

I find another important commonality in the fact that the integrative principles so important to the homebirthers were also much in evidence in the lives of some of the professionals. Their technologies of integration, as we saw earlier, included breastfeeding and bringing their children into the workplace both before and after birth. Most, even if they devalued feminine biological processes, did place high value on what they saw as the feminine qualities of nurturance and emotionality, and they sought to bring these qualities into the workplace in order to "humanize" the office environment.

Concomitantly, the separation so pervasive in the lives of the professionals was also an issue for the homebirthers, some of whom had to deal with the same issues of separation from their children during working hours, even when they were working at home. Ryla said:

> It's happened lots of times—I'll be seeing a client, and trying to come across like a professional, and then my two-year-old, who is supposed to be getting watched by his sister, will bang on the door and say, "Mommy, I pooped in the hall!" And I know it's because he wants my attention, and I feel just as guilty as if I had gone to the office—maybe more so because he's right there in front of me, and I'm telling him to go away.

Women's Perceptions of the Technocratic and Holistic Models of Birth and the Body Compared

The uterus is a muscular organ that is covered, partially, by peritoneum, or serosa. The cavity is lined by the endometrium. During pregnancy, the uterus serves for reception, implantation, retention, and nutrition of the conceptus, which it then expels during labor.

— Cunningham, MacDonald, and Gant, *Williams Obstetrics*

You can't take a woman and tear her apart—that's what the doctors do.

— Homebirth midwife

The table below presents a comparison of the basic tenets of the hegemonic technocratic model and the alternative, heretical holistic model as they have emerged from the words and behaviors of the women in this study.

Women's Perceptions of the Technocratic and Holistic Models of Birth Compared

The Technocratic Model of Birth	The Holistic Model of Birth
The body is imperfect, and separate from the self.	Self and body are One.
The body is mechanical—a vehicle, a tool for the self.	The body is an organism, intimately interconnected with mind and environment.
Life is controllable.	Life is not controllable.
The self should control the body.	The body cannot be controlled.
Pregnancy is out-of-control, and therefore unpleasant.	Pregnancy is uncontrollable and pleasurable.
The pregnant body is a vessel for the fetus, who is a separate being.	Mother and baby are essentially One—they form part of an integrated system that can only be harmed by dissection into parts.
Fetal growth is a mechanical process in which the mother is not actively involved.	The mother actively grows the baby.
The desires of the mother and the needs of the baby can and often do conflict during labor and birth.	The safety of the baby and the emotional needs of the mother are the same. The safest birth for the baby will be the one that provides the most nurturing environment for the mother.
Birth is a mechanical process.	Birth is hard work a woman does.
Technology is better than untrustworthy nature.	Nature is best, and can be trusted. Technology should support but not interfere.
The mind is more important than the body.	Mind and body are one—organically interconnected.
Active participation and control in life are good.	The most active participation can involve giving up control.
As long as a woman's mind is aware, she is an active participant in birth.	A woman gives birth with her whole being.
Pain is bad. Not to have to feel pain in labor is a modern woman's intrinsic right.	Pain is an integral part of the labor process. To eliminate that part interferes with the systemic whole.
Medical knowledge is authoritative.	Intuition/inner knowing are authoritative.
To be strong and powerful, one must be in control.	Strength and power come from letting go of control.

Body Image as a Template for the Future?

Nothing will have more of an impact on the future than medical science, with advances posing a series of ethical questions. Anyone thinking of starting a family will begin with a Sears catalogue of options: A woman wishing to postpone child-bearing for career development may want to freeze a few eggs for later use; a woman who is unable to conceive may want to "adopt" an embryo deposited by an anonymous donor at a frozen embryo bank, then carry it in her own body.
— *Life* magazine (February 1989:54)

Emily Martin saw the efforts of the middle-class women's health movement to regain control of birth as resulting in

> middle-class women becoming controlled themselves, being the agents of exerting control over themselves, as silent, except for certain controlled forms of breathing they perform in the public arena of the hospital. . . . In so doing they may be ignoring other aspects of their experiences, which are less easily articulated because they are (as our culture sees them) more physical and less controllable. Working-class women more readily articulate precisely these kinds of experiences: I am in pain, this hurts, it is enough to make me scream; I am not really in control of this situation, *and no one could be*. (1990:309)

Martin suggested that this situation mirrors social structures in the workplace, where:

> middle-class women more than working-class women advocate and practice "mind over matter" and seek mental concentration that does not allow the body to dictate events. . . . While resisting the medical ideology of reproduction, some middle-class women may be reproducing the ideology and practice of control, in this case exerting control over themselves. By enacting out-of-control behavior, some working-class women may be resisting both the treatment they expect from medical managers and middle-class ideology about the desirability of always being in control. That middle-class women find the idea of going out-of-control in labor repellent and even grotesque is evidence of an opposition among women that does not serve our common interests. (1990:310–311)

The opposition between home- and hospital birthers of the middle class over this same issue of control is equally dramatic, and we may equally well question whether it serves our common interest as women.

The professionals in my study insist on control, and they, like Martin's middle-class women, tend to be silent in the hospital: they do not scream out their pain; rather, they anesthetize it away. However, it does not look to them like they are being controlled by the medical establishment, but rather that *they are manipulating the technocratic resources of the medical establishment to control their own bodily experiences.* Martin suggests that such feel ings of being "empowered and in control" are illusory and that "losing control" in birth "can mean having one's body physically penetrated [via cesarean section]" (1990:309). But for these professional women (one of whom scheduled her cesarean to take place between conference calls with England and Japan), having a cesarean is not losing control but gaining it—given the models of reality they individually hold. Regardless of how they came to believe in the value of technocratic control, the fact that they do believe in and value such control is not an illusion, and their feelings of empowerment when they achieve such control through the agencies of the professionals they have hired for that purpose—their physicians—are not illusions either. Although I may personally perceive cesareans as disempowering for birthing women, as an anthropologist I know that those who participate most fully in a society's hegemonic core value system, as these women do, are most likely to be empowered by and to succeed within that system, as these women have.[2]

In "Society and Sex Roles," Ernestine Friedl postulates that

> in any society, status goes to those who control the distribution of valued goods and resources outside the family. . . . Only as managers, executives, and professionals are women in a position to trade goods and services, to do others favors, and therefore to obligate others to them. Only as controllers of valued resources can women achieve prestige, power, and equality. Within the household, women who bring in income from jobs are able to function on a more nearly equal basis with their husbands. (1990:218)

Certainly, these professional women confirm Friedl's hypotheses—they are highly successful in the wider society as controllers of valued goods and resources, including high levels of capital, and at home all but one reported that their marriages were extremely egalitarian. While the homebirthers in my study who worked from home certainly do not see themselves as unsuccessful, the criteria of the technocracy would judge them less so than the professionals, as they are not in general controllers of valued goods and resources (although they do enjoy egalitarian marriages with husbands who share the same alternative worldview as they).

Proponents of a paradigm tend to create the world in its image. Childbirth educators and midwives often speak of the "epidural epidemic." The deeper we probe into the worldviews of these professional women as they emerge in their descriptions of their beliefs about birth and their female bod-

[2] In "Media Representations of Pregnancy and Childbirth: An Analysis of Reality Television Programs in the United States," researchers Morris and McInerney (2010) described the results of their content analysis of 85 reality-based television shows depicting 123 births, aired in the US on Discovery Health and The Learning Channel in November 2007, concluding that "women's bodies were typically displayed as incapable of birthing a baby without medical intervention."

ies, the more we can understand why this is so. As the epidural numbs the birthing woman, eliminating the pain of childbirth, it also graphically demonstrates to her through her lived experience the truth of the Cartesian maxim that mind and body are separate, that the biological realm can be completely cut off from the realm of the intellect and the emotions. This microcosmic mirror of our technocratic society casts its reflection in ever-widening ripples in the pond of social life. As the drugged baby so mechanically birthed is carried off to the nursery to be separate from the mother, and spends much of infancy in cribs and plastic seats and carriers, so that same infant in later years will be carried off to day care and to school. Ours is a nation founded on principles of separation, and we enact and transmit those principles to each other in the spatial and interactional relational patterns we have developed between mind and body, mother and baby, and parents and child. Were the more technocratically-oriented women described in this chapter giving birth today, they would undoubtedly be separating themselves further from the birthing experience by texting, tweeting, and Facebooking throughout the process, as today's Millennials are so attached to doing.

Proponents of a paradigm tend also to envision the future in its image. When asked about her vision for the future of American birth, Joanne, the professional who did not want to "drop into biology," spoke of the benefits of genetic engineering, saying, "I think people in the future are going to expect medicine and science to have more answers." And Katie said, "I cannot envision how birth could be any different, except perhaps the drugs will be better and they will be able to measure the amounts more exactly."

The technocratic model's emphasis on separation potentiates various sorts of futuristic behavioral extremes in the cultural arena of birth. These technocratic extremes include, among many others: court-ordered cesareans—cases in which the mother refuses to have a cesarean but is forced to do so by the courts against her will (Jordan and Irwin 1989; Shearer 1989); surrogacy—a contractual arrangement in which the womb of one woman is rented to incubate someone else's child (Mondal et al. 2012); sex preselection—using various techniques to try to ensure that the baby will be a boy or a girl, using amniocentesis to determine which it is, and then aborting if it is not the desired sex (a practice extremely common in highly patriarchal societies such as India and China); genetic engineering—altering genes to select for certain desired traits or eliminate undesirable ones; and the development of artificial wombs that could grow a baby to term outside a woman's body. (It is worth remembering that such futuristic, cyborgian reproductive technologies are envisioned, invented, and "chosen" in a sociocultural context that values them more than the female bodies they act upon.)

This idea of the baby as separate, as the product of a mechanical process, is a very important metaphor for women because it implies that the technocracy ultimately can become the producer of that product, as of so many others. The current cultural debates over fetal vs. maternal rights dramatically illustrate how fundamental is this separation to technocratic notions of parenthood. Moreover, as Rothman (1989, 1992) has long pointed out, mind/body//mother/child separation forms the ideological basis of the new reproductive technologies, from amniocentesis to artificial wombs. As early as 1989, the February cover story of *Life* magazine, "The Future and You," predicted "Birth without Women":

> By the late 21st century, childbirth may not involve carrying at all—just an occasional visit to an incubator. There the fetus will be gestating in an artificial uterus under conditions simulated to re-create the mother's breathing patterns, her laughter and even her moments of emotional stress. (p. 55)

In contrast to such futuristic scenarios of separation, Tara's vision for the future makes an explicit connection between the ecological principles of the environmental movement and homebirth:

> How do we change this trend toward more drugs for birth, more machines? I think it starts with the way we raise our kids. I think the environmental movement could help as much as anything. That movement is in vogue, and it's nonpartisan—it's for everyone. It encourages us to love Mother Earth, and to teach our children—boys and girls—to be emotional, feeling, and caring. The environmental movement can help us to change our sex role stereotypes. Men have been moving in that direction, but society has not been very accepting. There is a passion and emotion that comes out in the environmental movement that both men and women feel and accept as good. And that will influence birth. It will take both parents seeing things differently to change birth. As men open up to their emotional, caring selves, they will begin to feel strongly about natural birth. Mother Earth has historically been seen as feminine. If we get back to caring about the Earth, being caretakers, it would be difficult not to translate that into other parts of our lives. Sooner or later people will ask themselves how they can give birth drugged and hooked up to machines, when they are trying to stop treating their own Mother Earth that way.

One of homebirthers in my study, Ryla—an ecofeminist like Tara—is engaged in research on water birth, and on birthing in the ocean with dolphins in order to tap the potential of interspecies communication—two futuristic extremes made possible by the holistic model's emphasis on interconnectedness. Other such extremes of interconnectedness include attempting to conceive babies consciously (Parvati-Baker 1986a, 1992) and working to enhance psychic communication between mother and child (Peterson 1981). Such holistically-oriented researchers are consciously attempting to counterbalance the disembodied future toward which the technocratic model seems inexorably to be leading us.

Extremes, on both ends of the spectrum, play an important role in defining the outer edges of the possible and the imagined. Most especially, those at the extreme of conceptual opposition to a society's hegemonic paradigm—the radical fringe—create much more room for growth and change within that society than would exist without them. How much more technocratic might hospital birth look, if no one in this country believed that mother and baby are One, that there is an inner knowing that can be tapped, that fulfilling the emotional needs of the mother is the best approach to the health of the child?

Because the technocratic paradigm *is* hegemonic, pervading medical practice and guiding almost all reproductive research, no middle-class woman who gives birth at home can fail to be aware that she is battling almost overwhelming social forces that would drive her to the hospital. The homebirthers in my study who espouse the holistic model do so in direct and very conscious opposition to the dominant technocratic model. They represent the 1% of American women who choose to give birth at home. I suggest that the importance to American society of this tiny percentage of alternative model women is tremendous, for they are holding open a giant conceptual space in which women and their babies can find metaphorical room to be more than mechanistic antagonists. Homebirthers I have interviewed use rich metaphors to describe pregnancy, labor, and birth that work to humanize, personalize, feminize, and naturalize the processes of procreation. They speak of mothers and babies as unified energy fields, coparticipants in the creative mysteries, entrained and joyous dancers in the rhythms and harmonies of life. They talk of labor as a river, as the ebb and flow of ocean waves, as ripened fruit falling in its own good time.

Jeannine Parvati-Baker, author of *Hygeia: A Woman's Herbal* (1978), *Conscious Conception* (1986a), *Prenatal Yoga* (1986b), and "The Shamanistic Dimensions of Childbirth" (1992), and self-acknowledged "Earth Mother" (now deceased) had this to say about being "on the radical fringe" (personal communication):

> Some years ago, I wrote a visualization . . . which led the participants in gradual steps to a door, and encouraged them to open it without giving any hints as to what might be on the other side. Experimenting, I tried it out on myself, and found that when I opened the door, I stepped out into the starry night sky, which began to swirl and swirl. . . . The next time someone told me that I "hang out on the radical fringe," something I've been hearing for most of my life, I suddenly saw that yes, I am on the fringe—on the fringe of the skirt of the goddess as she dances around the universe. That starry sky, that's the fringe of her skirt, and it swirls and swirls as she dances. And that's my place, and it's a wonderful place to be, full of movement and excitement and joy.

Homebirthers and their midwives in the United States have long been an endangered species, again, as they account, even today in 2017, for only 1.36% of American births. (As part of a fund raising effort a few years back, a group of local midwives sold T-shirts with whales stamped on the front; the caption underneath read "SAVE THE MIDWIVES!") Should they cease to exist, the options available in American society for thinking about and treating pregnancy, birth, and the female body would sharply decrease, and our society would be enormously impoverished. Should they thrive, we will continue to be enriched by their alternative visions and their enormous body of knowledge about how to facilitate and support normal physiologic birth.

As feminists, we fight for the right to make our bodies our own, to metaphorize, adorn, and technologize as we please. We are just beginning to guess at the cultural and individual impact of the symbolic messages today's professional women are sending through their symbolic placement of their bodies in relation to their families, and through their mental attitudes to the physical changes brought about by the biological processes of pregnancy, birth, and motherhood. The intensifying quest of many of these women for distance from these processes leads inevitably to the question: As women increasingly break out of the confines of the biological domain of motherhood, will/should our culture still define that domain as primarily belonging to women? What do we want? As we move further into the 21st century, will the options opened to us by our technology leave equal conceptual room for the women who want to *be* their bodies, as well as for the women for whom the body is only a vessel? As researchers like Ehrenreich and English (1973a, b), Corea (1985), Rothman (1982, 1989), and Spallone (1989) have shown, the patriarchy has been and is only too willing to relieve us of the necessity for our uniquely female biological processes. To what extent do we desire to give up those processes that since the beginning of the species have defined us as women, in order to compete with men on their terms and succeed?

In the new society we are making, will the homebirthers and the homeschoolers, the goddesses and the Earth Mothers, have equal opportunity to live out their choices alongside those who want to schedule their cesareans, and those who want their babies incubated in a test tube? I know that as anthropologists, my colleagues and I will continue to work to bring to consciousness the symbolic import of our unconscious behavior, to elucidate its cultural and individual ramifications, and to track the disappearance of old options and the opening of new ones. I hope that we can map the strategies, successes, and setbacks of those who try to have it all, and those who try to let it all go, and supply their accumulated wisdom of experience to ourselves and to the citizens of the future we are cumulatively trying to build.

Questions for Thought and Discussion

1. Why did Davis-Floyd conduct the study described in this chapter on these two particular groups of women? And why did she choose to focus on white middle-class women?

2. What did the notion of control mean to these two groups of women and how did their definitions and perceptions of "control" differ?
3. What are some of the differences in their perceptions of their bodies between these two groups?
4. Davis-Floyd conducted this research between 1988 and 1991. Do you think that these two types of women would respond differently to her questions today? Why or why not?
5. Can you personally relate to either of these two types of women? What kind of birth do you want for yourself?
6. Do you think that today's customs of texting, tweeting, instant messaging, Facebooking, etc during labor and birth are more likely to detract from, or enhance, the birthing woman's experience? Why or why not?

Recommended Films

Pregnant in America: produced by Steve Buonaguario, 2008. http://www.imdb.com/title/tt1231290/

Orgasmic Birth: produced by Debra Pascali-Bonaro. http://www.orgasmicbirth.com/ (Also available under the title *Organic Birth*)

The Face of Birth: Where the Personal Gets Political: produced in Australia. A film about families who choose to give birth at home and the midwives and health professionals who support them. Available at http://www.faceofbirth.com/. This film is accompanied by *Meet the Experts: Beyond the Face of Birth.*

It's My Body, My Baby, My Birth: A Film about Natural Childbirth: an educational childbirth film that tells the stories of seven mothers and their childbirth journeys. Available at www.ItsMyBodyMyBabyMyBirth.com

4

Medical Training as Technocratic Initiation

In most ways, medical education is more like high school than a graduate program. The emphasis is on learning mechanical tasks within a rigid structure rather than developing an inquiring mind. It is akin to eight to twelve years of boot camp.
— Terry Tyler, MD

Only a long and complex training process could produce individuals who have the ability to handle life-and-death situations adroitly, to ignore personal needs consistently while continuing to help others, and to suppress emotional response during the most intense situations. Medical training in the United States and elsewhere functions as an initiatory rite of passage, transforming medical students into doctors.[1] As such, it carries the burden, not only of transmitting knowledge and skills, but also of imbuing students with the values and beliefs basic to the technocratic paradigm of medicine. Across cultures and throughout history, humans have used similar kinds of rituals to bring about such transitions from one social status to another.

[1] In this chapter I focus on the *psychological transformation of medical students*, not on the process of medical training, which has been well and thoroughly described by numerous social scientists and physicians. See for excellent examples the works of Renée Fox (1957, 1980), Nancy Stoller Shaw (1974), Diana Scully (1980), Ann Oakley (1984), Howard Stein (1990), and Byron Good and Mary Jo DelVecchio Good (1993; see also Good 1995); as well as by physicians Cynthia Carver (1981) and Michelle Harrison (1982), medical anthropologist Melvin Konner (1987), and former social worker Charles LeBaron (1981), who have recorded their personal experiences of this process.

This chapter has been revised and updated from Chapter 2 of *From Doctor to Healer: The Paradigm Shift of Holistic Physicians* (1998) by Robbie Davis-Floyd and Gloria St. John. New Brunswick NJ: Rutgers University Press.

This chapter is based on interviews that I conducted with 12 obstetricians in 1987 and analyzed in depth in my article "Obstetric Training as a Rite of Passage" (1987c), on 40 interviews with humanistic and holistic physicians of varied specialties conducted by either myself or my colleague Gloria St. John between 1993 and 1995, fully described and analyzed in our coauthored book *From Doctor to Healer: The Transformative Journey* (1998), and on one interview I conducted with an obstetrician in 2016. All of these interviewees are from the US (see Chapter 5 for information on Brazilian OBs); many are currently still in practice.

Ritual and Rite in Medical Training

To recap from Chapter 2, a ritual, very simply, is a patterned, repetitive and symbolic enactment of a cultural belief or value (Davis-Floyd 2003 [1992]; Davis-Floyd and Laughlin 2016). Rituals often serve simultaneously as symbolic enactments of deep cultural beliefs and as techniques to achieve practical ends. In my analysis of medical training, for example, I will show that teaching techniques and technical routines serve significant ritual purposes above and beyond the communication of information and the "management" of illness. In all societies, individuals undergoing major culturally recognized life transitions must cross a "bridge" of rituals commonly known as a *rite of passage*. Rites of passage consist of three principal stages: *separation* of the participants from their preceding social status; a "liminal" (from the Latin *limens*, meaning a threshold) period of *transition* in which they have neither one status nor the other; and an *integration* phase in which they are absorbed into their new social state through various rituals of incorporation. For example, in the rite of passage that constitutes medical training in American society, the separation phase begins as soon as the initiate departs for medical school and gradually merges into the transitional phase, which lasts for seven full years—four years of medical school and at least three years of residency. This transitional or "liminal" phase of being "betwixt and between" is the most salient feature of all rites of passage, especially important in initiation rites. This phase, if the rite of passage is successful, creates a profound interior transformation in the initiate by means of the rituals that make up the rite. According to renowned ritual scholar Victor Turner (1979:238–239):

> It is the ritual and the esoteric teaching which . . . grows girls and makes men. . . . The arcane knowledge, or gnosis, obtained in the liminal period is felt to change the inmost nature of the neophyte, impressing him, as a seal impresses wax, with the characteristics of his new state. It is not a mere acquisition of knowledge, but a change in being.

In rites of initiation, the "gnosis" which so changes the neophytes' inmost nature usually consists of essential elements of the core value and belief system into which they are being initiated. One of the chief characteristics of the liminal or transitional period is the gradual psychological opening of the initiates to such new learning, ideally accompanied by the desired interior change. Many initiation rites involving major transitions into new social roles (for example, military basic training) achieve this opening through a combination of physical and mental hardships that break down the initiate's *belief system*—the internal mental structure of concepts and categories through which he or she perceives and interprets the world and his or her relationship to it. The breakdown of this belief system leaves the initiate profoundly receptive to new learning and to the construction of new categories. As Turner puts it, "The passivity of neophytes to their instructors, their malleability, which is increased by submission to ordeal, their reduction to a uniform condition, are signs of the process whereby they are ground down to be fashioned anew" (1979:239).

As rites of passage convey individuals from one social state to another, simultaneously inculcating them with the core value and belief system of the society or group, they also work to renew and revitalize that belief system to assure its perpetuation. The technomedical model is continually renewed and revitalized as it is taught to nascent physicians. Its perpetuation is vital to the perpetuation of the technocratic system as a whole. In all human societies, those in charge of the human body serve as society's representatives, responsible for inculcating the values of their culture into the bodies for whom they care. (This responsibility is implicit in their training and practice; it is rarely explicitly spelled out beyond their training, if they have it, in "patient education.") Thus the profound connections between technomedicine and technocratic society are reinforced through the rite of passage of medical training. In what follows, we will see how the above characteristics of ritual and rite are employed via what is known as the "hidden curriculum" of medical education to turn fledgling medical students into full-fledged physicians who first internalize, and then perpetuate, the core values of the technocracy.

Psychological Transformation in Medical School and Residency: Medical Training and Cognitive Narrowing

In every rite of passage, the initiates differ from one another in intellectual ability and complexity. Ritual deals with these differences by reducing all participants, at least temporarily, to the same simple cognitive level, which Davis-Floyd and Laughlin (2016) describe as "Stage One." A Stage One cognitive system is a closed system whose adherents try to make reality appear to conform to its picture.[2] Stage One thinking is black-and-white thinking in either/or patterns that make little allowance for the consideration of options or alternative views. Such cognitive reduction precedes the conceptual reorganization that accompanies true psychological transformation. In Turner's words, the initiate must be "ground down" in order to be "fashioned anew."

In initiatory rites of passage, the ritual techniques of hazing, strange-making, and symbolic inversion are employed with great effectiveness to achieve this grinding down. *Hazing* techniques, often used in fraternity and military initiation rites and induction into religious cults, involve wearing down and disorienting the initiate through exhaustingly repetitive activity (in basic training, repetitive exercises and drills; in fraternity pledge rites, receiving instructions to run to a certain place at a certain time, and once there, receiving instructions to frantically run to another place to avoid penalties, and so forth). *Strange-making* (Abrahams 1973) involves making the commonplace strange (e.g., shaving the heads of basic trainees or religious initiates and dressing them all alike so they will lose their sense of individual identity and familiarity with the world around them). *Symbolic inversion* means metaphorically turning things upside down and inside out, disrupting the order of everyday life to generate what Roger Abrahams (1973) called "the power attendant upon confusion" (see also Babcock 1978); this sort of disruption breaks habitual patterns of thinking and leaves initiates open to establishing new ones.

During medical school and again in residency, hazing, strange-making, and symbolic inversion are effectively employed. For example, medical school reduces to lowly status initiates formerly at the top of their class in college or already successful in another career. As one physician noted:

> The first two years of medical school are like backtracking. No fun. Your last two years in college, you tend to do more graduate-level work in smaller classes and you have more freedom about what you learn and how you learn it, and you are suddenly popped back into an environment like first-year basic science courses in college, where you kind of get what's thrown at you. . . . There's no freedom about what you learn—everybody learns the same thing.

First-year residents (formerly known as interns) must begin again at the bottom of the status hierarchy with enormous amounts of "scut work" to perform. Their lowered status is indicated by the language they and others often use to refer to themselves: "scuzz monkeys," "worms," and "moles" (Stein 1990:210).

[2] In *The Power of Ritual*, my coauthor Charles Laughlin and I describe four Stages of Cognition, ranging from the narrow tunnel vision of Stage One to the broad and fluid kinds of thinking we characterize as Stage Four. In anthropological terms, we characterize these as Stage 1: naïve realism/fundamentalism/fanaticism; Stage 2: ethnocentrism; Stage 3: cultural relativism; Stage 4: global humanism.

The first two years of medical school have traditionally been the same for all medical students, no matter what their eventual specialty: intensive study of the basic sciences—which include biochemistry, neurophysiology, anatomy, histology, and bacteriology—punctuated by countless quizzes and exams. Often taught by research scientists, not physicians, these courses are usually presented as pure science, divorced from any practical function. "Learning" biochemistry, for example, often requires endless rote memorization of chemical formulas, with little or no sense of why or how these might be useful to a physician. In *Gentle Vengeance: An Account of the First Year of Harvard Medical School*, Charles LeBaron recalls:

> Introductory lectures on the "Embden-Myerhof Glycolytic Pathway." . . . What is it? Are we synthesizing something, breaking it down? Does it take place in the ocean, outer space, crayfish, where? Does it start things off, end them? In short, what's it all about? Silly concerns. Just plunge right in and start getting it all down cold:
>
>> Rabbit muscle adolase—Class I, Type A, MW 160,000, four subunits of MW 40,000; Formula: Alpha-2, Beta-2, but isozymes of varying ratio Alpha/Beta are found. . . . See handout. Consider reaction in direction of synthesis of hexose-P. (1981:62–63)

The apparent irrelevance of much of this material to clinical medical work is a source of great discontent to many medical students, especially to those who entered medical school with ideals of helping humanity. As one physician noted,

> Most of us look on the basic sciences as something you put up with until you get to the real heart of the issue. I don't know why they even had a lot of the courses. We took bioengineering and biostatistics. Even a lot of biochemistry is extremely detailed and really has no relevance. The Krebs cycle is a classic example—a biochemical cycle where you have to learn all these enzymes and then when you get through you never use it. My sister in med school now tells me the same thing. She can't understand why she is going through all these detailed analyses of DNA structures and things like that.

The enormous quantity of much of this irritatingly irrelevant material adds to its effectiveness as a hazing technique. One physician's assessment is:

> Medical school is not difficult in terms of what you have to learn—there's just so much of it. You go through, in a six-week course, a thousand-page book. The sheer bulk of information is phenomenal. You have pop quizzes in two or three courses every day the first year. We'd get up around six, attend classes till 5, go home and eat, then head back to school and be in anatomy lab working with a cadaver, or something, until one or two in the morning, and then go home and get a couple of hours sleep and then go out again. And you did that virtually day in and day out for four years, except for vacations.

Alex Cadoux added:

> Much of medicine was treating numbers, not people. What counted was your class rank, and where was your internship. All the external parameters. I guess I still harbor anger at myself for buying into this system hook, line, and sinker. There were points of interest, points of joy in learning. But they were fairly rare, because there wasn't enough time to digest the information. We were constantly cramming down the volumes that we were responsible for. . . . It was high volume learning, not integrated.

One result of such an overload of information—which one physician described as "like trying to drink water from a fire hose"—is the increasing isolation of the student-initiates. It is characteristic of rites of passage that the initiates are separated as a group from the rest of society, in order to ensure their removal from the everyday world. This social separation is prerequisite to achieving the necessary cognitive retrogression, as Jack Mansberger explained:

> Little do you realize that when you get to the next step, it's going to be just as bad as the one before it, or worse. And then all you want to do is finish that one. So you lose all sight of what you really want, and of what you enjoy. I mean, I used to love to go backpacking, I used to love the woods. And there's no time to do that. You become totally isolated. It's what the system does—is take up all your time. And that indoctrinates you that the system is the only thing in the world that's important. It's not necessarily caring for patients or love or anything like that. It's just the system, that's it. So you're indoctrinated in that, and you lose the entire rest of the world.

In the first two years of medical school, pressures of threat and uncertainty mount. A competitive emphasis on grades and tests, the unpredictability of pop quizzes, the overwhelming bulk of the work at hand, and the increasing isolation—all combine to reduce the initiates' range of cognitive functioning. It is not that medical students become less intelligent; rather, the span of their intellectual capacities and concerns becomes constrained. A kind of tunnel vision develops: the cognitive overload that first- and second-year medical students experience forces them to focus only on what is immediately in front of them. They become progressively less capable of self-reflection and of the psychological distance from the socialization process that such self-awareness might have helped them to achieve. The positive side of this cognitive narrowing, as Bethany Hays pointed out, is that "you become able to focus on a problem with many variables, under intense pressure, and to solve it without becoming mired down in personal issues—a great skill at three in the morning when someone is bleeding to death." The down side, Hays continues, "is that you learn to problem-solve under pressure in purely technomedical terms. If a solution coming out of some other model might have been better, you're not going to find it." When one is totally immersed in one model of reality to the exclusion of everything else, one can easily lose sight of the importance, even the existence, of other ways of thinking and being. As Karin Montero put it, "I worked so hard, I was so busy, that I didn't think very much."

Redundancy and Emotional Numbing as Transformative Techniques in Medical Training

For maximum effectiveness, a ritual will focus on sending one basic set of symbolic messages, which it repeats over and over again in different forms. Symbols work through the right hemisphere of the brain; we thus receive their messages as a gestalt that is physically felt through the body and the emotions, often bypassing the intellect. Repetition and the hazing process of physical exhaustion, begun during medical school and intensified during residency, work together to ensure that the resident will internalize the set, established routines of standard medical practice—and the separation-based core value system that underlies them—so thoroughly that she can perform them on automatic pilot. Obstetrician Bethany Hays explained, "As senior residents at Baylor, we knew that we had done more twins, more breech deliveries, more c-sections, more complicated forceps than anybody out in practice. We were the experts by the time we finished that residency. The price we paid for that was that we were exhausted; we didn't have time to think about what we were doing: it was just do it, and do it, and do it some more."

Many hospitals require their residents to perform repetitive and redundant daily chores that have little to do with training to be a physician. These include delivering lab specimens, carting patients around, starting IV lines, drawing blood, and doing record keeping. This "scut work" occupies a quarter to a third of residents' time, the equivalent of six months out of a four-year residency, or about eight hours out of a 36-hour shift (Duncan 1993:64). In addition to its effectiveness as a hazing technique, the tradition of using residents to perform this scut work saves hospitals and attending physicians millions of dollars a year. Residents, typically paid well below minimum wage, often make less per hour than nurses, physician's assistants, and orderlies. Not only does this system provide financial benefits to the hospitals, it also works to ensure that when residents, drastically underpaid and exploited for years, finally enter private practice, they will feel entitled to the same high fees as their former exploiters and thus will help to perpetuate the profit orientation of the technomedical system (Duncan 1993:65).

In the haze of cognitive overload and physical exhaustion that characterizes medical school and residency, most students gradually lose sight of the idealistic goals they may have had on entering. If the rite of passage is successful, the new goals medical students eventually develop will be structured in accordance with the values of the dominant medical system. This process is aptly summarized by a resident:

> Most of us went into medical school with pretty humanitarian ideals. I know I did. But the whole process of medical education makes you inhuman. . . . I've seen people devastated when they didn't know *an* answer. . . . The whole thing can get you pretty warped. I think that's where the feelings begin that somebody owes you something, 'cause you really, you know, you've blocked out a good part of your life. People lost boyfriends and girlfriends, fiancées and marriages. There were a couple of attempted suicides. . . . So you forget about the rest of life. By the time you get to residency, you end up not caring about anything beyond the latest techniques you can master and how sophisticated the tests are that you can perform.

For many physicians-in-training, an emotional numbing accompanies the psychological transformation this resident describes. Emotions can be inconvenient in medical school: they can interfere with one's ability to dispassionately dissect a cadaver, grasp the beating heart of a dog minutes before its death, absorb enormous amounts of decontextualized information, and treat the many tragic figures who present themselves for care. Gradually, many medical students and residents begin to learn to cut themselves off from their feelings. Jack Mansberger explained:

> After a while, you don't even feel, because you put such a tremendous emotional box around yourself. Particularly in my field, surgery, you know, the long hard hours, the whole bit. You're not supposed to be emotional. Trauma cases come in—there's no room for emotion and all that. So you build this tremendous wall around yourself to protect yourself and keep yourself going. You actually lost sight of where you really were, and the box becomes so thick and heavy. It's what you carry around. It's not until later on, when the weight of that box is so tremendous that it about does you in, that you realize what you've been doing the whole time. And of course your family suffers and everybody else around you suffers.
>
> Q: What were you boxing yourself in from? What would the emotions have been if you had stopped to feel them?
>
> I think there would have been a lot of fear, a lot of pain, all that kind of stuff. I mean, you're dealing with people who are dying left and right. Awful scenarios. I mean, just really difficult things to deal with and nobody ever talks about it at all. You just keep going. Just don't stop. It's like if you ever stop you'll get done in. If you stop and reflect on what you're doing, that'll be the end of it—you'll fall back down the hill. The only way to keep going is to keep going up the hill. Because everybody else is going with blinders on, but that's the only thing you can do. If you take them off, you might just quit. You might just say, "I'm going to go and do something else—this is ridiculous!"

Bethany Hays echoed his commentary. When I asked her, "How did you feel about residency while you were experiencing it?" she replied:

> I was brain dead, so I really didn't have a feeling about it. I just wanted to be done because they kept telling me that next year would be better—you know, "Don't worry, because next year will be better!" It took me a long time to figure it out, but by the time I was a senior resident, I knew that was a lie, that it was never going to be better. And it took me another 15 years to figure out why.
>
> Q: Why?
>
> A: Because what they were teaching was incomplete. It had no connections. . . . like in college, the philosophy majors took pure philosophy—Descartes, Locke, Kant, etcetera—but I was interested in the philosophy of art, of music, of science. . . . I was interested in where philosophy interfaced with other disciplines, because any subject in the center of that subject gets detached from other disciplines. Higher mathematics could exist in a vacuum; it's *applied* mathematics that gets things done. And the same is true of medicine. If medicine is being practiced in a vacuum, without regard to what we are doing, why heal people? Why bother? There's no point in pretending we can keep people from dying. So why bother? If you bother, it must have to do with the fact that those people are in relationships with other people, or are not done learning what they are here to learn. It's all connected. And it's those connections that my medical training just completely ignored.

Ignoring such connections by presenting enormous quantities of information out of meaningful context enhances the left-brained, linear focus of medical training and works to shut down the gestalt-oriented right hemisphere, which is also the processor of the emotions. Such disconnected teaching, in combination with physical exhaustion, information overload, and the repetitive redundancy of many medical tasks, can emotionally numb initiates and regress them away from higher-level, integrative thought. They will develop of a kind of narrow tunnel vision in which the gnosis of medicine, separate from all other realities, becomes all important.

Cognitive Transformation: Learning "The Way"

Cognitive transformation occurs in ritual when "symbol and object seem to fuse and are experienced as a perfectly undifferentiated whole . . . and insight, belief and emotion are called into play, altering our conceptions . . . at a stroke" (Moore and Myerhoff 1977:13). A 63-year-old obstetrician presented the outcome of such transformative learning:

> I think my training was valuable. The people who trained us, and their philosophy, were unbeatable. Dr. Pritchard—he was *the* man in obstetrics [when I trained with him]. And his philosophy was one of teaching one way to do it, and that was *his* way. And it was basically the right way. . . . I like the set hard way. I like the riverbanks that confine you in a direction. Later on . . . you can incorporate a little bit of this or that as things change, but you learn one thing real well, and that's *the* way.

In medical schools and hospital units, this cognitive transformation of the initiates—this perceptual fusion with "the way"—occurs when *reality as presented by the technocratic model gradually becomes one with reality as the initiate perceives it.* Training programs in other fields may also be focused on "the way" to repair an engine, try a case, or polish a gem. But in medical education, the student, like the Marine in boot camp or the religious novice, is "decontextualized"—removed from the normal life context and outside interests that could leaven the initiation process. Thus the projection of "the way" to practice medicine tends to merge in the initiate's psyche with the exclusion of other ways. Christiane Northrup illustrates the extent of this exclusion when she describes her OB training: "I would say we're taught that this baby is basically just a tumor to be cut out. I was so steeped in the training that I didn't begin to see or appreciate the miracle that the body is, particularly in birth."

As we have seen, the intellectual overload of the first two years plays a significant role in this transformational process, despite the fact that most of the content of the courses is quickly forgotten; said one physician, "I was thinking yesterday that I must be a lot dumber than I was when I went to medical school, because I don't remember any of the stuff that we learned. You remember the things that you use clinically, that's all." In contrast, physicians-to-be spend most of the last two years of medical school, and all four years of residency, in just the sort of embodied hands-on experiential learning that *is* remembered (Jordan 1993:ch 7). A practicing obstetrician recalled:

> I had delivered maybe 30 babies as a medical student. When I was a first-year resident . . . on my first day I was thrown in as the Chief of Labor and Delivery. I had an intern and six medical students under me. A lady came in off the elevator abrupting [the placenta was in the process of peeling away from the inner wall of her uterus]; we had to do an emergency cesarean on her. I had never even seen one, much less done one! And I had to go in there, scared. Well, the second-year resident comes in and walks me through it. It's a "see one, do one, teach one" program, and that's how medical schools are generally run. Somebody shows you how; they walk you through it once or twice. And the next few times, you do it, with them still watching you and guiding you. You do that a few times, and then you start teaching others. And that's the basic philosophy of how you learn. It's not a bad system. I don't know of anything that can replace it. And you learn pretty quick!

Given the effectiveness for learning of this sort of embodied, apprenticeship-style involvement, we might well ask why the first two years of medical school consist primarily of intellectual overload? A rite-of-passage perspective reveals a function, if not a purpose, underlying this educational method. Two years of nothing but science, besides serving to separate the nascent physician from the person that she was, also serve very effectively to separate her from the people whom she will treat. Before she begins to deal with real people as patients, she learns conceptual distance from them.

For example, to study the basic sciences is to be taught to think of the body as a machine. During anatomy lab, medical students dissect the body's muscle groups, organs, and vasculature in finer and finer detail. Discussing the effects of this process, one student noted, "I've had some real perception changes of people. We all have this sort of thing—I'm good at tennis, say, or something else, and therefore, I'm good. I started realizing more and more, I can't help but think of us as machines. And there's none of this individuality and goodness; it's just whether or not you synapse quickly" (quoted in Good and Good 1993:96). As Howard Stein puts it, "In biomedical training, the body is a lifeless machine before 'it' is a person. Death and deconstruction precede, and set the tone for, life" (1990:186). Charles LeBaron elaborates:

> I held the slide up against the light again. Yes, that had once been someone's finger. It had felt coffee cups and pieces of paper and buttons, scalded itself, shook hands, gestured in excitement, caressed faces. Now it lived between pieces of glass in a box. A small chill ran through me. "Strange," I said. "Yeah, isn't it? Here's a piece of penis. A little later, you'll get to a salivary gland from someone's tongue." I looked at him, my eyes widening. Phil shrugged. "After a while, you just don't think about it anymore." I started again, a little more slowly. If this was human flesh, however sliced, dried, or stained, I should at least show it the courtesy of adequate attention. Soon people began to leave for lunch. It was almost one, I was hungry, and another class started at one-thirty. I sped up: esophagus, testicle, intestine. . . . Where are those crazy terminal bars they said I should see? The heck with them. . . . I'm getting something to eat. You get used to things fast around here, I thought as I locked up the microscope. (LeBaron 1981:40)[3]

Growing detachment from both the diseases studied and the people who have them leads fairly rapidly, in the first year of medical school, to the development of cynicism and intellectual arrogance. LeBaron documents this process, describing one of his first-year Harvard class' rare contacts with an actual patient, a multiple sclerosis victim. The class' first reaction was dismay at the actual physical presence of a "CPC—clinical-pathological correlation," as disease victims were named, but soon:

> "Shit, I'd love to do a coronal section on his frontal lobe," said someone behind me. "You'd see demyelinated plaques the size of golf balls." Some

[3] Charles LeBaron was a social worker in the New York hospital system for 12 years before he entered Harvard Medical School at the age of 34. His book, *Gentle Vengeance: An Account of the First Year at Harvard Medical School* (1981), perceptively and insightfully chronicles his experiences during his first year at Harvard in 1979, before any attempt had been made to create the present, more humanistically-oriented "New Pathways" program there. See https://hms.harvard.edu/departments/medical-education/md-programs/new-pathway-np

> knowing snickers. People hadn't started off talking that way; initially everyone had approached our occasional CPC sessions with an almost reverential awe—the word actually made flesh. But now after a year of dog labs, corpses, continual memorization, and no patients, that kind of conversation was part of the background noise. And those expressions of flippancy, cynicism, the sarcastic smiles that had been so conspicuous by their absence back at orientation were already starting to spread through the class like some sinister psychological tide. (LeBaron 1981:213)

The objectification of the patient and the alienation of practitioner from patient so evident in the above quotation are the philosophical correlates of the Cartesian separation of mind and body. This belief in mind/body separation, inherent in the scientific medical view, does not permit the interaction of individual consciousness with the molecules and atoms that comprise the stuff of "scientific" inquiry; thus, as physician Cynthia Carver (1981:132) notes, it is easy to leave people out of the medico-scientific equation:

> The first two years of medical school . . . are not taught in a framework of how *people* function. The students are taught about bodies as though the minds, emotions, and lives associated with those bodies were irrelevant. They are also taught about hundreds of pathological conditions and processes as though they were all equal: equal in importance, equal in outcome, equal in incidence.

Teaching about pathological conditions as if all were equal in importance and incidence presents medical students with the very false impression that learning about rare pathologies is just as important in patient care as studying more common conditions. Most medical schools withhold actual clinical experience, which could teach students very differently, until after the initiates have internalized the basic attitudes and values underlying this scientific worldview. As resident Paulanne Balch explained:

> Medical school is so sterile and abstracted from the person. It's a process that really begins the first day of medical school. You begin by learning about a disassembled set of organ systems. That's about the most integrated it gets. You learn about the digestive system, the circulatory system, the nervous system. You learn about the different body parts and processes, and how they work together, and how to break down information a patient might give you as to which system is involved. Then you develop a treatment program based on the results of your diagnosis. Notice I have not spoken a word about the person. And the crisis, if it occurs for you, is when you sit down with a person to solve a problem they have, and you don't have any tools from your training to recognize the fullness of what a human being is.

Although clinical experience early in medical training has the potential to bring students and patients closer together, in many medical schools it begins in the second semester of the second year and seems designed to intensify psychological distance. Because this clinical work consists primarily of the highly routinized tasks of doing physicals and taking medical histories, it tends to widen the gap between medical students and the people they are going to school to learn to heal, encouraging them to regard these individuals as "cases"—"the gall bladder in 133" or "the kidney case in 304." This objectification of the patient is further intensified in residency, as this second-year resident suggests:

> As interns, we lose why we went into medicine—whatever humanistic interest we had. It's very hard to sit there and listen to someone tell his life story when you've got six other admissions, bloods to draw, you've got to be up all night. Every second you spend being compassionate means that much less time to sleep. So you become very efficient at not really listening to people—just getting the information you need, and shutting them off. (quoted in Harwood 1984:70)

With this internalization of "scientific objectivity," initiates have the opportunity to find a sense of individual identity within the medical paradigm through clinical rotations that expose them to the practice and procedures of various medical specialties, where the highest value tends to be placed on the acquisition of technological and surgical skills. The second two years of medical school allow the overwhelmed student to associate with and seek approval from the masters of the craft. Whisked through the various departments of the hospital—itself the cathedral of technology—students are understandably hungry for the excitement and adrenaline rush provided by the drama of the ER, the intensity of the ICU, and the theater of the OR. With just a few weeks in every department, it is no wonder that the slow pace of, say, an outpatient department fails to capture their imaginations. Applying cream to eczema, prescribing an antibiotic for a strep throat infection—these mundane treatments just don't measure up to the thrill of bringing life back from the brink, whether in birth or near-death. The value of taking a thorough and time-consuming patient history pales in comparison to the frenzy of caring for accident victims or the drama of participating in organ transplants.

Psychologically, medical students are seeking approval and nurturing with the only receptors available—the brain and adrenals. Is it fascinating, high-tech, new? Is it exciting? Will it give me an edge, a high? The process of rotation does far more than expose doctors-to-be to techniques, patients, and the wonders of technology; it exposes them to doctors from whom they will learn the finer points of conduct, ethics, and behavior on which to model their future selves. The cathedral is full of priests. The high priests conducted the ceremonies of the first two years; now the clergy move in for the final preparation for ordination.

Mental overload and increasing levels of physical exhaustion as residency proceeds ensure that rarely, in the course of seven long years, is there an opportunity to reflect, to integrate, assimilate, or contextualize the information that has been force fed through intellectual, physical, social, and cultural channels. As one doctor summed up the cognitive transformation that occurs, "It doesn't seem to matter—male or female, young or old, wealthy or poor—it is only the most unusual individual who comes through a residency program as anything less than a technological clone. This rite of passage that you are talking about is an assembly line to the adoration of technology." And *as you learn, so shall you practice*—unless you make concerted attempts to change.

Gender and Medical Initiation

Before the Industrial Revolution, healing in the Western world was primarily women's work. The technomedical system was created by men; its creation encompassed four centuries of active repression of female healers in the West and the deliberate stamping out of their knowledge and traditions. This repression continued on into 20th century America. The Flexner Report of 1910, a study of various types of medical training available at the time that was funded by the Carnegie Foundation and the government and supported by the AMA, resulted not only in the closing of homeopathic and naturopathic schools of medicine but also in the closing of the separate medical schools for women that had been established in the 1800s. It took 50 more years for women to be able to enter male medical schools in any significant numbers; when they got in, they found themselves confronting a medical system based on intensely patriarchal principles and values.

In the early 1960s, the population of physician-trainees was 90% white and male; by 1993, it had changed to 30% women and 18% minorities (Duncan 1993:63). The American Medical Association predicted that by 2010, 30% of US doctors would be women, compared to 19% in 1995. That prediction has now been surpassed; today in 2017, around 47% of both medical students and residents are women (yet women constitute only 22% of tenured medical professors; https://www.aamc.org/members/gwims/statistics/). As more women enter medicine, the question arises: is it changing them, or are they changing it?

Modern medical education is conducted within a realm where masculinist beliefs predominate. Its rituals of hazing, emotional deadening, and physical suffering are typical of male initiation rituals around the world, from the ancient Spartans to the contemporary Marines. The feeling here is that in order to leave one way of being and enter a new one (as in leaving the world of childhood to become a man), the initiates must sever all connections with their prior life. This kind of left-brained, separation-based thinking is not found in female rites of initiation, which tend across cultures to be connection-based, to celebrate a woman's ability to grow and change while still remaining connected to her kith and kin (Farrer 1980; Lincoln 1981; Davis-

Floyd and Laughlin 2016).[4] Psychologist Carol Gilligan (1993) has shown that this kind of connection has long characterized the upbringing of American women.

Thus it is to be expected that women would have an especially difficult time accepting their medical training and its underlying values and worldview, which fail to recognize the personal, an area where women often excel. The medical system's unwillingness to acknowledge feeling and value relationships, the realm of "the feminine," was the underlying cause of the suffering that the women physicians interviewed particularly expressed. Ann McCombs said that she "found medical training offensive intellectually and . . . in the area of relationships—being a female in a predominantly male system." The devaluation of the personal that often typifies medical training can be devastating to women students. "The interaction I had with my patients," reports one female physician, "the appreciation they had for me and the fun and enjoyment of being a helping, caring person carried me through years of frustration with the profession. I felt I was in a hostile environment and didn't know where I fit, but at least there was something positive and right happening with my patients. When this was no longer happening, there was little to make it seem worthwhile" (Julia Hall, quoted in *MetaPhysicians' Tales,* Tyler and St John 1989).

A coping strategy that obstetrician Christiane Northrup found useful was to consciously defer gratification—for years. She could accept her "average" academic performance, knowing she excelled in intuitive and relational skills: "I just knew that my ability to find out what was going on with a patient was not average. But I also knew this ability was completely invisible in that world. It wasn't seen or honored. I would do no harm, I would do no harm. I would learn my skills, and then when the time came, when it mattered, I would add this other stuff I was doing—when it was my turn." And indeed she did, becoming one of the most renowned holistic practitioners and speakers in the US and internationally, as well as author of *Women's Bodies, Women's Wisdom* (2010 [1994])—a holistic medical guide for women often referred to as "the bible of women's health care"—and many other highly popular publications.

Although women have achieved parity in the profession as students and as practicing physicians, many are scarred by the stress and lack of self-expression they endured as women—on top of all the other pressures the sys-

[4] It has been suggested that because the corpus callosum, which plays a major role in conveying information between hemispheres, is significantly larger in women, they are less able than men to maintain emotional detachment. In other words, while men can compartmentalize, engaging in left-brained rational thinking that completely excludes the emotions, women are more likely to think and feel at the same time, making decisions and taking actions in a more integrated, whole-brained way. However, the whole brain is involved in all brain functions, and the corpus callosum can be deliberately developed in either sex (see Davis-Floyd and Laughlin 2016: Ch 2).

tem imposes. They told of eagerly awaiting the day they could bring their total being to bear in their work, but fearing the loss of their feminine abilities along the way as the unrelenting pressure of the system brought more and more conformity to the masculinist norm. Several female interviewees expressed their anger and outrage at a system of training that barely recognized and in no way accommodated their roles as mothers. Bethany Hays recounts "marching into the office of the chairman" of her ob-gyn department at Baylor prior to applying for internship, and asking:

> "What concessions are you willing to make for women in your program?" And he said, "Um, concessions?" And I said, "Well, you know, like the pediatricians have shared and part-time residencies. They can take time off if they have kids, they get leaves of absence if they want to have babies. You know, I'm married now, and I don't intend to wait until I'm 40 to have my first baby, and if you want real women in your program, some of them are going to want to have children. And so I want to know what your plan is for that?" And he was dumbfounded. It had never occurred to him—it didn't have to because they had never had any women in the program. So he said, "Well, uh, uh, I guess if you want to have a baby the third year, you could be on pathology the last three months." And that was it, and I thought "Oh, my God."

The women medical students and physicians I interviewed seemed more troubled than many of their male colleagues by the high degree of personal imbalance required by their profession. Although some of the men interviewed commented on the grueling conditions of medical school, none touched on the sense of being personally out of balance the way women did:

> I found medical training extremely difficult. When I finished training I was in a very vulnerable state. It was a real soul-destroying experience. One of the things I found difficult was how little respect there was for the need to balance. I need balance. My life was one-sided and unhealthy. It really bothered me. I went to faculty members and asked for advice on this situation. They advised me to be unhealthy for three years and then become healthy. "Get balanced later." This was totally unacceptable to me. (Marilyn Levinson, quoted in Tyler and St. John 1989)

Several women described themselves as "ill" during and after medical training. This was often not the type of illness that could be diagnosed and treated, but rather a kinesthetic sense of the effects of unrelenting stress, sleep deprivation, adrenaline states, and social deprivation. Rebecca Lawrence found herself "becoming more physically and emotionally spent. I felt ill most of the time, not with any one symptom, but just sick. I'd wake up in the morning with a damn-it-all attitude, feeling too sick to eat." Marilyn Levinson was "sick continuously for two years. It started with some type of pneumonia and then bronchitis, bronchitis, bronchitis."

A fourth year female medical student told us in a letter she sent:

> By the third year of medical school, I found myself in a severe depression and sleeping for ten hours a day. Everything I knew about life and living, everything I believed in, was being trampled and pissed on every single day of my medical school experience. Love, joy, deep caring, touch, relationship, individualized care—these had no place. It made me sick, physically and emotionally. I could handle the assault on my body, but the continuous assault on my spirit was too painful to bear. So I took a year off, hoping that by the time I came back I would have found the inner strength to continue while protecting my soul.

Like this student, Rebecca Lawrence also took a year off to recover some balance, but lost it almost immediately upon returning to training. "It sure was difficult. I didn't feel my approach was recognized, validated or supported. I started to get real tired again, and when that happened, my desire to be creative with my patients decreased. I started doing the bare essentials again. I fulfilled the requirements to make my supervisors happy, but it wasn't making *me* happy." In a blog (July 15, 2016), Jamie Riches, DO, wrote the following in response to the suicide of one of her residency colleagues:

> The Intern Health Study, a longitudinal study of depression among interns nationwide, estimated that "suicide rates among physicians are something like 40 to 70 percent higher in males and 130 to 300 percent higher in women." Statistical estimates state that as many as 400 physicians commit suicide every year. Three young men and women leapt to their deaths in one city, in 16 months. We are not experiencing a tragic event; we are experiencing a harrowing trend. What can we do?

She goes on to discuss the intense stresses of residency and to critique the insistence of her superiors that those devastated by the suicide of their colleague and friend should develop "resilience" and get immediately back to work. She describes that those who did take "sick days" to deal with their grief were punished later on by having to make them up before they were allowed to graduate from their program. In response to her question: "What can we do?" she suggests the following:

1. Eliminate the word "burnout" from the lexicon: Not only does burnout minimize the severity of depression, detachment, and (at extremis) suicidal ideation among health-care professionals (HCPs), it implies that those suffering post-trauma have some inherent flaw or weakness that impairs their ability to remain functional. This mindset removes the onus from the system.
2. End the stigma: Remove the question, "Have you ever sought treatment for any mental illness?" from the job applications. We should encourage residents, physicians at all levels, and other HCPs to actively seek out cognitive therapy as we do vaccines or PPDs.

3. Decide what graduate education is: If residents are primarily learners, we must protect their time and use it solely for educational (both clinical and didactic) purposes and not to provide underpaid labor to perform all tasks for which the hospital is at a loss, no matter how menial. If residents are employees, we must provide adequate pay for educational level, protect sick leave, and outline contractual responsibilities before enrolling in the agreement.
4. Stop penalizing unwellness: Physicians and HCPs are as human as our patients. We are not immune to everything. There will be times when we will be ill, physically and emotionally. We will need time and space to heal.
5. Structure the system in a way that minimizes fear of retaliation: If the person creating or enforcing destructive policies is the same person who needs to write the words "excellent candidate" on the letter of recommendation that carries the weight of your future career opportunities, your best and worst interests are one and the same.
6. Embrace our own fallibility: Learn to be comfortable with imperfection. Let us have an equal respect for our accomplishments and failures. Employ mentors who set this example.
7. Accept that medicine is not martyrdom: The work does not stop. Let it not deplete us. Let us take care of each other and ourselves and not give away everything that we need. (The entire blog can be found at https://resident360.nejm.org/content_items/what-is-resilience.)

Although Riches does not mention gender, her words carry highly "feminine" nuances, including a desire to make the system more compassionate. That she feels the need to offer this advice in 2016 tells me that not much has changed in medical training since my colleague Gloria St. John and I conducted most of the interviews on which this chapter is based during the late 1980s and 1990s (Davis-Floyd 1987a; Davis-Floyd and St. John 1998).

As we discovered from those interviews, female interviewees tended to be acutely aware of the moral ambivalence of their position in a system that forces them to cause pain to their patients, often for no apparent benefit. Their attempts to mitigate that pain through emotional nurturance were apt to incur the wrath of the system, so they had to cultivate deviousness in order to be able to practice the kind of medicine they cared about. Rebecca Lawrence said, "I did provide good eye contact with my patients, and did a little caring touch, so my personality did some good. They seemed to like the personal interaction, though it was real basic. I would cross out appointments in my book or put in fake names so I would have more time for people, manipulating the system as best I could. But I was basically in a survival mode most of the time."

Some women, like Rebecca Lawrence, risked their careers in subtle and invisible ways to make situations more comfortable for their patients. Others, like Chris Northrup, sometimes confronted the system head-on:

> I had the idea that when I'd be alone with the patient, I'd try to learn what was really going on. I knew many times that the treatment wouldn't be successful because the person didn't want to live. There isn't any receptor site for that information in allopathic medicine. I'd go to tumor conferences every Wednesday, and the guys would present the patient: Forty-eight year old multipara, tumor in the pelvis, diagnosed by local MD, stage two pap. . . . Then they'd talk about what kind of cancer she had, what stage it was in, and the specialists would talk about the treatment they were going to give her. You never, ever heard about who this person was. And I'd bring it up. That was stupid, like taking the Star of David into a fundamentalist Christian church. But I knew in myself that I had something to offer and something to say that wasn't being recognized.

One of Northrup's anecdotes illustrates how patriarchal values cross gender lines, in this case being invoked by women. She describes her OB residency as characterized by technologically assisted births. After finally gaining permission from her supervisor to attend some women without the use of electronic fetal monitors, she found that the nursing staff was often unwilling to cooperate, fearing that the outcomes would be bad.

Many women in touch with their capacities for intuition, sensitivity, and empathy were acutely aware that these were neither acknowledged nor valued in their training. Some, like Northrup, had the confidence and self-esteem to know that, one day, they would be able to create a kind of practice in which where these were valued. Others went forward with agonizing doubt about their ability to find fulfillment. Although male students and doctors also suffer in high-pressure and impersonal situations, the women seemed to suffer doubly because they doubted they would ever be valued for who they were. One woman physician particularly warned against the idea that women could change medicine or medical training: "I see a lot of women making the mistake of thinking that, when they are in the belly of the beast, they are going to change the beast. It does not work." Bethany Hays, who calls technomedicine "the prototype addictive organization," described the pain of finding out that she could not change "the beast":

> I tried for 15 years to change the way OB was done at Baylor, to make birth more humane for women. I felt like I was beating my head against the wall and I couldn't figure out why I couldn't seem to make a difference. I thought there was something wrong with *me*. Then Polly Perez handed me a manuscript one day. It was your [Robbie's] dissertation, before it even got published. You were talking about birth as a rite of passage that indoctrinates women with the core values of American culture, and I suddenly realized that it wasn't me, it was the *culture*! I was trying to change an entire culture, and of course it was so much bigger than me that I couldn't make a dent.

Some women coped by choosing a specialty that allowed for a more holistic treatment of the patient. For example, Sandra Kamiak spurned a specialty in internal medicine in favor of psychiatry to avoid the impersonal handling of patients. "People are broken down into parts," she noted in her interview. "It's mechanical. I felt at first that I was going to go into internal medicine, but thought that I would not have enough time with a patient. With ten minutes for an exam, you just don't have time to deal with all the stuff that's going on emotionally. You could do an x-ray or throw a pill at a person, but it didn't seem to be adequate."

The first generations of women to graduate from medical schools as a distinct minority often coped by becoming overachievers. As Bethany Hays put it:

> In medical school I just wanted to prove that I could do as good as the guys. I wanted to be the best man for the job, and so, when things happened to me because I was a woman, I always assumed it was because I wasn't doing a good enough job. And so I worked very hard. Like most women, I did twice as much work to get half as much credit. I knew that to actually be given concessions because I was pregnant would be like being given second class citizenship. I would not have been able to have any power in the program. And so I worked very hard all through my pregnancy up until the day I delivered.

Some women, fearing they would be labeled "soft," "not tough enough," overcompensated by becoming not only better, but also more technocratic—more aggressive, more interventionist, more mechanistic—than their male counterparts. During my research on obstetrics from the 1980s to the present, I often heard labor and delivery nurses voice the complaint that the new women physicians were "worse than the men" when it came to ordering unnecessary interventions. Now that the numbers were evening, female students did not necessarily feel the same compulsions to beat the men at their own game. Nevertheless, many still felt that their educational process was a continual trade-off of their inner reality for outer rewards.

It is unfair to imply that men make medical school bad and difficult and that all women suffer. The individual men or women involved are not the problem: they are simply participants in a system that is closed, dominant, and derived from a larger system where the same patriarchal/technocratic values prevail. Patriarchal values still characterize Western civilization, and the concomitant devaluation of the feminine has produced many social ills (e.g., Eisler 1995). Achieving inner and outer balance—the challenge and opportunity of the times—means balancing one's character and practice between aggressive intervention and patience, objectivity and relationship, analysis and intuition. Both men and women physicians face a great deal of confusion if they begin to value the feminine principle in life as well as in medicine. Many of them initially despair of finding any relational way to practice medicine as they have been trained. The gift of such despair is an ability to shift perspective and activate the feminine principle—regardless of the gender of the doctor. The "feminine" qualities of trust, patience, relationship, and surrender then become allies in the search for a new way.

Maintaining Psychological Distance

Human beings are not automatons; rites of passage can fail in their goal of transmitting the core value and belief system of a given society to the initiate. While most of the 40 physicians in our primary study did buy into the medical system during their training "hook, line, and sinker," as one of them put it, some managed to maintain a high degree of distance between their psyches and beliefs and the intensive initiation process to which they were exposed.

An instance of the hook, line, and sinker school was a physician whom I asked, "Why do medical students not see patients until late in the second year?" She responded, "I don't know. Mostly it's because you have to have some of the other background before you start playing like you're a doctor. You have to have some basics to work on, and you really have to go back to basic sciences and learn principles about why things work a certain way before you can build clinical medicine onto that." This physician demonstrates the effectiveness of her socialization through her acceptance of the science-before-patients structure of her medical school training.

In contrast, a holistic physician demonstrated the difference that psychological distance can make: "As it is now, the basic sciences really get you off the track of what you're there for. Most of us went in with pretty high humanitarian ideals, but by the time you get through the basic science years, most of the people in my class had developed a pretty cynical attitude. If we could have taken clinical rotations and seen patients early on in medical school, we would have come out with a lot better attitude and a better idea of the purpose of the basic sciences."

How did this physician manage to maintain enough psychological distance from his socialization process to be able to analyze it in this highly reflexive way? Realizing early on that his family would suffer considerably if he did not spend *some* time with them, he made a commitment to take off one night a week for that purpose, accepting in advance that it would mean being "a few answers short" on the next day's test: "It was a trade-off, but I think worthwhile in the long run, because I knew that my family would be with me a lot longer than medical school. That difference, whether it's a maturity level or not, was missing in a lot of people. I was older, about 27; most start at 21 or 22." The cognitive separation achieved by this conscious decision not to participate in the competitive values inherent in medical education was intensified by his first child's birth—an overly medicalized and very unhappy event that occurred while he was in medical school. "When my wife and I kind of figured out that things didn't have to be that way, I guess it made us both into crusaders."

As physician Cynthia Carver pointed out, the medical school selection process ensures the admission of students with highly competitive instincts and a strong scientific bent, who "generally went straight through, from high school to college to medical school, [managing] to reach the age of 21 without having experienced anything much other than academic life" (1981:129; see also Stein 1990:180). Students selected *out* by this process include those who, "despite being as bright as the high mark getters, allow themselves to be 'distracted' by . . . volunteer work, music, art, literature" and other careers (Carver 1981:129).

Those interviewees who resisted their technomedical socialization during training were able to do so for a variety of reasons. The ones who entered medical school later in life discovered that their life experience gave them a distinct advantage in this endeavor. Paulanne Balch began medical training after a long and successful business career. In response to the question, "Did you feel part of the group while you were in medical school?" she answered, "No, because I'm old enough to be the mother of some of them. There was a group of us who were over 40. We were united by our awareness of a lot of the crap that we were being fed . . . and of the hazing aspects." Others found maintaining a range of outside interests to be essential, as was the case with Dubravka Milas (personal communication): "As a second-year medical student, I have found that it's so important to get involved in other things besides school—work in a clinic, volunteer for a program that needs your help. If you don't do it now in medical school, you won't do it later either. I'm really finding that to be true. The people who are willing to reach out, they start doing it in their first year. And those that don't, they never do reach out, and so they are the ones who get tunnel vision and get eaten up by the system."

Finding himself unable to maintain outside interests, Peter Grote took a radical step:

> While I was in medical school, I felt that my focus was getting too narrow because I wasn't taking the time to do any other sorts of things. I looked at the people I was surrounded with and saw that most everybody was in the same boat—very narrow in their life experiences and their focus. I saw that those people who did other things for a number of years before going on to medical school were bringing a greater wealth of knowledge and a better attitude and approach to things. So I decided, in the middle of medical school, to take a year off. . . . I got myself involved in a program that summer called Crossroads to Africa. I went to Africa with a small group of other people who were also in medical or nursing school. We went to a town where there was no medical care at all. We set up a little clinic and spent two months there treating people and trying to teach two native nurses from the area some things they could keep doing after we left.
>
> Q. What effects did that experience have on you?

> It had a lot of effects. One was opening my eyes to other cultures. Another was opening my eyes to the benefits of a broader, public health approach to medical care over and above a narrow high-tech approach. I was also very impressed by how happy people were with what in our view was so little. And how willing they were to share everything they had.

Exposure to other ways of healing is a common catalyst for the paradigm shift made by holistic physicians (see Chapter 5), usually after they complete their medical training. In this case, such exposure gave Peter Grote a cognitive distance from his medical socialization that broadened his vision beyond technomedicine's narrow bounds.

The distancing factors for Barry Elson included yoga training and vegetarianism. Here is how Elson discovered that the emperor had no clothes:

> One unsettling thing about my medical school was that here we had this huge faculty, multi-million dollar buildings, etcetera, and not a single course on nutrition. I wanted to learn some nutrition so I went to the director of basic sciences education and asked, and he said I'd have to get other students interested in taking it. So I passed a petition around and got a whole bunch of people to sign it, and he said, "Well, it's great that everybody wants to take it, but we don't have anybody to teach it." So I went around to the faculty and I found a gastroenterologist here, a biochemist there, an anatomist there, and we set up an elective. And the first session, here was the gastroenterologist teaching that white bread was better for you than whole wheat bread because it had more vitamins injected in it, and that this whole "health food" thing was completely wrong. And that was in the early seventies. Now, of course, even the federal government recognizes that whole grains are good for you. And I realized that I was dealing with incredible ignorance at a very basic level by narrowly specialized people who didn't know anything about other fields at all. So in a sense I had created a monster, because it reinforced the delivery of all kinds of misinformation. At that point I just threw up my hands.
>
> Q: Why did *you* know about nutrition?
>
> A. I had been studying yoga for awhile, and was a vegetarian as a result of that. Over the years I learned about nutrition from other vegetarians, and then started reading voraciously.

Elson's commitment to the holistic philosophy he expressed through yoga and vegetarianism was so deep that it almost ended his medical training. Ultimately he found that a clear vision of his purpose for being there was essential to his ability to stay the course:

> I went into medical school firmly committed to holistic medicine—I actually thought I had coined the word. I found myself using it in college. Now I realize I must have seen it before that—it was just coming

into use in the late sixties. That was definitely my orientation . . . nutrition, stress management, and working with the *whole* person in a collaborative relationship. So the third and fourth years of medical school were particularly ironic and bizarre for me because I'd find myself in a hospital, supposedly a place for helping people get better, and a diabetic, for example, would be getting white bread with caffeinated coffee and sugar—which causes an immediate increase in blood sugar, which puts added stress on the patient's metabolism of glucose, which was already impaired! Basic principles of nutrition were being ignored. The person as a whole, of course, was also being ignored.

And you get poked and prodded by 18 medical students, 16 residents by the time you get out of there. I couldn't image a hospital as being any place to heal from anything and of course, we know that's often true. We know an overwhelming percentage of hospital days are spent from misprescribed medicines and many surgeries are done to correct previous surgeries. We know that there's an enormous iatrogenic realm that hospitals are palaces to . . .

So during my training I was a stranger in a strange land. . . . Part way through medical school I seriously considered dropping out. . . . For a while I thought about becoming a naturopath so I'd only be doing things I really believed in.

Q: So why did you decide to stay?

I had a vision about what I was doing on the planet. . . . I confronted something very basic about where I was going and what I was doing, and I realized that what I needed to do was go back and play the game some more and become a doctor. . . . I came to understand that my purpose on the planet is . . . to be a "healer" and by that I don't mean someone who does something *to* someone else, but someone who helps other people heal themselves. I had a very clear vision that that's why I am here, and that vision sustained me during the rest of my training.

Such clarity of vision is a tremendous boon to those who manage to achieve it during or prior to their medical training. In an interesting twist, Elson discovered that some of the medical education he was resisting as abstract and irrelevant turned out to be essential to the kind of holistic healing he later came to practice. Many physicians have used the Krebs cycle as an example of how boring, abstruse, and archaic medical education can be. Yet as Barry Elson explains, he and Alan Gaby (author of the authoritative textbook *Nutritional Medicine*) have "rediscovered" it in their practice of medical nutrition:

In the kind of medicine that Alan and I practice, the Krebs cycle and the biochemical intricacies of human metabolism are absolutely essential. They give us a key to nutritionally unlock the door to healing a wide range of chronic illnesses. It's particularly ironic for me, because here I was this philosophy/psychology holistic kind of guy in the first two

> years and I was one of those people who said, "I don't need to know this biochemistry. . . . I need to relate to my patients."
>
> But where I was completely wrong was that I was making the assumption that the doctors I was going to be learning from knew what they were talking about when it came to treating metabolic disorders appropriately. Their solutions were to throw drugs at them. My solution now is to find a way to nutritionally speed up those enzyme processes that are lagging, so the body can function more efficiently and heal itself. And the Krebs cycle is an essential part of that. It's a completely different paradigm. . . . I think that's an analogy for what we try to do interpersonally in holistic medicine—it's a whole synergistic model, rather than an analytic one.

The reason why Elson originally missed the importance of the Krebs cycle no doubt had much to do with how it was taught. As noted earlier, much of the information in the basic science courses is taught as if it had no connection to anything beyond itself. In a conversation with a fellow student, Charles LeBaron (1981:107–109) elaborated:

> You know, I spent three years working in an institution for the retarded . . . and there was never a time there that was as intellectually deadening as now. . . . Look at biochem—I counted seven separate stages in that pyrimidine synthesis. What's it all mean? Why are we memorizing it? . . . When I was studying physics back in night school, we calculated the mass of the Milky Way, did all sorts of problems with harmonic motion, nodes and antinodes, blackbody radiation, quantum energy levels. . . . I can't see how it has any practical value. But it seemed to me that measuring the mass of a galaxy was fun, revealed some principles about natural phenomena, and shows how accessible immense and faraway objects could be to mathematical analysis. So I know why I was there. . . . Memorizing the seven steps of the pyrimidine synthesis just to memorize them doesn't give me any sense that I'm doing anything but wasting my time and developing a contempt for the subject matter and the people who are teaching me.

To this tirade, LeBaron's classmate responded, "Maybe there's a theoretic significance that you don't see?" LeBaron answered, "So why don't they point it out?" and she replied, "Perhaps they assume we see it." LeBaron (1981:109–110) replied:

> Fine, let's say it's of tremendous significance. . . . Let me give you an analogy. The rose window in the north face of Chartres Cathedral is extraordinarily complex and beautiful. When I visited Chartres, the guide turned his back to the rose window, faced us, and proceeded to describe in exact detail each image on each shard of glass, the symbolism of the colors, the mosaic pattern of the panes. . . . He had dedicated his life to studying it. If, instead of explaining the rose window to us,

> he'd forced us to try and memorize all those images and recite them back by rote, the whole thing would have been worthless and unpleasant. At the very best, we could only have parroted what he'd said himself. Now, let's say one of these cycles is a rose window of biochemistry. Should we just memorize it, recite it, and forget it? Or should we be taught how to understand its meaning and roles and interaction in life?

After the final lecture in LeBaron's first-year biochemistry class, the instructor put down his pointer, shut off the slides, and summed up his impression of the science that he had made his lifework:

> [The instructor said] "The extraordinary fact about living creatures, living processes, is the structure, the order they manifest in the face of disorder. Each process is interlocked, each life depends on another, the prey upon the predator, the predator upon the prey, cycle upon cycle, pathway branching upon pathway in a web of inconceivable beauty. We don't exist as units alone in an inanimate world but as part of that intricate web. It is this sense of location in the midst of loneliness, repose in the midst of chaos, that constitutes the aesthetic and the real reason for the study of the chemistry of living things."
>
> [I] sat there stricken as people filed out, hurrying off to the library. I thought again about the rose window at Chartres. . . . You son of a bitch, I thought. . . . I can understand being so immersed in the day-to-day world of test tube research that nothing larger ever invades the mind. But if you *know*, if you see that beauty, how could you defile it by teaching it to us in this way? (LeBaron1981:136–37)

The sort of disconnected teaching that so wounded LeBaron's soul is an accurate reflection of the separation-based worldview that, since the early 1900s, medical training has been designed to perpetuate. Those who resist internalizing this worldview during medical training form a ready pool of candidates for expansion into holistic practice. (See Chapter 1 for a description of the technocratic, humanistic, and holistic models of medicine.)

Trends in Medical Education: "Walking between the Worlds"

Although all of our interviewees took issue with the attitudes and values that underlay their medical training, most were unequivocal in their appreciation of the knowledge, skills, and experience they gained. In particular, those students who had ferreted out more progressive medical training situations found much to appreciate. Deborah Malka found that "the University of New Mexico had one of the finest programs in the state. Students learned in tutorial style in small groups of six instead of large lecture classes. We learned by case study approach"—a patient-oriented teaching tool. Anu de Monterice discovered Case Western Reserve to be "a very progressive school. Dr. Spock was there. They tried to integrate the curriculum, using clinical experience earlier, which is unusual. Then they tied the systems together. Quite a good education." What Ann McCombs loved about McMasters, an experimental medical training program in Canada, was that "it was set up to teach you to think, the way law school teaches you to think. It's not about how much factual information you've got, it's about what you can do with it. Because when that factual information becomes obsolete, you need to be able to bring in another set of facts and use them. What you have to learn is problem solving, and that's a lifelong skill."

A second reason for valuing medical education was the feeling that it lent credibility to physicians' future work within the holistic realm. Christiane Northrup found that she "liked the grounding of it. I like the tradition of medicine, the whole of learning those skills, learning how to get someone out of trouble. It gave me the underpinnings and the tradition to say what I am now saying with more authority than if I had not gone through that. I know what I'm talking about, and I believe people listen in a different way than they would if I had not had that training." Bethany Hays said that her medical training gave her "the technical skill and knowledge to be able to sort of walk between the worlds. I managed to do medicine differently because I did it so well. They couldn't criticize; they couldn't question my outcomes. Believe me, they watched; they scrutinized. If I had had bad outcomes, I'd have been buried long ago." Ed Neal also noted the benefits of having "the good housekeeping stamp of approval. I don't have to fight with someone if I want to do acupuncture or something. Power comes from my medical training. Power is not a bad thing. . . . It's good to be able to stand up and say to my colleagues that people have souls. And they listen." Neal appreciated the rigors of his medical training, recognizing the character-forging worth of the long hours and difficult work:

> I'm proud to be an MD. The best thing about the training is not the treatments you learn, which are not very effective in primary care. But I'm really proud of having done the work. It's hard work. What was really of value was being in the fire. It was very grounding that way. When I work with alternative practitioners, sometimes it seems a little fluffy because they haven't seen people puke blood at three in the morning, when things aren't pretty, or spiritual; when you connect with life and death and pain and suffering.

Our interviewees agreed that the challenge in medical training is to keep what is worthwhile in the current system while reshaping its underlying core value system. Cadavers can be dissected with respect or with disdain; patients can be appreciated as individuals or treated perfunctorily. The physicians we interviewed, most of whom completed their medical education in the 1970s and 1980s, were reporting on their socialization into a paradigm of medical education that is currently undergoing some modification in response to sociocultural influences. In the prime of their life careers, they and their cohorts wield powerful influence over current developments in medicine. Fortunately, the medical care system is responding to pressures from patients to place a higher value on qualities such as equality, communication, and noninvasive techniques.

Terry Tyler asks, "Is the pain of medical education a necessary initiation? For most doctors there is no transcendence of the pain, or of the ego. A deliberate initiation needs to be carried out with a great deal of love. Then there is the possibility of transcendence. My hope is that there will be an upswelling of protest from people going through the medical training process. Perhaps they will say, 'We need to be whole. We need to be healed in order to be healers.'"

A look at developing trends shows some important shifts in that direction. First is a recognition that *physicians benefit from earlier exposure to clinical experience.* I have suggested a strong correlation between delaying actual contact with patients and the unconscious adoption of technocratic values. Some medical schools have begun to incorporate patient care into the first-year curriculum, beginning on day one. One impact of a curriculum that integrates clinical experience with basic science is a renewal of interest in primary care. During the 1980s the number of doctors entering primary care dropped 14% as the trend toward specialization gained ground. However, this trend seemed to be reversing in the 1990s as more medical students became aware of the need for primary care physicians. A surprising finding in our interviews with holistic doctors was how many of them had considered choosing surgery as their specialty, yet a serendipitous event like the location of the residency, a family obligation, or the Vietnam War intervened and pushed them into primary care.

Of the 40 primary interviewees for *From Doctor to Healer,* 20 were board-certified as primary care physicians. Primary care is defined as first-line care and is provided by the physician who is first consulted when a problem is suspected or develops. Many times warm and long-term relationships develop between primary care doctors and their patients, in contrast to the impersonal interactions often characteristic of patient/specialist relationships.

My own primary GP and I have been together for over 30 years, and sometimes I think he understands me better than many of my friends. His name is Ted Edwards. He was one of the first presidents of the American Holistic Medical Association (AHMA) and has always practiced a judicious combination of allopathic and holistic medicine, combined with a truly humanistic touch. Once I was referred to a new specialist by another doctor for my osteoarthritis; this new physician took one look at some test results, concluded that I had rheumatoid arthritis—though I had none of the symptoms—and prescribed a very aggressive medication that I was to take daily. I went straight to Ted and have never seen him so angry—he exclaimed in fury, "How can some doctor straight out of residency prescribe these pills for you based on a number on a page? They would have destroyed your metabolism!" He held my shoulders, looked me in the eye, and proclaimed with utter certainty, "You do *not* have rheumatoid arthritis, so stop worrying about it!" I've never been so relieved nor felt so reassured, not to mention loved. This interaction taught me firsthand what the ideal physician–patient relationship can be. Yet, all too often, patients do not have access to this kind of care.

"The time is ripe for change because all parties—students, faculty, and the public—agree the system isn't working," said former Surgeon General C. Everett Koop, who introduced a new approach to medical training at Dartmouth Medical School. Dartmouth requires first-year medical students to do a seven-week primary care rotation with a doctor in the community and to assume responsibility for the care of a family during that time. They experience the humanistic rewards of primary care firsthand at an impressionable stage, before the seduction of technology has swayed them. "Most people feel there is a tremendous information overload during the first two years of medical school," said Dr. Jonas Schulman, formerly the award-winning associate dean of education at Emory University's School of Medicine in Atlanta, as reported in the *San Francisco Examiner*, October 4, 1992. "What all of us are trying to do is get students involved with patients early, before they are able to visualize them as diseases."

A related benefit of this trend is a conscious attempt in some schools to model communication skills to medical students in the hope that they will develop more effective styles as practitioners. The strategy involves acceptance of students' emotions, rather than repression, and a conscious rejection of the emotional deadening that accompanies traditional medical education, as the same issue of the *Examiner* reveals in a report on a Dartmouth anatomy class: "Nervous students in surgical gloves and aprons filed into a fluorescent-lit laboratory and lined up alongside steel tables where cadavers lay ready for dissection. Instead of feeling pressured to maintain a stoic composure, these first-year medical students were encouraged to cry, laugh, faint, or leave the room if they wanted to. None did, but many said they appreciated the 'permission' to do so."

In contrast, here is Terry Tyler's experience of his medical anatomy class during the 1970s:

> The first week of medical school, we were required to dissect a fetus. We were arranged in teams of four around a dissecting table with the cadaver on it, all mummified in gauze bandages and stinking of formaldehyde. On that first day we were faced with a fetus which had been placed on top of the cadaver. Our group had a full term baby which had been stillborn. The very first thing we were to do was to take a meat cleaver and do a saggital section through the head of this fetus. That is we were to cut its head in half from front to back. Out of that class of 85 students, six did not return the next day. I think they might have made the best doctors.

With that suggestion, Tyler acknowledged the importance of feeling and compassion in medical practice. Dr. Koop echoed this sentiment, as the July 3, 1994, *San Francisco Examiner* reported, suggesting that technology, which in many ways has undermined the interpersonal realm of healing, can also be part of its reestablishment:

> Suppose you're a third-year student working in the clinic. You see a patient who had a major convulsion yesterday—the first one of his life. He asks you: 'What's wrong with me? Will it happen again? Is it curable?' Well, a third-year student knows nothing about that. But, with software that connects us to the National Library of Medicine, he can punch "grand mal seizure" into the computer and get facts on the prognosis, therapy, and likely recurrence. He'll learn a little bit, retain some of the specific knowledge; but he'll get experience in problem-solving and listening to patients that will be more important than memorization.

The scenario in which technology frees a doctor to focus on the interpersonal aspects of a medical interview fulfills a prediction John Naisbitt made in *Megatrends* (1980) that at the turn of the century the blending of "high-tech and high-touch" would reintroduce the personal element into a culture he foresaw as increasingly alienated by technology.

Growing public awareness of the abuses of residency and the danger posed to patients by exhausted residents who fall asleep during surgery, prescribe the wrong medication, or write down the wrong information in the chart sparked calls for more humane hours and more time off for residents. Many are on call every other night, while working 36-hour shifts every other day. A study compared a group of post-call residents who had slept approximately 30 minutes in the preceding 36 hours with a non-postcall group of residents who were not fatigued. While manual dexterity, reaction time, and short-term memory were relatively unchanged by sleep loss, the study found, creative thinking suffered appreciably, as well as originality, verbal fluency, motivation, and the ability to maintain constant vigilance (Nelson et al. 1995). The then-director of the residency program of the neurology department at Baylor Medical Center in Houston, Dr. Cliff Gooch, noted:

> In order to make residency less intensive, it is necessary to hire more people to do the work that residents have done. Some places have done that, and I think it's a positive step in the right direction. What's working against that, though, are the HMOs, which are really causing the financial crunch that medicine finds itself in now. . . . In an ideal world, residents would have exactly the right balance of supervised experience and autonomy [and] would be freed from doing a lot of the more mundane tasks that are not really necessary to their training. [Scut work is] part and parcel of residency training now in public hospitals, because they don't have enough money to pay enough people to do those things . . . you really want to give the resident what they need without taking undue advantage of them. (quoted in Flint 1996:12)

Another trend in medical education is increasing willingness to both conduct research and offer courses in alternative medicine. Harvard Medical School, for example, endowed a Mind/Body Medical Institute Chair, the first in the field of behavioral medicine. During the period of fieldwork for this study, Dr. Herbert Benson, who conducted the research behind the "relaxation response," held that chair. Harvard Professor David Eisenberg, who long taught a course in alternative medicine, strongly advocated the rigorous evaluation of alternative therapies in testimony before a Senate subcommittee in 1993 and stated that "research centers should be built in the midst of our most respected medical institutions to insure credibility and fair-mindedness" (1996:22). By 1997, the NIH's new Office of Alternative Medicine had funded ten such centers across the country in well-respected universities from Stanford in California to Columbia in New York.

I had the opportunity to teach such a course at Baylor Medical School in 1999, the first of its kind at that institution. The medical anthropology students I had taught at Rice University who went on to Baylor recruited me to teach that course after managing to convince their professors that it would be a good idea. I designed it around having local holistic physicians come every week to describe their practices, which were all radically different from the technocratic norm. I vividly remember one holistic ophthalmologist describing to my class how he had managed to reduce the number of drugs he used during and after certain eye operations to two. Yet when he had given a talk to current residents in ophthalmology, they had dismissed this achievement as "ridiculous," telling him that they were being taught to prescribe 15 or more drugs for the same procedures! I was happy to be told that the course continued to be taught at Baylor after my departure. Offering a course is not the same as requiring one; nevertheless the increase in the number and availability of these courses certainly points to the expansion of medical education beyond the boundaries of the technocratic paradigm. Many of these classes are introductory or survey, clearly not designed to provide medical students with skills in alternative techniques, but their existence indicates a new level of responsiveness, not just to students, but to the overall health care environment. The *Journal of Alternative and Complementary Medicine* (http://www.liebertpub.com/overview/journal-of-alternative-and-complementary-medicine-the/26/) annually publishes a full listing of all courses in alternative medicine taught in US medical schools. For information about degrees in complementary and alternative medicine, see http://www.healthcarestudies.com/Masters-Degree/Alternative-Medicine/.

The market and the need are huge: the 2012 National Health Interview Survey, which was conducted by the National Center for Health Statistics, part of the Centers for Disease Control and Prevention, gathered information on 88,962 American adults and 17,321 children. The survey found that 33.2% of adults in the United States aged 18 years and over and 11.6% of children age 4 to 17 years had used some form of complementary health approach in the previous 12 months. The percentages of adults and children using complementary approaches were similar to those in previous surveys (https://nccih.nih.gov/sites/nccam.nih.gov/files/NCCIH_2016_Strategic_Plan.pdf, see p. 7). The ongoing increase in the use of complementary and alternative therapies is an excellent example of a successful social movement; once its users passed the 20% tipping point, it became unstoppable. It's problem is its name: to call all such holistic therapies "complementary" or "alternative" reinforces the hegemony of technomedicine, which is why many CAM users and practitioners call their field "holistic," "integrative," or "functional" medicine (see Chapter 1).

Conclusion: Hope for the Future?

In this chapter, I have shown how initiation into the technomedical or technocratic model is accomplished through rituals that effect a psychological transformation of student to physician, a transformation that generally takes place in alignment with the core value system of technomedicine. At the end of this seven-year-long rite of passage (and sometimes more for certain specialties), the student-initiate is admitted into the ranks of one of the most prestigious and powerful professional groups in our society. The new doctor goes forward, fully imbued with the values and capable of using the arsenal of techniques available in the technomedical paradigm.

That paradigm has resulted in many dramatic improvements in diagnosis and treatment of illness and disease; it has also left many patients angry and alienated by its cold and impersonal treatment and has been unable to help them with many of their illnesses. Its emphasis on aggressive intervention has done a great deal of harm, and its high costs have become a major problem in the American economy. Many physicians themselves remain far

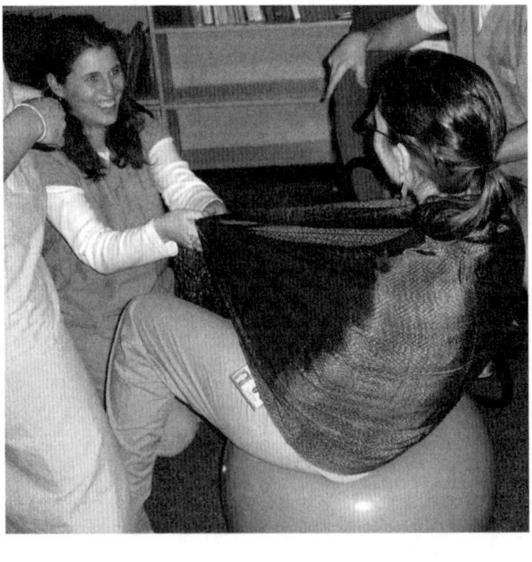

Medical students at Bellevue Hospital in New York learning doula labor support techniques in a class taught by famed doula trainer Debra Pascali-Bonaro, who also teaches such classes at Columbia University and the University of Pennsylvania, as well as around the world. The rebozo, a type of Mexican shawl, has multiple uses for labor support. Many medical students, as well as nursing and midwifery students, take this course, as pain-relieving doula techniques can be helpful to many patients besides laboring women. Photo by Debra Pascali-Bonaro from satisfied with the limitations and Stage One nature cognitive narrowing of their technomedical training. And general agreement exists in the health care field that the hard edges of technomedicine must be softened. The humanistic and holistic (and "functional") models of care described in Chapter 1, and the increasing number of practitioners espousing them, offer great hope for continuing movement in this direction, as I will more fully describe in the following chapter.

Questions for Thought and Discussion

1. Why does Davis-Floyd refer to medical training as "technocratic initiation"?
2. What are some key features of initiatory rites of passage and how are they manifested in medical schools and residencies?
3. Why does the author suggest that seeing patients earlier in medical school can benefit medical students?
4. What roles do you see for "complementary and alternative" or "integrative" medicine in medical training?

Recommended Film

The Business of Being Born: produced by Ricki Lake and Abby Epstein. http://www.thebusinessofbeingborn.com/ While not specifically about medical training, this film does include a very revealing interview with a group of ob/gyn residents during which they freely admit that they have almost no exposure to normal physiologic birth during their training.

Acknowledgements

I wish to express deep appreciation to Gloria St. John, coauthor of *From Doctor to Healer: The Transformative Journey*, for allowing me to adapt much of our mutual work for this chapter, and to my student intern Christina Weis for her invaluable help in updating the references.

5

The Paradigm Shift of Humanistic and Holistic Obstetricians

The "Good Guys and Girls" of Brazil

with Eugenia Georges

Question: Where does your passion come from?

João Batista: From my heart. I believe in justice and rights, and women in Brazil have neither, and their rights are most violated during birth, even the rich ones. It's ironic that the rich women have the worst treatment and they believe they have the best. . . . I want every OB professor to teach this to his residents: The woman is the center of care!

Throughout Latin America, "humanization" is the unifying concept around which social movements to demedicalize and transform childbirth have coalesced.[1] In the 1980s, feminist, environmentalist, human rights, and other oppositional movements began to proliferate in the democratizing after-

This chapter has been significantly expanded and updated from the original version, "Humanistic Obstetrics in Brazil: A Revolution in Maternity Care," by Eugenia Georges and Robbie Davis-Floyd. In *The Routledge Handboook of Medical Anthropology,* 2016, eds. Lenore Manderson, Anita Hardon, and Elizabeth Cartwright. London and New York: Routledge, pp. 340–345.

math of authoritarian rule. Since then, Brazilian humanization activists, like their counterparts in these movements in other countries, have engaged in ongoing political struggles to produce new meanings and cultural categories with which to challenge dominant medical discourses (Alvarez, Dagnino, and Escobar 1998). Although a diverse project, humanization at its core is grounded in the principle that safe, respectful, and supportive maternity care, free of unnecessary medical interventions, is a *woman's human right as a citizen of the nation*. Following this logic, unnecessary obstetrical interventions have come to be redefined as a category of violence against women—"obstetrical violence." In 2010, for example, Venezuela became the first nation in the world to recognize obstetrical violence as a legal category and punishable offence (the law exists, but to our knowledge has never been implemented). To ensure that such unnecessary interventions are eliminated, the humanization movement also insists that care of mother and infant consist exclusively of "best practices" that are supported by up-to-date, evidence-based medicine. Thus, the objectives of humanization are simultaneously ethical (promoting the view of women as persons with the right to respect and autonomy and of doctors as committed to protecting those rights) and instrumental (improving outcomes for mother and infant).

Brazilian birth activists, including a significant number of obstetricians, have long been in the forefront of attempts to humanize birth practices. In 1993, ReHuNa (*Rede pela Humanização do Parto e Nacimento*—the Network for the Humanization of Childbirth), was officially formed as an NGO to advocate for a woman's right to a humane and respectful childbirth experience grounded in scientifically sound practices. ReHuNa is composed predominantly of obstetrician-gynecologists, public health doctors, nurses, professional midwives, and other highly educated professionals. Their dual identities as professional experts and movement activists have enabled many ReHuNa members to move between the state sector and civil society and participate in the democratic institutions constructed to bridge them (Schild 1998:96).

In this chapter, we focus on a group of humanistic obstetricians, almost all of whom are members—and some, founders—of ReHuNa, describing their motivations to change the way they practiced and their processes of transformation, and noting their personal and political involvement in the wider social movement for the reform of maternity care in Brazil.

[1] Davis-Floyd has described the spread of this movement all over Latin America, as well as 21 essential characteristics of a social movement to humanize birth, in an article called "Changing Childbirth: The Latin American Example" (2007); available from Midwifery Today or on her website, www.davis-floyd.com

Humanizing Self and Practice: Becoming a "Good Guy or Girl"

Robbie's idea for this research project began in November of 2000, when she was invited to deliver a keynote speech at ReHuNa's first International Conference on the Humanization of Childbirth held in Fortaleza, Brazil. The conference was predominantly funded by the Japan International Cooperation Agency (JICA), which has close ties to many projects in Brazil, and was cosponsored by many other agencies and local and national ministries. Around 600 attendees were initially expected, but as Day One of the Congress progressed, the auditorium kept filling up until there was standing room only—in the end, over 1,800 attendees had registered and everyone there realized they were witnessing the full-fledged emergence of a national and international social movement for the humanization of birth.

As Robbie turned to step down from the podium after her talk (on "The Technocratic, Humanistic, and Holistic Paradigms of Birth and Health Care"—the subject of Chapter 1), she found a group of handsome young men waiting for her, all enthusiastically holding copies of her books for her to sign. "Who are you?" she asked. "We are the good guys!" was their response. "The bad guys are the ones who do the routine cesareans. We are humanistic and holistic OBs who work hard to put the woman first! We have read all your books and we try to put your ideas into practice." Beyond delighted, Robbie happily signed the books but had no time in the moment to find out who these OBs were—what were their names, where did they live, how did they practice, and most of all, why did they choose to practice holistically in a country with one of the highest cesarean rates in the world? Eventually, Robbie, joined by Nia (Eugenia Georges), undertook a research project to answer these questions; in 2011 and 2012 we interviewed 32 of these "good guys and girls" (as they happily continue to call themselves) at great length, in some of the cities in which they live and practice.

We found that most of them practiced in relative isolation, with little support and lots of ostracism from their technocratic colleagues. For many of them, "feeling alone and lonely" as they struggled to educate themselves about new approaches was one of the most difficult challenges they faced. So why did they persevere? From the quotation with which we began this chapter, and from these obstetricians' mode of self-identification, we gain glimpses of their deeply ethical engagement as they attempted to refashion themselves and their practices according to models alternative and oppositional to those of the powerful biomedical institutions that had shaped them as professionals. They identify themselves as the "good" doctors who struggle for justice and rights for women during childbirth. Here, we trace the transformative trajectories of some of the humanistic and holistic obstetricians who have been pioneers in radically reshaping how women are cared for during childbirth. These physicians have also been involved as organizers, leaders, or sympathetic supporters in the broader social movement to rethink and reinvent the cultural management of childbirth in Brazil. We explore how and why these doctors, trained and credentialed in high-status and authoritative modes of knowledge and practice, undertook the decision to reject their deeply embodied technomedical expertise and retrain themselves in less-prestigious, professionally stigmatized and even, in the Brazilian context, sometimes legally persecuted, holistic approaches.

We found it helpful to approach the process of self-transformation as an ethical project in which, according to Foucault, "the subject actively constitutes itself in an active fashion" through the application of technologies of the self that help guide him through the process (1973:296). As Foucault also argues, the ethical practice of self-transformation requires an "open territory," that is, a social and political context that, although never fully removed from domination, does offer an array of "ethical interstices" or gaps that allow for critically rethinking common sense habits of thought and practice. The obstetricians we spoke with came of age in the distinctive Brazilian context of the 1980s and 1990s, a period of democratizing transition from military to civilian regimes in which such interstices became available. We examine the processes by which the doctors we studied managed to refashion their subjectivities and craft themselves into different sorts of "humanized" professionals. What narratives, discourses, norms, and techniques have they deployed to guide their transformation and stay the course in the face of the criticism and opprobrium of their colleagues?

About Our Interviewees

The 32 obstetricians we interviewed are a cosmopolitan and diverse group. Half were women and half were men. For some, the preponderance and clarity of the scientific evidence in favor of supporting normal, physiological birth was most important in their decision to transform their practices; for others, it was allegiance to humanistic values rooted in their intersecting affiliations with feminism, left-wing politics, liberation theology, environmentalism, traditional medicine and midwifery, as well as a variety of New Age or older spiritual beliefs. Despite their differences, however, they typically shared an ethos that blended, or at least honored, all these dimensions to varying degrees. Some of our interlocutors had private practices that catered to a select group of highly motivated, middle-class women—those who, in one doctor's words, were "100% to 10,000% committed to normal birth." This group of our interviewees attended homebirths almost exclusively and had cesarean rates of 7–10%. Others had cesarean rates of 14–30% because they chose to care for all who came to them, believing that every woman has the right to a humanized birth, whether that is a natural birth at home or in hospital, or a scheduled CS. Others worked in the public health system providing care mainly for poor women who had no other options. In addition to working in public or private practice, some of our interviewees occupied salaried government positions, including influential positions in the Ministry of Health; others held faculty positions at some of Brazil's most prestigious universities.

For example, two of our interviewees, Dr. Ivo Lopez de Oliveira and Dr. João Batista (whom we quote at the beginning of this chapter), work as clinical directors of Hospital Sofia Feldman in the city of Belo Horizonte, state of Minas Gerais. Sofia Feldman is a high-risk center, providing tertiary-level care available to all women in the state. More than 50 nurse-midwives practice there, along with 20 OBs and 14 doulas, who are provided by the hospital for those women who bring no companion. They have very low rates of forceps, vacuum extraction, and episiotomy (around 8% for each); electronic fetal monitoring is used only intermittently; delayed cord-clamping and vertical births are the norm. Needless to say, Sofia Feldman is widely regarded as an exemplar of sustainable humanistic practice in the international childbirth movement. In December 2012, Director João Batista stated:

> Our cesarean rate is 24%, the lowest rate in Minas Gerais and one of the lowest in Brazil—but last year it was only 20%—it went up 4% in one year! That year there was a huge increase in high-risk women sent to us from all over the state. We are a high-risk hospital with a 42-bed NICU—the biggest one in the state, including malformations, et cetera—

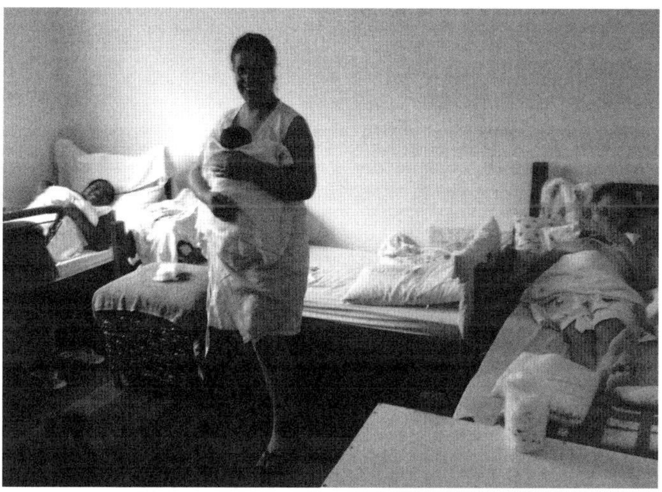

Women who were in high-risk pregnancy situations. They are from other cities or towns in the state of Minas Gerais who were transferred to Hospital Sofia Feldman weeks before birth and can stay for a week or two afterward in shared rooms with their babies always present. Mothers and babies are never separated in this hospital unless the baby is truly ill and needs NICU care. And even in the Sofia Feldman NICU, mothers and their babies are together as much as possible with the widespread use of "kangaroo care."

> so our PNMR [perinatal mortality rate] is 14.4/1000. Ten percent of our babies are preterm. More than 50% of the babies here are from other cities. Maybe we are doing the best we can. Hypertension, preterm labor, premature rupture of membranes are the most common—hypertension is the really big one, a lot of preeclampsia. If they come to us early, we can stop it, but most are sent late.

When we asked João, "Are you afraid of birth?" he responded, "No. I am afraid of not doing all I can for women."

Tools and Resources for Self-Transformation 1: Guidance from Books and Films

Working in relative isolation because they did not know of each other at the time they began their new trajectories (mostly during the late 1980s and the 1990s), these humanistic and often holistic OBs undertook a process of self-education to effect their personal and professional transformations. Still, in almost all instances, this process was profoundly influenced and guided by a common corpus of resources that served as guides. Particularly influential were texts written by international advocates of childbirth reform. Among the authors they most frequently cited were the French doctors and reformers Frederick Leboyer and Michel Odent (whom one doctor described as "open[ing] new doors of perception for me about the miracle of birth" [Jones 2009:277]), the Uruguayan obstetrician Roberto Caldeyro-Barcia, British authors and activists Sheila Kitzinger and Janet Balaskas, and the American writers Marsden Wagner, Penny Simkin, Marshall Klaus, Ina May Gaskin, Henci Goer, Elizabeth Davis, and Robbie Davis-Floyd. Melania Amorim explained:

> I started my Masters of Science Program [in 1993]. And I was introduced to evidence-based medicine. I also had to read philosophy of science and I was introduced to Thomas Kuhn and research on scientific revolutions. And I began to think, "Oh! It can be different." And I started to read about the [standard obstetrical] procedures . . . and I could realize that they were not necessary! That there was *no evidence* to support my practice. But I couldn't realize, why, with so much evidence against these procedures, they always have been performed by other obstetricians. . . . And so finally I encountered Robbie's book *Birth as an American Rite of Passage*, and I could understand what evidence-based medicine didn't explain—why these procedures have been maintained for decades with no scientific evidence—because they are rituals that reflect deep cultural values. And that's why her book changed my life. Because before I had books, I was changing my practice, but I didn't understand *why* all the others continued to maintain the old procedures.

The critiques of conventional childbirth our interviewees pored over and took to heart have deep domestic roots as well. Moysés Paciornik's book

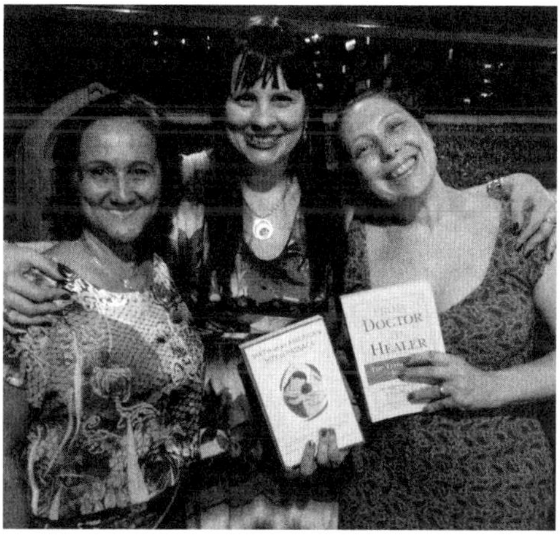

Three of our holistic OB interviewees—Edilsa Pinhiero de Araujo, Melania Amorim, and Leila Katz—displaying their copies of the two of Davis-Floyd's books that they found most helpful and influential. They said that her first book, *Birth as an American Rite of Passage*, had taught them that they needed to change, and *From Doctor to Healer* had shown them how. [Author's note: It is a distinct thrill for an anthropologist to find her work actually useful to and applied by practitioners.]

Aprenda a Nascer e a Viver com os Indios (*Learn How to Give Birth with the Indians)* and classic film *Birth in the Squatting Position*, released in 1979, have had a significant impact on alternative birth activists, not only in Brazil, but internationally as well. Paciornik also designed his own birthing chairs to simulate the benefits of the squatting position (*parto salvagem,* "savage birth") that he used in his private hospital in Curitiba and sold to other obstetricians and hospitals throughout Brazil (for the equivalent of around $200 USD). Hugo Sabatino, a respected professor of obstetrics at UNICAMP, was also one of the early pioneers whose teachings and writings on squatting birth were highly influential in stimulating the movement for humanized birth. And the early work during the 1970s and 1980s of Dr. José Galba de Araújo in the state of Ceara in humanizing hospital birth and providing support to the rural midwives in his catchment area was so influential that today ReHuNa gives an annual award in his name to a hospital that has made the greatest strides toward humanization in that year. (See Chapter 9 for a full description of Dr. Galba's work.)

Not only did the texts and individuals we mention above serve as exemplars, but also some of their international authors, such as Odent, Marsden Wagner (now deceased), Davis-Floyd, and Gaskin, themselves developed close ties to the humanization movement, visiting Brazil on numerous occasions, offering workshops, attending conferences, and delivering keynote speeches.

Tools and Resources for Self-Transformation 2: Guidance from Midwives

Another source of guidance in reshaping our interviewees' views toward childbirth was the recuperation/revaluation of the figure of the midwife. Among at least some activist sectors, the contributions of traditional midwives and their premedical practices were recognized, and occasionally even romanticized, as part of the more general valorization of the experiences of subaltern and indigenous women (Tornquist 2004:62). By 1970, schools that had trained direct-entry professional midwives, called *obstetrizes*, had been shut down and were replaced by nurse-midwifery programs. Yet nurse-midwives have made few inroads into Brazilian birthing culture to date—they still attend only 9% of Brazilian births. Meanwhile, the *obstetriz* has been reinvented in a relatively new direct-entry program at the University of São Paulo.

Yet until recent times (and still today in some rural areas, most especially the Amazon region), indigenous midwives still attend childbirth. Some of the older OBs we interviewed acknowledged the midwives who had assisted their mothers in childbirth and expressed respect and appreciation for their skills, as did others who were raised in rural areas and had witnessed the midwife-assisted homebirths of relatives. Two of our interviewees, Claudio Paciornik (son of Moysés) and Bernadette Boussada, had in fact learned directly from traditional midwives. Claudio and his father spent years observing the birth practices of the Kaigang and Guarani tribes on tribal reserves in Ibirama and Xanxare in South Brazil during the 1970s. Bernadette, in contrast, met traditional midwives for the first time when she was assigned after residency to a hospital in the remote city of Coração de Jesus in Minas Gerais for one year (1997–1998). She was the only OB in the only maternity hospital there. There were three *parteiras tradicionais* working in that hospital as auxiliary nurses; they became both her assistants and her guides. She told us that the two most important things the traditional midwives taught her were (1) respect for the woman, and (2) respect for the physiology of birth. She watched them treating women with kindness, attending labor without interfering, and using movement, upright positions, squatting, no episiotomy, and so forth. She slowly started to practice more and more like they did. The first

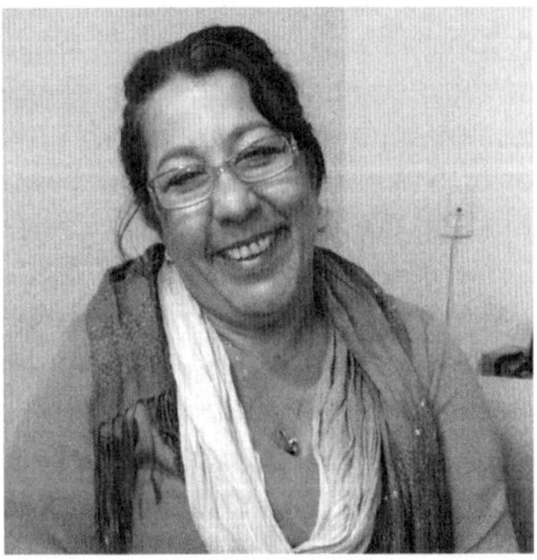

Bernadette Boussada, exclaiming, "Yes, I am afraid of birth. But I am a woman of courage!" In her hospital practice, Bernadette keeps all the women she is responsible for—often five at a time—in one room where she attends them during labor and receives their babies. She stays until they have all given birth and does not allow any other practitioners in the room, to preserve the holistic integrity of the space. She told us that her patients post their positive birth experiences widely on Facebook and thereby are changing the conversation around birth in their city of San Sebastio. Her personal CS rate is 10% while that of her hospital is over 70%.

intervention she gave up was the Kristeller maneuver (pushing on the abdomen), then forced pushing (yelling at the woman to "Push, push!"), then episiotomy, "then all the rest of it all at once!"

In addition to their support of the remaining indigenous midwives in Brazil, all of our interviewees believe that, ideally, professional midwives should be the primary birth attendants in Brazil—indeed, in every country—because, again ideally, midwives are or should be the experts in normal physiological birth. When there are professional midwives in their cities, our interviewees are generally happy to work with them as a team, support them however they can, and back them up when needed (see Jones 2009). They often wistfully lament the small number of Brazilian nurse-midwives (called *enfermeiras obstetras*) and the even smaller number of *obstetrizes* (all recent graduates from the direct-entry midwifery program at the University of São Paulo). All of our interviewees wish that there were thousands of professional midwives in their country, and many actively work to create new midwifery programs within universities, to support and expand the existing ones, and to develop birth centers in which the "midwifery model of care" can be actively implemented. In the meantime, they try themselves to practice the midwifery model (which is based on keeping the woman at the center and on understanding and facilitating normal physiological birth with a minimum of interventions; see Chapter 11). For example, Carla Polido noted:

> After concluding my master's degree I began to teach at the new medical school. I found out about humanization—it hit me like a bomb—I couldn't think of anything else! This friend of mine was the first step—she was an obstetric nurse and now she is a nurse-midwife. [She taught me about normal birth and now] I attend homebirths with her.

Those who do have professional midwives in their communities not only support these midwives but also receive support and encouragement from those midwives and from the doulas as well—in fact, given their general ostracism by their technocratic colleagues, these OBs generally receive their primary emotional and psychological support from their local midwives, doulas, and birth activists. Some call themselves "midwife-obstetricians," yet Carla noted, "I would like to say I'm a midwife, but I can't say that because I have this little monster in my head saying, 'Oh shouldn't I do an episiotomy?' I'm an obstetrician, I'm a teacher."

Tools and Resources for Self-Transformation 3: The Importance of Doulas

Doulas have long existed in Brazil, and the doula movement there is growing. Perhaps the very first Brazilian doula is Maria de Lourdes da Silva Teixeira, affectionately known as Fadynha (Little Fairy). In practice for over 28 years supporting hundreds of women during labor and birth, Fadynha is also one of the founders of the humanization movement in Brazil and an active member of ReHuNa; she has organized many conferences herself and spoken at many others, and in recent years has also become a doula trainer. The doula movement in Brazil was given a huge boost in January of 2003 when Debra Pascali-Bonaro, a renowned doula and doula trainer from New Jersey, was brought to Brazil by humanistic OB Maria Helena da Silva Bastos—Robbie had connected them, suggesting to Maria Helena that she bring Debra to develop doula programs for Brazil. Humanistic OB Marcos Diaz, another interviewee, helped to start the first doula program at the Municipal Secretariat of Rio de Janeiro at the Leila Diniz Hospital, a large public maternity hospital attending 300–400 births per month. Until 1998 this was the only public hospital in Rio that allowed a laboring woman to bring a family member or friend. For the program, Fadynha and Maria Helena recruited volunteers from community centers to be trained as doulas, naming their program *Amigas na Luz* (Friends in Light). Resistant at first, the doctors and nurses at that hospital quickly warmed to the doulas as they proved their abilities to soothe and support birthing mothers, and women increasingly began to ask for these hospital-provided doulas at their births.

Ricardo Jones, Christina Guimares, and the Mystery of Page 128

Meanwhile, far away in the south of Brazil, in the town of Porto Alegre, obstetrician Ricardo Jones had already made his paradigm shift and was working hard to keep reducing his intervention rates, as he found, over and over, that *the less he intervened, the better were his outcomes*. But despite his efforts, he could not get his cesarean rate below 25%. His goal was the 10–15% rate long recommended by the WHO. Frustrated and unsure as to why he seemed unable to lower that rate, one day while attending a course in homeopathy in Buenos Aires he entered a bookstore and a book seemed, as he recounts, to fall off a shelf right into his hands, open to page 128. The book was the famous *Birth Reborn* (1994), by world-famous holistic obstetrician Michel Odent, and the full-page picture on that page captivated Ric's attention: it showed a midwife at Pithiviers, the hospital in France where Odent first began attending water births, in a full-bodied embrace with a naked laboring woman. "Well," thought Ric, "if that's what it takes to get my cesarean rate down, I'm never going to succeed—I'm a Brazilian male, and if I tried to do that, my client's husband would kill me!"

Some weeks later, a beautiful woman named Christina Guimares came to Ric to ask him to attend her natural childbirth in the hospital, which he did. Two weeks after the successful birth, she came back into his office for a postnatal exam and announced, "You need me and I need you and we are going to work together!" "Oh?" said Ric. "And what is it that you do?" "I'm a doula," she replied; Ric's answer, of course (this was many years ago), was "What's a doula?" As soon as she explained the doula's role in birth, Ric immediately saw that here was the answer to what he had been thinking of as "the mystery of page 128." He felt that, as a man, he could not embrace a naked woman who was not his wife, but Christina as a doula could do precisely that and much more.

As Ric describes in his beautifully written chapter "Teamwork" in *Birth Models That Work*, he and Christina began to work together almost immediately. Remember we mentioned that Christina is beautiful? Well, Ric's wife Zeza began to get a bit jealous when her husband began to head off to births at 2 AM in the company of this lovely woman, so she started going with them and soon became hooked on birth herself. Already a trained pediatric nurse, it took her only one year to complete a nurse-midwifery program, and so the three became a team—the doctor, the midwife, and the doula. This teamwork model they created together carried on for several decades (until Ricardo retired from active practice in 2016).

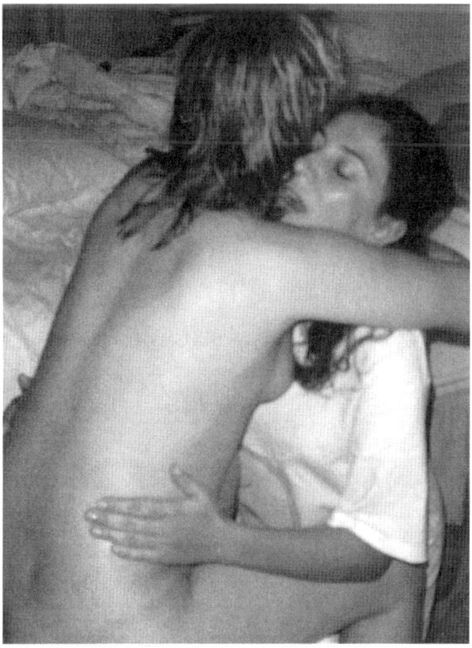

Christina solving the mystery of page 128. Photo by Ricardo Jones

After Christina married and moved away, Ric

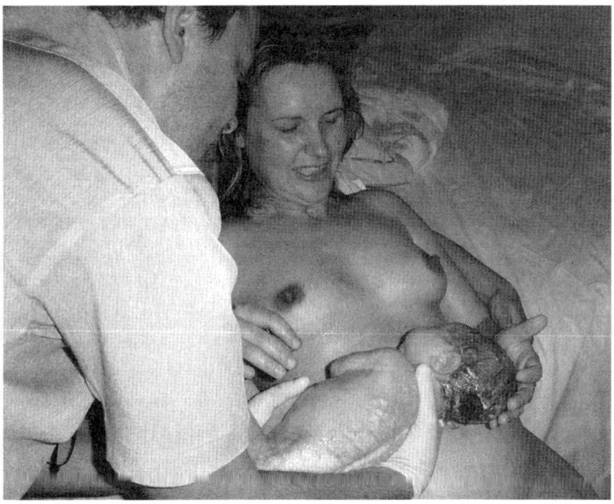

The birth outcome: Ric gently places the baby on the mother's abdomen immediately after birth. Passing through the birth canal and then being put in immediate contact with the mother ensures that the baby's body will colonize with its mother's internal flora, which will help to increase its natural immunities—what is called the "microbiome" (Harman and Wakeford 2017). Photo by Zeza Jones

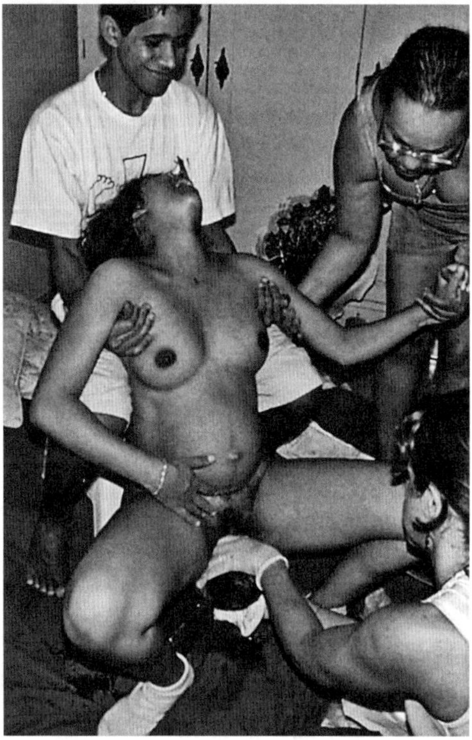

The birth, with Zeza receiving the baby while the husband and the doula support the mother in this physiologically beneficial upright position. Photo by Ricardo Jones

and Zeza trained other doulas; part of the doulas' job was to arrive at the home of the laboring couple shortly after labor began. If it was a planned homebirth, the doula was the one to advise the midwife and doctor when they should come. If a transport and a cesarean were required, Ric performed the CS, providing complete continuity of care. If a planned hospital birth, the doula provided support during early labor and then accompanied the couple to the hospital, where they were met by Ric and Zeza and cared for by the team. To preserve the integrity of what Ric terms "the psychosphere" of birth, they did not allow any other hospital practitioners into the birthing room (except the pediatrician, who has to come in by law after the baby is born). By the time Ric retired, over half of their births were homebirths, and Ric's cesarean rate had long stood at the 15% that had always been his goal.

Ric believes that midwives and doulas should be the primary attendants at birth; he only used to go to homebirths to provide legal protection for the team. There he mostly confined his role to taking photos and afterward creating a beautiful slide show of the labor and birth, set to the music of the couple's favorite song, as a special gift. The day after the birth, the team would go to the couple's home to give them the DVD and they all would watch the slide show together.

The Benefits of Doula Support

As we noted, most of our holistic interviewees are the only such doctors in their city; they receive little to no support from other OBs, but lots of support from midwives (where they exist), birth activists, and most especially from the doulas who often work with or for them. Many told us that they

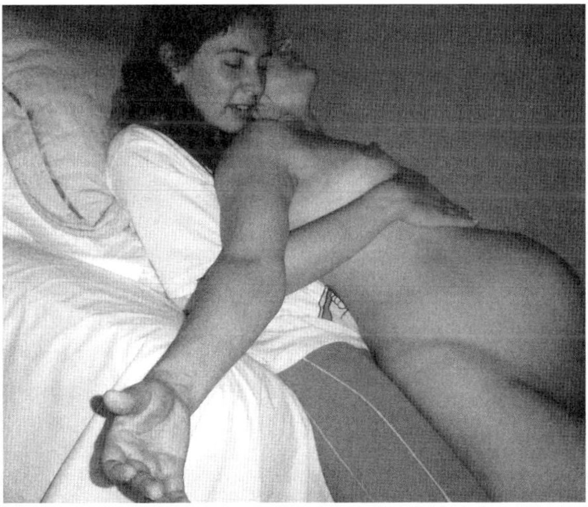

Full-bodied, full-on doula care by Brazilian doula Christina Guimares. Photo by Ricardo Jones

could not practice as holistically as they do without the doulas who are there for that one-on-one continuous support long proven to be extremely beneficial. Doulas help reduce the amount of pain women experience, help women cope with that pain, alleviate their anxieties, and deal with the emotional issues that often emerge during labor, thereby shortening the length of labor and reducing the number of interventions performed. For example, a meta-analysis of 12 randomized controlled trials on the effects of the doula's presence (Scott, Klaus, and Klaus 1999) showed that support from a doula resulted in:

- 51% reduction in cesarean births
- 25% reduction in labor length (average of 98 minutes)
- 35% reduction in analgesia
- 71% reduction in oxytocin augmentation
- 57% reduction in use of forceps/vacuum (See also Kennell et al 1991; Scott, Berkowitz and Klaus 1999; Hodnett et al. 2003; and http://www.childbirthconnection.org/giving-birth/labor-support/resources/)

Tools and Resources for Self-Transformation 4: Social Movements and Networks

In addition to books, midwives, and doulas, our interviewees credited ReHuNa (which, again, some of them were instrumental in founding) and other activist networks as critical sources of knowledge, support, and guidance. Many of them met each other for the first time at ReHuNa conferences and were beyond delighted to discover that they were part of a community of like-minded alternative practitioners previously unknown to them. Today,

Brazil's "good guy and girl" OBs keep in regular touch via Facebook and other social media, where they engage in vigorous dialogues and debates over such issues as whether it is wise and safe to assist a woman with two or more previous cesareans to give birth vaginally, how best to turn a breech baby, and what constitutes optimal nutrition during labor, among other issues. Melania Amorim described her discovery of the Internet chat group *Parto Nosso* (Our Birth) as "magic. . . . It was a revolution in our life because you could find persons whose thoughts were similar to ours. We were not crazy. We were accepted, we were stimulated." When they experience ostracism or outright persecution from their technocratic colleagues (often called *cesaristas* for their routine use of cesareans, as opposed to *vaginalistas*—another term by which our good guy interviewees identify themselves), they turn to these activist networks for both advice and support.

The Process of Transformation

Pivot Points

Ricardo Jones: The Epiphany

One bright day in the first year of Dr. Ricardo Jones' obstetric residency, a nurse came bounding in to the residents' lounge where he was hanging out with his colleagues, saying directly to him, "Please doctor, come quickly—there is a woman who has just come in from the street with no prior prenatal care and she is having her baby in the emergency room!" Realizing that in that moment he was the senior resident in the room, Ric rushed downstairs to the ER. Pushing the door open, he was shocked to see the delivery table empty, and turned angrily toward the nurse, thinking she was playing a trick on him. "No doctor," said the nurse, "please push the door further!" And there Ric was horrified to see a peasant woman squatting on the floor in the corner of the room. He yelled at her to stand up immediately and get onto the table, but, as he told me years later, "she was in another world, and she simply looked right through me, as if I were made of glass." Lifting up her skirt, Ric saw the baby's head crowning. No time even to put on gloves, so he knelt down and caught the slippery body with his bare hands, handing the baby off to the nurse as quickly as possible with a shudder of disgust—he had never before touched a newborn without wearing gloves. Then he scolded the woman, who continued to "look right through me," for making such a bloody mess on the floor as the placenta emerged. The baby was whisked off to the NICU because it was considered "contaminated" by its birth on the floor, while the mother, who finally did climb onto the table, was rolled away to a postpartum recovery ward.

All day Ric felt bothered by that birth but couldn't pinpoint why, until later in the afternoon the nurse exclaimed to him, "Doctor, what a good thing you were there! Only think what might have happened had you not been there!" And suddenly it hit him with the force of a strong blow that if he had not been there, that mother would in fact have had a perfect birth. She would have caught her own baby; she had not needed him for anything—indeed, everything he had done was to spoil, not enhance, her birth experience. And with that realization began his decades-long journey from technocratic to holistic practice, which he has beautifully described (in Portuguese) in his books *Memoirs of a Man Made of Glass* (Jones 2010) and *Entre as Orelhas: Historias do Parto* (*Between the Ears: Birth Stories*) (Jones 2012), and in English in his chapter "Teamwork: An Obstetrician, a Midwife, and a Doula in Brazil" in *Birth Models That Work* (Jones 2009).

Roxana Knobel: The Evidence

During her residency, Roxana Knobel, an obstetrician from Florianopolis, read a study about the iatrogenic effects of episiotomies to enlarge the perineum during birth; she found the evidence so compelling that she immediately stopped performing them. And just as immediately, her colleagues and superiors began to chastise her for that. This chastisement for stopping what she now understood to be a completely unnecessary procedure in the vast majority of cases made her suspicious of everything else she was being taught, so she began to read more studies until she finally understood the detriments she was causing to the normal physiologic process of birth with all those interventions. Once she was in private practice, she completed her paradigm shift and continues to practice holistically to this day.

Paulo Batistuta: The First Vertical Birth

Paulo Batistuta's turning point came when he accepted a scholarship to study normal birth in Sweden. Having performed over a thousand cesareans by then, he realized he knew little about normal birth and decided to take this opportunity to learn. In Sweden he watched midwives attend normal births but never did so himself. Upon his return, he was approached by a French woman who informed him in no uncertain terms that she wanted "a vertical birth." Feeling empowered by his experiences in Sweden, he agreed, and was a bit shocked during labor to find himself on the floor underneath the laboring woman attempting to ascertain her cervical dilation, at her request, but was unable to interpret what his fingers were feeling as he had never before performed a vaginal exam "from below." His experience shows us how deeply embodied medical knowledge becomes; his fingers, used to assessing cervical dilation "from above," simply did not know what they were feeling in that unfamiliar position. The birth turned out very well, and he was hooked, quickly becoming an expert on normal birth and empowering his clients in turn to birth on their own, as beautifully illustrated in his DVD *Sagrado*.

"Step by Step" along the Transformation Spectrum

As we came to understand during our interview process, even for our interlocutors like Ric, Roxana, and Paulo, whose narratives of transformation highlight a pivot point—an "aha moment" in which their perspectives abruptly shifted—changing their day-to-day practice was in almost all cases a slow and painful process that required the conscious choice to dissociate themselves from their habitual forms of thinking and acting. Changing deeply embodied knowledge and habits typically occurred "step by step, step by step" (Paulo Batistuta) and could take years to complete. As Ric eloquently put it, "between rationality and fear, there was a considerable space still to cross" (Jones 2009:292).

For many, the episiotomy was one of the hardest routines to give up. Carla Polido noted:

> [As a student at UNICAMP] I saw squatting births with Dr. Hugo [Sabatino] but it didn't influence me—the other professors said he was a lunatic, "That's for savages!" At the time I also thought that those women were too demanding. Today I *want* women to have demands, but at the time, I was Dr. House—I was *the boss*. We didn't value the woman, we thought that *we* were the stars of the show, not her. From there was a whole process, one birth after another. The toughest thing for me to stop doing was the episiotomy. I had this fear of the perineum blowing up!

The step-by-step nature of this process was further elaborated by Marilena Pereira. Even once convinced that a procedure was unnecessary, finally relinquishing it was sometimes still a struggle, as Marilena described:

> I filled in at the last moment for a colleague to do a homebirth, but I arrived late, just as the woman was giving birth. . . . I didn't do anything; she was doing it all. I had the intuition to shut my mouth, not to tell her what to do. That's when the light went on for me, when I understood what was happening. [Yet] many times, I still couldn't believe it would be OK not to cut. When the birth would start, I'd say to myself, "It's going to tear, it's going to tear," and I would cut. Sometimes I would succeed in not cutting, but I was afraid, really afraid, so many times I would cut. [It took me] the next two years to give up doing episiotomies.

Yet give them up they did, soon discovering that upright positions were much more likely to prevent vaginal tears. Attending women who are upright—sitting on a birthing chair or ball, squatting, standing—of course requires the OB to be below her, perhaps sitting on a low stool or kneeling in front of the laboring mother. This sort of status reversal was a challenge for some, while others took to it easily. Quick to go was the routine use of pitocin to speed labor; hard to learn was the patience it takes to attend births without artificially rushing the process. Helio Bergo noted:

> When I started with squatting birth, with the woman in vertical position, I saw that there was no need any more for forceps and other aggressive and

> invasive methods. Because this is natural! . . . Little by little I was learning to watch the rhythms and this is what enchanted me. Do not intervene. [Just] watch. I would just be there, observing and learning. I learned in this way, from attending homebirths. To respect the rhythm was the hardest thing to learn. And it's what brought me the most benefits. When I learned how to do that, things became easy. But it was hard to let go, to respect the rhythm, to not intervene. Because there are moments when, without any doubt, it is necessary to intervene. To know, to decide which moment it is, without intervening prematurely, is difficult.

During residency, Carla Daher found herself shocked and horrified that thirsty laboring women were not allowed to drink even though they were working so hard and sweating. She began to offer them water during labor, and then to encourage them to move around and walk. Like Helio, she learned from a sympathetic colleague "to be patient, to just watch women work, to be nice." She gave up manual extraction of the placenta because she saw it as "unnecessary and cruel." As a result, her OB chief called her practice "messy" and so made sure she was the only resident in her cohort who was not hired by the hospital from which she graduated. (She went into private practice.)

For our interviewees, giving up routine interventions meant placing great emphasis on treating their patients as individuals, which in turn entailed getting to know them as such. Banished were the five-minute standard question and answer sessions, which they replaced with prenatal visits lasting an hour or more, with childbirth education classes they often taught themselves, and with discussion sessions in which their patients could come together in groups and ask all the questions they wished. Those in private practice made conscious decisions to limit the number of patients they accepted in order to be able to provide the high-quality humanistic care they now offered. They found themselves happy to accept lower salaries (and often ostracism from their technocratic colleagues) as a small price to pay for the much greater levels of satisfaction they experienced via providing that high-quality care (see Manaham 2011).

On the spectrum technocratic–humanistic–holistic, all of our interviewees placed themselves very much on the right-hand side of humanism (keeping the focus on the woman, treating her with kindness and respect, paying attention to her nutrition), merging into holism (perceiving the body as energy and birth as a spiritual process) (see Chapter 1). Some vacillated between the two terms; for example, João Batista noted:

> I don't consider myself a holistic OB, but Andrea [one of the Sofia Feldman midwives] is. She is holistic—she believes in energy, in everything that's supernatural. Sometimes I believe, sometimes I don't—I'm in the middle. She is a spiritualist. I don't consider myself one—but my wife says I am. Sometimes I'm technocratic because I need to be. Most of the time I'm a humanist, sometimes I'm holistic too.

Conclusion: The Obstetric Backlash and Positive Change

Although their numbers are relatively small, the OBs we discuss in this chapter have managed to provide options for humanistic maternity care in nearly every major city in Brazil. Sadly, most of them no longer are able to offer the homebirth option due to some recent highly restrictive regulations from CREMERJ (the Medical Board of the State of Rio de Janeiro). Ricardo Jones (personal communication 2016) has summarized these regulations for us as follows:

- Article 1. The participation of doctors in the so-called domiciliary actions related to birth and perinatal assistance is forbidden.
- Article 2. Doctors are forbidden from providing supervision to other professionals attending home births.
- Article 3. An exception can be made in the case of an obstetric emergency/urgency, but notification to the Medical Board of Rio de Janeiro (CREMERJ) is compulsory.
- Article 4. When obstetricians working on shift in the hospital assist in births transported to hospitals from homes or birth centers, they must report that assistance to CREMERJ.
- Article 5. Non-compliance with these resolutions is considered an ethical infraction and can result in disciplinary action.

These regulations were generated by CREMERJ in 2014 as part of a strong technomedical backlash against the movement for the humanization of birth, which was given huge impetus by a film, *O Renacimento do Parto* (described below). This film was shown in movie theaters all over the country and helped to generate huge marches supporting the humanization of birth around Brazil. Strictly speaking, these regulations are not legally binding but have been influential enough to make most obstetricians afraid of attending homebirths (Rattner 2017; Jones forthcoming). So as of 2014, most of the homebirths in Brazil are perforce attended by midwives—either nurse-midwives (*enfermeiras obstetras*) or direct-entry (non-nurse) midwives (*obstetrizes*). As we mentioned above, collectively these professional midwives attend around 9% of births nationwide, mostly in hospitals but sometimes in homes and birth centers. The "good guy and girl" OBs back these midwives up when possible, and a very few of them still do attend homebirths. They have also succeeded in creating a few institutionalized humanistic practices in Brazil such as Hospital Sofia Feldman and the Maternity Department of the University of Santa Catarina. As Carlos Miner noted:

> Some of our residents are from Santa Catarina, and there I think they are a little more advanced. They told me that they had two hospitals, one very humanized and one they call a "butchery." And there are very old doctors there that are . . . practicing that kind of obstetrics of 50 years

ago and they are not changing. . . . Last night I was on duty . . . with some residents who were my students two or three years ago and they accepted everything, they were practicing like me, and so I think there is going to be a change.

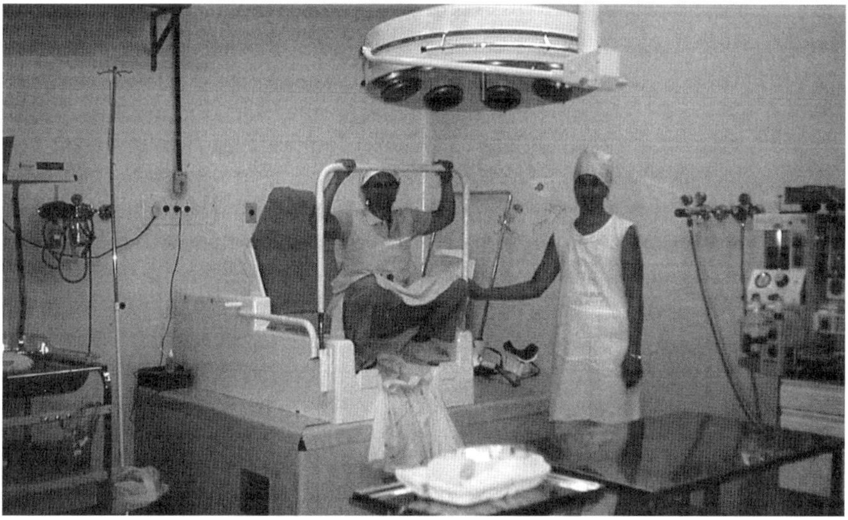

A nurse-midwife in the maternity ward at the University Hospital of Santa Catarina (where midwives attend the majority of births, referring only the high-risk ones to the OBs) demonstrating the use of their specially designed upright birthing chair (which can also lie down flat so mothers can rest when they wish to). Normatively, this and all their other birthing beds/chairs are placed upright to encourage women to take that position. The indentation at the front of the chair is for birthing the baby onto a warm plastic hot water bottle with a towel covering it, to keep the baby warm and with the sensation of floating until the mother is ready to bend down and pick up her newborn. It is important to note that many mothers just need a minute or two to themselves to recover from the intensity of the birth experience. This kind of squatting position allows them to do that, reaching down to stroke and then slowly pick up their babies when they are ready. Photo by Marcos Leite

As we previously mentioned, some of our interviewees, along with others of their humanistic colleagues, have been appointed to influential positions in the Ministry of Health where they can promote large-scale policy change. Some are also instrumental in *Rede Cegonha* (the Stork Network)—a sweeping program inaugurated in 2011 by then-newly elected President Dilma Rousseff to transform maternal health care delivery throughout the nation's Unified Health System (SUS), within which 76% of Brazilian births take place (SUS n.d:10). This program is designed to address issues such as maternal mortality and the nation's cesarean rate—which in 2013 was 56.7%, with a range of about 40% in the public sector up to 85% in the private sector—by replacing the intensely technocratic model of maternity care that has dominated Brazilian obstetrical practice since the 1970s with a humanized paradigm.

As a way to synthesize the concept of humanization as applied to childbirth, Ric (Jones 2012:223) noted that the humanized birth is characterized by:

1. The protagonism it gives to women, without which we would be merely further entrenching, in this modern era, the dependence of women on men imposed over millennia by patriarchy;
2. An integrative and interdisciplinary view of birth focused on a deep understanding of the characteristics of the biological process and its emotional, social, cultural, and spiritual aspects, which must all be equally valued and attended to;
3. A visceral connection with evidence-based medicine, making clear that the humanization of childbirth movement, which nowadays has spread all over the world, works under the aegis of reason.

Ric's objective in creating the above synthesis was to offer a simple vision of the movement's proposals. "More than general indignation at the excess of intervention," he said, "we needed a very clear idea of what we wanted for birth."

Questions for Thought and Discussion

1. What were some of the primary motivations of the humanistic/holistic obstetricians described in this chapter to change their practice model?
2. How did they go about this process of change?
3. What sort of repercussions from the obstetric establishment did they experience as a result?
4. Why did they persevere anyway?

Recommended Films

O Renacimento do Parto (The Rebirth of Birth, or ***Birth Reborn)***: produced by Érica de Paula and Eduardo Chauvet, 2013. This film showed in movie theaters all over Brazil for five months and was viewed by over 30,000 people. It played a major role in moving forward the humanization of birth movement in Brazil. Davis-Floyd is one of the interviewees in this film, as are Ricardo Jones and others of our "good guys and girls" interviewees. It was this film that generated the backlash from CREMERJ (mentioned above) and led to regulations prohibiting all OBs from attending homebirths. (http://tumeloyissakhar.blogspot.com/2015/10/watch-birth-reborn-online-2013-full.html)

Violência Obstétrica—A voz das brasileiras (Obstetric Violence: The Voice of Brazilian Women): (2012). Available at https://www.youtube.com/watch?v=eg0uvonF25M (A subtitled version in English is available.)

Sagrado (Sacred): produced by Paulo Batistuta, available at http://www.maternidadeativa.com.br/videos.html or www.paulobatistuta.com.br

This gorgeous video shows a series of holistic, sexual, even orgasmic hospital births attended by obstetrician Paulo Batistuta. English subtitles available.

Birth in the Squatting Position: produced by Moysés and Claudio Paciornik, 1979. This historic film, one of the first to be made on normal birth, shows a series of births in the squatting position taking place in the clinic originally built and run by Brazilian obstetric pioneer Moysés Paciornik, and now operated by his son Claudio Paciornik. Available at http://www.worldcat.org/title/birth-in-the-squatting-position/oclc/23748796

Nacer con amor cambia el mundo: produced by Diego Alarcon MD. A series of 40 short documentaries about birth at *Clinica La Primavera*, a private and highly humanistic maternity hospital in Quito, Ecuador. Available at midwiferytoday.com

Why Not Home? The Surprising Birth Choices of Doctors and Nurses: producer/director Jessica Moore. This film focuses on hospital birth providers who choose homebirth with the goal of moving toward improvements to maternity care in hospitals and at home. http://www.whynothome.com/

Birthing in Peace: produced by British midwife Peggy Oolsthorn. This 32-minute film documents the successful fusion of traditional and biomedical obstetrical systems achieved by Brazilian obstetrician Dr. Galba Araujo, who organized the building of maternity clinics throughout northeastern Brazil, staffing them with local midwives who were given biomedical training but were strongly encouraged to continue with their traditional style of birth: the mother labors while walking or resting in hammocks and gives birth upright on a birthing stool with little or no insertion of hands into the vagina; after birth, the baby stays with the mother. Such practices, continued in the clinics, kept infection and mortality low, and were incorporated by Dr. Galba as far as possible into hospital practice in Fortaleza, Ceara, where he was director of obstetrics. http://www.worldcat.org/title/birthing-in-peace/oclc/36410096

PART TWO

Midwives, Culture, Ideologies, and Birth

6

American Midwifery

A Brief Anthropological Overview

Why I Wrote This Chapter: A Public Lack of Understanding of the Complexities of American Midwifery

In 2006, *Mainstreaming Midwives: The Politics of Change* was published, coedited by myself and Christine Barbara Johnson. Christine had served as an expert consultant on a project exploring how online health care information influences ideas and behaviors (Johnson and Galvin 2001). Christine wanted to explore this question in relation to public knowledge about midwives. She and her team created a website containing information about both nurse- and non-nurse (direct-entry) midwives, along with a questionnaire that was filled out by 100 women about what they had learned about American midwives from the site. The respondents reported that, while before this project they would not have considered using a midwife, after learning more about midwives, now they would. Yet despite the extensive information provided about the differences between types of midwives,

> the women in the study were not able to discriminate between them, but rather combined them into one indistinguishable category. We found that the idea of using a midwife was so novel that the information about the differences between the two types of midwives . . . was not retained. This was a big surprise to us as our study population was highly educated and able to readily grasp conceptual information. We hypothesized that the novelty of seeing midwives as viable options caused the majority of women in our study to reach saturation at this point, and the difference between the two types of midwives became excess information. (Davis-Floyd and Johnson 2006:16)

In light of this general public ignorance about the complexities of American midwifery, I wrote this chapter for this book because American midwifery is complex and I believe that students, the general public, and policy makers, as well as midwives themselves and other health-care practitioners should be able to understand its complexities. Understanding US midwifery is key to helping women make truly informed choices about the kind of childbirth they wish to have and the best practitioner(s) to attend them. It is also key for obstetricians, many of whom encounter midwives at some point in their careers, to legislators seeking to understand and vote appropriately on various types of proposed legislation involving various types of midwives, and to policy-makers involved in health care reform. This brief synopsis is necessarily oversimplified due to space limitations. I intend it simply to provide a general overview of American midwifery for those unfamiliar with its variations. Full descriptions of the political, educational, and practice variations in American midwifery can be found in *Mainstreaming Midwives*, in *Midwifery and Childbirth in America* by Judith Rooks (1997), in *Paths to Becoming a Midwife: Getting an Education*, edited by Jan Tritten and Kelley Meyer (2010), and in *A History of Midwifery in the United States: The Midwife Said "Fear Not"* by Helen Varney and Joyce Thompson (2016). For an understanding of the many midwifery organizations' (quite confusing) acronyms, please see the Glossary I have provided at the end of this article.

A Short History of American Midwifery

The word "midwife" came into use in Middle English around 1100–1500, with *mid* meaning "with" and *wif* meaning "woman"—a midwife is "with woman." That ancient definition and its emotion-laden meaning are the reasons contemporary midwives have consistently refused to change their English name, even though midwives in other countries have adopted more professional-sounding labels in their respective languages than the old traditional names by which they used to be called—for example, *parteira* (*parto* means birth; *a parteira* is someone who attends births) in Brazilian Portuguese was changed to *obstetriz* or, for nurse-midwives, *enfermeira obstetra* (nurse-obstetrician). In the early 20th century, with the rise of modern medicine, midwifery became unpopular in the US. Physicians, especially obstetricians, believed that women were too uneducated and incompetent to attend births and did not want competition from midwives for their lucrative obstetrical practices. Perhaps most significant was their desire for obstetrics to become recognized as a medical specialty and to obtain the right to educate residents. To accomplish this goal, OBs needed to take the births away from midwives, into whose hands were born over 50% of all newborns in 1900. At the time, GPs managed most of the rest (Litoff 1978; Ettinger 2006; anon. rev'r. 2017).

Thousands of immigrant midwives in the Northeast (many of whom had been professionally trained in European midwifery schools), along with the legendary black granny midwives of the South, the Latina *parteras* of the Southwest, and Native American midwives around the country, were phased or forced out of service. At this point, childbirth was increasingly seen as not as a natural process but as a dangerous, potentially pathological condition; homebirth began to disappear as increasing numbers of women moved to the hospital to give birth. Modern medicine's interventions to assist in or force childbirth included forceps, episiotomies, and anesthetics (and, very rarely, cesareans), and only trained physicians could provide such practices. Women were given little to no control in childbirth and could not be attended by anyone but hospital staff. By the 1960s, the vast majority of American women gave birth in hospitals; that rate has long stood at 99%. (The cesarean rate in those days was around 6%; obstetricians had many hands-on skills [for delivering, for examples, breeches and twins] that they are not learning today.) In 2013, 90.3% of birthing women were attended by physicians (Martin et al. 2015).

The Development and Growth of Nurse-Midwifery

In 1925, an American woman named Mary Breckinridge, who had studied both nursing and midwifery in Europe, brought professionally trained British nurse-midwives to the US and opened the first American nurse-midwifery service in Hyden, Kentucky—the Frontier Nursing Service. In 1939, FNS started the School of Midwifery and Family Nursing, which now functions as the Frontier Nursing University. Breckinridge had made a careful survey of the needs of the Appalachian poor—whom few doctors wished to serve—and concluded that the British combination of public health nursing and midwifery was ideal to meet them. Nurse-midwives soon began studying and working in New York as well, serving the urban poor. By 1955, nurse-midwives had created a professional organization, the American College of Nurse-Midwives (ACNM). One of its sister organizations—the Accreditation Commission for Midwifery Education (ACME)—accredits all US nurse-midwifery educational programs

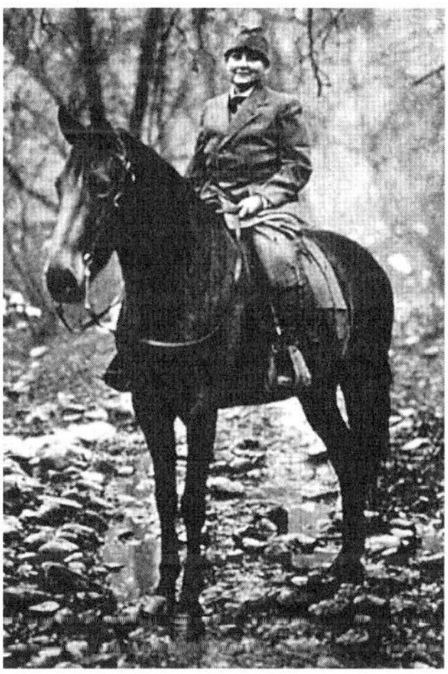

Nurse-midwife Mary Breckinridge on horseback in Hyden County, Kentucky, serving the needs of the rural poor during the late 1920s. Photographer unknown

(which must be based in or affiliated with a college or university), while another, the American Midwifery Certification Board (AMCB), administers a national examination and certification as a Certified Nurse-Midwife (CNM or Certified Midwife CM—see below).

While early American nurse-midwives had practiced almost entirely outside the hospital (except for the small hospital at Frontier), CNMs managed to gain admission into some central-city hospitals in the Northeast during the 1950s, where they were welcomed by exhausted obstetricians coping with the full effects of the baby boom. Today the vast majority of the county's 7,500 or so practicing CNMs attend births in hospitals; around 500 of them attend births in homes and birth centers (Lisa Kane Low, ACNM president, personal correspondence, August 2016). Although they are increasingly sought out by middle-class women for the humanistic quality of their care and their efforts to minimize interventions during labor, CNMs' primary motivations have always included serving the urban and rural poor. Their great secret is that—although it is generally supposed that they attend only normal, low-risk births—due to their care of impoverished women, they often attend or co-manage higher-risk women as well. The national certification exam to confer the CNM credential was instituted by ACNM in 1971 (www.midwife.org). CNMs have been legal and licensed in all states since the early 1980s (Lisa Kane Low, personal correspondence, August 2016).

Most CNMs have kept careful statistics on their practice outcomes, which have consistently been excellent. It has long been known that midwives are less likely than OBs to use interventions like labor induction and cesarean section (CS) (which is 50% more costly than vaginal delivery and carries far greater risks). A study called "State Scope of Practice Laws, Nurse-Midwifery Workforce, and Childbirth Procedures and Outcomes" (Yang, Attanasio, and Kozhimammil 2016) that analyzed data on 12 million US births between 2009 and 2011 found that *midwifery autonomy is key to midwifery outcomes*. Women in the 22 states that allow CNMs to practice autonomously (with no required physician supervision or contractual practice agreements with MDs) have a 60% greater chance of having CNM-attended births, as well as 13% lower odds of cesareans and preterm births, and 11% lower odds of low-birthweight newborns than the 28 states that do not allow autonomous practice.

Perhaps one factor slowing CNMs' growth is the extensive education they must attain, which includes a Master's degree and can be very costly; many CNMs graduate with debts of $60,000 or more. In 2005, as the ACNM celebrated its 50th anniversary, CNMs attended only 8% of American births; in 2013, they still attended only 8.2% (Martin et al. 2015). Yet their numbers are growing: by 2015 new data showed that they had reached attendance at 11.9% of American births (Declerq 2015). Critical mass is generally thought to be around 20%—once a profession reaches that level, it is pretty much unstoppable in terms of its continued growth and cultural success.

Yet according to researchers at the Rensselaer Polytechnic Institute (2011):

> When just 10% of the population holds an unshakable belief, their belief will always be adopted by the majority of the society. The scientists, who are members of the Social Cognitive Networks Academic Research Center (SCNARC) at Rensselaer, used computational and analytical methods to discover the tipping point where a minority belief becomes the majority opinion.

If this information is accurate, then it is happy news to me that CNMs have already passed that tipping point, as they now attend almost 12% of US births, and the consumers who utilize their services believe in them deeply. Yet there is still a long way to go to reach the around 80% of births that CNMs should be attending. The major factor impeding nurse-midwives' further growth is physician resistance to the economic competition they present. Over the many years of my fieldwork with midwives, I noted a consistent trend: when CNMs practicing in hospitals reached attendance at around 30% of the births, they often were fired or had their privileges and/or scope of practice restricted, because the obstetricians did not appreciate the competition and because hospitals tend to make less money from midwifery care, since, as noted above, midwives tend to use fewer costly interventions. Said a CNM in my own home town of Austin, Texas:

> We practiced as a group at the two biggest hospitals in town for years with no problems as our practice slowly grew. We didn't think much about how much we were growing—we just knew we kept getting busier and we liked it that way. Then one day out of nowhere the corporation both hospitals belonged to invoked some archaic rule in the bylaws from the 1930s that an OB had to be within 100 feet of any midwife attending a birth. Then they said they couldn't afford to have OBs just hanging around like that and just like that they closed our practices, so Austin went from having plenty of CNMs working in hospitals to having none, practically overnight. We were bewildered—our outcomes had been really good—until we ran the numbers and realized we had gone beyond that 30% point and the docs felt that we were taking too many patients away from them.

Such mass closings of CNM hospital-based practices have often resulted in various kinds of consumer protests, from letter-writing campaigns to creating documentaries to marching in the streets, usually to no avail. (One notable exception to the 30% hospital "rule" is New Mexico, where CNMs have long attended around 27% of births statewide, with higher percentages in some hospitals, perhaps presaging changes to come in other states [Lisa Kane Low, personal correspondence, August 2016].) And Austin now has CNM hospital-based practices again, after some decades without; it is also a mecca for birth centers and homebirth midwives, whom we will discuss in the following section.

The Lay Midwifery Movement and the Creation of the CPM

> Lay midwife to Robbie, 1991: Nurse-midwives don't understand the difference in the models of care. They think they are preserving midwifery. They cry in meetings because of the restrictive care they have to give, but they don't see that they could support us to keep giving the kind of care they wish they could give. They are oppressed by an oppressive system. . . . They have been co-opted by the oppressor. The way they practice makes me sick! They spend so little time with their clients compared to us, and they way overuse interventions because the system makes them. But they get to care for more women than I do, and I'm jealous of that.
>
> Nurse-midwife to Robbie, 1991: Lay midwives are selling themselves, women in general, and the profession of midwifery short by accepting an education that society regards as inferior. They make all of us look bad. No obstetrician would practice without degrees! Why should women accept anything less? But when I see their videos, I admit I am jealous of the beautiful births they do—we rarely see births like that in our hospital.
>
> Lay midwife to nurse-midwife, 1991: OK, when I try to put myself in your world, I see how much you do manage to do for women in spite of the price you have to pay, and you are there in the hospital where most women are and they need you. I think you are too much of a medical model, but I'm glad you're there. At least you give a lot better care than OBs!
>
> Nurse-midwife to lay midwife, 1991: OK, sometimes I get women I can't help—women who really want a homebirth or birth-center birth but are slightly post-dates. I'm bound by protocols to induce them at 42 weeks. You will let them go much longer than I can. I am secretly grateful that I can tell them about you. I'm scared of you but sometimes I'm glad you're there. But how do I know you're qualified? Anyone can hang out a shingle and call herself a midwife!
>
> [These quotations are amalgamated from my Wenner Gren-funded interviews with hundreds of midwives in 1996–2000. See Acknowledgements for a description of that research.]

During the 1970s, the growth of the North American counterculture was accompanied by an increased interest in homebirth. A new category of white, mostly middle-class "lay" midwives arose to serve the mostly white, middle-class women who were rejecting hospital births with their often-harmful and unnecessary interventions. In 1981, Sister Angela Murdaugh, who was ACNM president at the time, wanted to be "in dialogue with lay midwives" and so invited some lay midwifery leaders to come to a meeting at ACNM headquarters in Washington DC, where she asked them to create an official organization that ACNM could be in dialogue with (interview with Sister Angela, 1996).

And so, at the 1982 ACNM conference, American lay midwives (and some CNMs) created a new organization, the Midwives Alliance of North America (MANA), eventually outlining voluntary standards of practice, a code of ethics, and a set of core competencies (modeled on ACNM's core competencies in the hope of achieving eventual unification). MANA was inclusive, welcoming all midwives as members, including many CNMs—for several decades, one-third of MANA's membership consisted of CNMs, usually those supportive of or attending home- or birth-center births. Until recently, voting membership in MANA required nothing more than the statement that one is a midwife, a fact that subjected the lay midwives who founded it to a great deal of criticism from physicians and nurse-midwives who believed deeply in the need for formal, accredited educational programs and nationally recognized credentials. Recently MANA has changed its requirements; it now only accepts credentialed midwives as voting members; other midwives, as well as doulas and activists (and social scientists), can be affiliated members.

During the 1980s, lay midwives achieved legal status and licensure in California, New Mexico, Oregon, Texas, Florida, New Hampshire, Vermont, and a few other states—a process of professionalization that became a primary catalyst for their rejection of the term "lay" in favor of the more professional term "direct-entry." The former "lay" midwives interpreted this term as meaning that the student enters directly into *any type* of midwifery education without passing through nursing first, whereas the nurse-midwives thought it should mean direct-entry into *only university-based* programs. Those dual meanings of the term created a great many misunderstandings between the two organizations, especially during the creation of the CM (see below).

Between 1990 and 1993, the Carnegie Foundation sponsored a series of meetings between nurse- and "lay" midwifery leaders called the Interorganizational Working Group (IWG), in the hope that these leaders could come to consensus on creating a unified midwifery profession in the US. That goal was not achieved due to their inability to agree on appropriate educational routes, yet the MANA members who had participated heard from the CNM participants over and over the very true accusation that "anyone can hang out a shingle and call herself a midwife." And so the MANA participants left those meetings with a clear sense of mission to create a national certification for formerly lay midwives to prove that they had achieved a requisite degree of knowledge, skills, and practice.

Soon most MANA members came to agree that there was a need for at least a voluntary national credential. This credential was developed in 1994 by the North American Registry of Midwives (NARM, a daughter organization of MANA), and called the "Certified Professional Midwife" (CPM). Its requirements were refined over the years as the NARM board developed its knowledge of testing and its requirements for CPM certification. CPMs can train as midwives through self-study, apprenticeship, formal private vocational schools, or the few college/university programs available to them. As of 2017, about half of CPMs still learn primarily via apprenticeship and do not graduate from accredited midwifery schools; the other half graduate from formal programs while also completing apprenticeships. Currently, there are ten midwifery schools accredited by the Midwifery Education Accreditation Council (MEAC). Some of these vocational "schools" are actually colleges that issue bachelor's and master's degrees (such as the National College of Midwifery, the Midwives College of Utah, Bastyr University in Kenmore Washington, and Southwestern Tech in Wisconsin) (Cheyney et al. 2015; Ida Darragh, NARM board chair, personal communication, 2016; www.meac.org).

After many uphill battles, sometimes lasting over 10 years per state, CPMs are now licensed and regulated in 30 states, and unregulated in all other states and the District of Columbia. In these "a-legal" and "illegal" states, CPMs have no legal protection; penalties for practice range from misdemeanors to Class C felonies. I know of no CPMs allowed to practice in hospitals in any state; their practice arena is births at home and in birth centers.

CPMs have long been engaged in trying to achieve licensure and regulation in almost all of the states where they are not currently regulated—a lengthy and costly process that is often unsuccessful or that results in a problematic compromise (as in Indiana, for example, where the CPMs had to accept highly restrictive regulations). Because medical professionals or others—who do not recognize the midwifery model of care as a valid, evidence-based system of knowledge in its own right—often have the power to set regulatory standards, they sometimes impose severe and inappropriate limitations on midwives' scope of practice. Thus some direct-entry homebirth midwives prefer to practice outside the law, often calling themselves "plain midwives," "community midwives," or "traditional midwives." However, the arrests and prosecutions of dozens of unlicensed homebirth midwives in various states from the 1970s to the present have convinced most direct-entry midwives of the need for the professional recognition that accompanies legalization and licensure. It is better after all, they reason, to lose one's license after a problematic birth than to go to jail for practicing a profession without a license.

The American College of Obstetrics and Gynecology (ACOG) has often denounced the variations in practice and regulations among CPMs across states, while at the same time opposing legalization of CPMs in most of the states where they are still fighting for it. Via this opposition, ACOG officials are working against the standardization of CPM education, practice, and regulation that ACOG itself keeps calling for—an ideologically fraught conundrum and a truly dysfunctional situation that puts both CPMs and the mothers they attend at risk in states where they are denied the legislative right to practice and to be licensed and regulated—a vital first step in becoming a full-fledged part of the maternity care system. Where midwives are not legally recognized, they often cannot obtain needed emergency medications (like anti-hemorrhagic drugs) or tests for their clients like ultrasounds, and they run the risk of persecution should they accompany a client to the hospital during transport—a time when it is critically necessary that the homebirth midwives communicate with hospital personnel to ensure they have the necessary information to care appropriately for the mother and baby. (See Chapter 10, this volume and Cheyney et al. 2014 for analyses of the problems with home-to-hospital transport and their solutions). Midwives also know that some of the mothers who ask them to attend their births will give birth unassisted if they do not, so they bear the tensions and difficulties of lack of licensure to serve the women who deeply want their out-of-hospital care.

Much to their chagrin, CPMs' primary clients are still middle- or upper-class white women. This concern has long been addressed by the International Center for Traditional Childbearing (ICTC), which has often served as the voice of minority midwives and midwives of color. Moving to stress the needs of minority women and midwives on many fronts—for example, MANA's 2104 and 2015 conferences were filled with lectures and workshops on race, ethnicity, and social injustice (see Oparah and Bonaparte 2016)—both MANA and ACNM members are making active efforts to include more midwives of color in their ranks and to serve poor and minority women, often by providing a cash-pay discount for un- or under-insured clients or by providing care *pro bono* (see Joseph forthcoming). While most CNMs are paid through health insurance, CPMs are able to be paid via insurance only in some states.

Two Direct-Entry Certifications: The Creation of the CM

Between 1994 and 1996, ACNM developed its own direct-entry credential, the Certified Midwife (CM), in the hope of relieving women desiring to be midwives of having to go through nursing training, but would still go through university-based midwifery training identical to that of the CNM. (See May and Davis-Floyd 2006 for a full description of the original creation of the CM in New York and the disputes that arose over the differing definitions of the term "direct-entry.") As of mid-2016, only 102 CMs had been certified (Lisa Kane Low, ACNM president, personal correspondence, August 2016), as only two educational programs are available to prepare CMs (one at the State University of New York [SUNY] Brooklyn in New York City and one at the Midwifery Institute in Philadelphia). CMs are at present (2017) only legal, licensed, and regulated in five states—New York, Rhode Island, New Jersey, Delaware, and Maine. During lengthy interviews with two of the prime movers in the creation of the CM, Dorothea Lange and Elaine Mielcarski, they told me that they intended this certification to "open up" hospital-based midwifery by dropping the nursing requirement. Most university midwifery programs are located within schools of nursing, which are not generally interested in offering a non-nursing-based curriculum; there are still so few

CMs because there are still so few programs for educating them, and, disappointingly, funds for creating CM programs in other university arenas (such as medical schools or schools of public health) have not been forthcoming.

National Recognition: Certification, Accreditation, and the ICM Standards

Regarding the much older credential, the CNM, by 2016, over 11,000 CNMs had been certified since the ACNM's inception in 1955; the ACNM does not have data on how many are currently in practice, but, again, an educated estimate is around 7,500. Regarding the much more recent CPM credential, since November 1994 almost 3,000 CPMs have been certified. In 2016, 2,019 had current certifications (Ida Darragh, NARM board chair, personal communication, August 2016) and are attending around 1.3% of US births—far from the tipping point needed to reach full cultural assimilation. Achieving legalization and licensure in the 20 remaining states and growing the number of programs leading to CPM credentialing are essential steps for further growth, as is educating the public and the OBs about the safety of planned, midwife-attended homebirth.

The two relatively new direct-entry certifications signify the desire of many American women (and a few men) who wish to be midwives to avoid the cost in time and money to receive degrees in nursing—a profession they do not wish to practice—and as well to avoid the subordinated identity of the nursing role in order to develop an autonomous midwifery identity. The existence of two direct-entry certifications also signifies midwifery leaders' inability to agree on a unified set of criteria for midwifery education and practice. All three certifications—the CNM, CM, and CPM—are accredited by the National Commission for Certifying Agencies (the accrediting arm of the Institute of Credentialing Excellence [ICE]), which recognizes both NARM and the AMCB as valid certification agencies. Likewise, both MEAC and ACME are recognized by the federal government as valid accrediting agencies. This recognition means that all schools accredited by either agency are federally recognized, and thus their students are eligible for federal education loans; it also means that students graduating from all such accredited schools who obtain licensure in their states meet the international definition of a midwife, which reads:

> A midwife is a person who has successfully completed a midwifery education programme that is duly recognized in the country where it is located and that is based on the ICM Essential Competencies for Basic Midwifery Practice and the framework of the ICM Global Standards for Midwifery Education; who has acquired the requisite qualifications to be registered and/or legally licensed to practice midwifery and use the title

> "midwife"; and who demonstrates competency in the practice of midwifery. (http://www.internationalmidwives.org/assets/uploads/documents/Definition%20of%20the%20Midwife%20-%202011.pdf)

CPMs who do not graduate from a MEAC-accredited school do not meet that international definition and so are not recognized by the ACNM and ACOG as "midwives," but rather are coded as "traditional birth attendants" (TBAs). Nevertheless, many primarily apprenticeship-trained CPMs are licensed and practicing legally in states where they, via their own very determined lobbying, have achieved licensure and regulation. As previously noted, about half of today's new CPMs attend MEAC-accredited schools. The other half learn via a non-accredited formal program or by apprenticeship with senior midwives (or both), and go through NARM's Portfolio Evaluation Process (PEP), during which experienced midwives document and attest that the student applying to take the NARM written and skills examinations has met all of the clinical experience requirements to quality as a CPM. According to CPM Melissa Cheyney (personal communication 2017), "almost all CPMs apprentice because that is how we get our numbers so we can apply to sit for the NARM exam. The question is did they also graduate from a MEAC school or did they do the PEP process?" The answer to that question makes all the difference in whether the graduates meet the international definition or not. (See www.narm.org for full information.) As Cheyney et al. (2015:2) explain (I will paraphrase here), NARM's approach to certification of CPMs relies on highly flexible, competency-based pathways that require students to obtain essential knowledge, skills, and experience, but allow them to do so through a variety of means, including accredited or non-accredited brick-and-mortar schools, accredited or non-accredited distance-learning programs, self-study, apprenticeship with one or more senior midwifery preceptors, and/or internship at one or more birth centers. This competency-based approach focuses on *what has been learned* independently of how or where it was learned, and of course also on whether a candidate can successfully apply appropriate knowledge and skills in various clinical encounters. This competency-based focus is premised on both ideological and practical reasons. The practical reason is to ameliorate a key barrier to training described by prospective CPMs: there are only ten formal MEAC-accredited schools that can graduate CPMs and these are expensive relative to the income a CPM can generate, whereas non-accredited schools, apprenticeships, and internships in birth centers are more accessible. (To become MEAC-accredited is both a time-consuming and expensive process, so these accredited schools have to charge more to be able to afford obtaining and keeping their MEAC accreditation, which must be renewed every three years.)

I fully describe the ideological basis for keeping open the time-honored apprenticeship route in Chapter 8; I will provide a brief summary here in a quotation from that chapter:

> [Homebirth midwives value apprenticeship] for the connective and embodied experiential learning it provides. Apprenticeship training is a thoroughly individualized process, the shape and nature of which depends on the relationship that develops between apprentice and mentor. When it is successful, the apprentice–mentor relationship provides a supportive and nurturant educational context within which the apprentice can learn about pregnancy and birth through the immediacy of touch and experience, and can supplement that embodied knowledge with reading and long discussion with her mentor and others.
>
> Apprentices accompany their mentors to homebirths, witnessing woman after woman give birth successfully on her own, and developing comprehension of the normal birth process. Where hospital training tends to focus on pathology and generate a fear-based approach to birth, homebirth apprentice training generates trust. Midwives who fundamentally trust birth are more likely to be able to create an atmosphere within which women can find their power and trust themselves to give birth.

Apprenticeship training is certainly not exclusive to CPMs; the university educations obtained by CNMs/CMs contain long periods of "preceptorship" during which the student works hands-on and one-on-one with one or more clinical preceptors. The difference is that CNMs and CPMs trained in accredited programs do a great deal of didactic studying and class attendance (in person or online) as well; such studies are organized into categories, such as prenatal, intrapartum, and postpartum care, as are CNM/CM preceptorships, while purely apprentice-trained midwives tend to do their reading after they are confronted with an issue they need to learn how to deal with while attending births during their apprenticeships. For example, they see and help their preceptor midwife deal with a hemorrhage; then they go and read everything they can about hemorrhage because they now fully understand how frightening it can be and how badly they need to know how to manage it. Another difference is that CPMs tend to work with only one or two preceptors during their entire three years or so of apprenticeship, which can be both an advantage (preceptor and student get to know each other deeply, so the preceptor can tell in which areas a student still needs training, or just more self-confidence) and a disadvantage (the student is limited to learning only what those one or two preceptors know). In contrast, CNMs/CMs will work with a variety of different preceptors during their training—that also has both advantages (the students are exposed to different approaches) and disadvantages (they don't get to know each other deeply, so the preceptors may not be able to pinpoint the student's weaker areas).

CNM/CM education is also based on experiential learning and students are expected to conduct research based on what they experience in the clinical setting and bring cases to class for discussion.

> This is the basis for our modular and problem-based learning curriculum. The goal of both educational models is to develop practitioners who will

> return time and again to the literature to understand clinical situations they experience for the first time when in practice. Practitioners are confronted with new situations after 100 births, and after 1,000 births, and so on. Midwives keep researching and learning throughout their career. (anon rev'r. 2017)

Prospective student CPMs often cobble together as much attendance at accredited programs as they can afford or geography will allow with long stints as apprentices or interns or attendance at less expensive, non-accredited schools. Once again, from NARM's point of view, it's *what they know and can do that counts*, not where or how they learned it. With this viewpoint ACNM ideologically disagrees; its leaders generally would prefer that MEAC-accredited programs be the only valid routes to national certification and the right to call oneself a midwife. *It is precisely this disagreement over what constitutes appropriate educational routes that prevents the unification of American midwifery*, at least at this time of writing (2017). The other inhibiting factor to unification is the scope of practice differences between CNMs/CMs, who are trained and certified to offer well-woman gynecologic and primary health care from puberty to old age, and CPMs, whose training focuses on the perinatal period (though it can also include well-woman gynecologic care, and many CPMs do offer that in their practices). However, some progress toward this goal of eventual unification or at least complementary and collaborative practice has been made with the formation of a group called US MERA, which I will discuss below.

Midwifery Differences and Commonalities: Working towards a More Unified Future?

In spite of their differences, American midwives of all types share multiple commonalities. Dr. Caroline Peterson (2010) has argued that "a comparison of CPM certification requirements with those of CNMs/CMs indicates that both branches of professional midwifery in the US utilize similar core competencies; have established similar clinical training requirements; and use examinations nearly identical in terms of content, structure, and depth and breadth of knowledge required." US midwives in general ground themselves ideologically in the "midwifery model of care," which focuses on the normalcy of pregnancy and birth and emphasizes caring for the emotional and physical well-being of the expectant mother, providing her with all relevant information, minimizing medical interventions, and detecting any abnormalities that should lead the midwife to consult a physician and together with the mother develop a plan of care (http://cfmidwifery.org/mmoc/; see also Rothman 1982; Rooks 1999; and Chapter 11, this volume).

Presently, more and more American women are interested in using a midwife during childbirth instead of a physician; by 2014, midwives cumulatively attended 9.1% of American births (up from 2% in 1979) and today, as previously noted and referenced, that figure is up to around 13%—around 12% for CNMs and 1% for CPMs. Many women who choose hospital birth wish for the compassionate and respectful care that midwives provide and for the much greater time intervals their CNMs spend with them relative to the average obstetrician. Of US women, 1.36% choose to have children in the comfort of their own homes and in freestanding birth centers away from what they perceive as the risks and dangers of hospital intervention (MacDorman, Declerq, and Matthews 2013) and to enjoy the lengthy pre- and postnatal visits and checkups CPMs (and also CNMs and CMs who attend out-of-hospital births) provide, which often last well over an hour. These women believe—and scientific evidence shows—that homebirths by healthy pregnant women with no known high-risk factors attended by well-educated midwives are safe, that natural childbirth results in fewer injuries to mother and child, and that midwives are the best attendants for such births (Malloy 2010; Cox et al. 2013; Jackson, Lang, and Swartz 2003; Johantgen et al. 2012; Stapleton, Osborne, and Illuzzi 2013; ACNM Position Statement 2014; ACNM Home Birth Clinical Bulletin 2016).

As a result, there has long been a large base of consumers working as part of a full-fledged social movement to support midwives of all types, but most especially those who attend homebirths, as they are generally the most marginalized and least understood by the medical profession. In every state where CPMs have achieved licensure and regulation, consumers have played a significant role in those achievements, from lobbying legislators to packing legislative halls when midwifery bills are up for discussion. The national spokesgroup for this consumer movement has long been Citizens for Midwifery (CfM) and now is spearheaded by a group called The Big Push.

Contemporary American midwives—CNMs, CMs and CPMs—are educated in the anatomy and physiology of pregnancy, labor and birth, nutrition during pregnancy, and many other aspects of the care of normal pregnancy and birth; they are also often specialists in herbalism, homeopathy, and other holistic modalities. Again, CNMs/CMs and some CPMs also provide well-woman care across women's life spectrum. Homebirth midwives and midwives who work in freestanding birth centers are highly skilled at identifying risk factors that might preclude an out-of-hospital birth or require transport to a hospital during labor. *Studies of American midwifery outcomes for all three types of certified midwives show excellent results in or out of the hospital—about the same as those of obstetricians attending low-risk births, yet with far fewer in-stances of iatrogenic damage, due to their efforts to minimize interventions in birth.*[1,2] As one of ACNM's conference advertisements stated, "Whether you wish to give birth at home, in a birth center, or in the hospital, you're in better hands with a midwife!"

Midwifery in the US is not an integrated profession—that is, it is not a profession in which all members are fully integrated into our health care system nor go through the same standardized educational processes—as it is in places where it works best, such as New Zealand, the Netherlands, the Scandinavian countries, the UK, and some Canadian provinces. As a longtime midwifery advocate and supporter, I look forward to the day when all three certifications—CNM, CM, and CPM—are legally recognized in all 50 states, are fully insurance-reimbursed, and agree on educational standards based on those set by the International Confederation of Midwives (ICM). At present, 99.5% of CPMs meet the ICM's standards for completion

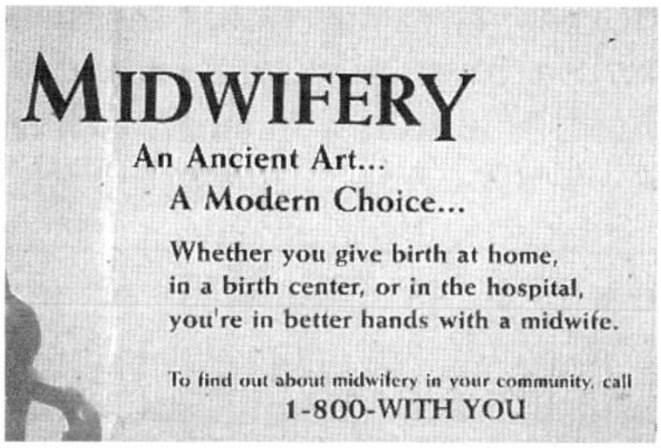

Poster advertisement displayed in buses and other places all over Boston in tandem with the 1996 ACNM conference held there.

[1] These are the primary studies showing the excellent outcomes achieved by CPMs; I summarize their findings here because so many people—practitioners and the general public alike, believe homebirth to be both risky and irresponsible—a selfish choice made by the mother, who is often believed to be placing her desire for the best possible birth experience over the safety of her unborn baby. The results of these studies show that in fact, what is best for the mother is generally best for the baby as well:

Johnson, K. C., and B. A. Daviss. 2005. "Outcomes of Planned Home Births with Certified Professional Midwives: Large Prospective Study in North America." *British Medical Journal* 330(1416). doi:10.1136/bmj.330.7505.1416. This study contains the results of data collected from all 350 CPMs in practice in the year 2000; they were required by NARM to submit data for every birth they attended during that year in order to be eligible for recertification. Its results were so good that many midwifery critics pointed out that the 350 CPMs who participated were usually very experienced midwives with many years of practice under their belts. So the study described just below was conducted on births attended by CPMs between the years 2004 and 2007, who include many recently certified midwives; the results of the two studies are nearly identical, showing consistency and continuity in the results achieved by Certified Professional Midwives.

Cheyney, M., M. Bovbjerg, C. Everson, W. Gordon, D. Hannibal, and S. Vedam. 2014. "Outcomes of Care for 16,984 Planned Home Births in the United States: The Midwives Alliance of North America Statistics Project, 2004–2009." *Journal of Midwifery & Women's Health* 59(1): 17–27. The results of this study were as follows: Among 16,924 women who planned homebirths at the onset of labor, 89.1% gave birth at home. The majority of intrapartum transfers were for failure to progress, and only 4.5% of the total sample required oxytocin augmentation and/or epidural analgesia. The rates of spontaneous vaginal birth was 93.6%, assisted vaginal birth 1.2%, and cesarean 5.2%. Of the 1054 women who attempted a vaginal birth after cesarean (VBAC), 87% were successful. Low Apgar scores (< 7) occurred in 1.5% of newborns. Postpartum maternal (1.5%) and neonatal (0.9%) transfers were infrequent. The majority (86%) of newborns were exclusively breastfeeding at 6 weeks of age. Excluding lethal anomalies, the intrapartum, early neonatal, and late neonatal mortality rates were 1.30, 0.41, and 0.35 per 1000, respectively.

of secondary education, while 61% meet ICM midwifery educational requirements; the day may come when all of the CPMs meet those requirements.

American women are increasingly choosing midwifery care, and the (3 types of) certified midwives who attend them, all of whom work hard to achieve these certifications, should have full legal recognition and the support of the state midwifery boards that are created to regulate and serve them where they are legal and licensed, as all certified midwives deserve to be. And all three types of certified midwives wish these boards to consist primarily of midwives who understand midwifery practice and the evidence-based knowledge system of the midwifery model of care. They all also want to be able to practice autonomously, without requirements for physician backup or supervision. These shared commonalities are helping midwives to make progress toward those idealistic goals; in the past, as documented in *Mainstreaming Midwives: The Politics of Change* (Davis-Floyd and Johnson 2006), internecine warfare often characterized the interrelationships of the various midwifery organizations.

[2] These are the primary recent studies showing the excellent outcomes that CMNs also consistently achieve, and have been achieving for decades.

ACNM (American College of Nurse-Midwives). 2012. *Issue Brief: Where Midwives Work*. Silver Spring, MD: American College of Nurse- Midwives. Available at: http://www.midwife.org/ACNM/files/ACNMLibraryData/UPLOADFILENAME/000000000277/Where%20Midwives%20Work%20June2012.pdf. Accessed April 28, 2014.

Cox, K. J., R. Schlegel, P. Payne, D. Teaf, and L. Albers. 2013. "Outcomes of Planned Home Births Attended by Certified Nurse-Midwives in South-Eastern Pennsylvania, 1983–2008." *Journal of Midwifery and Women's Health* 58(2): 145–149. doi:10.1111/j.1542-2011.2012.00217.x.

Declerq, Eugene. 2012. "Trends in Midwife-Attended Births in the United States: 1989–2009." *Journal of Midwifery and Women's Health* 57(4): 321–326.

Jackson, D. J., J. M. Lang, W. H. Swartz, et al. 2003. "Outcomes, Safety, and Resource Utilization in a Collaborative Care Birth Center Program Compared with Traditional Physician-Based Perinatal Care." *Am J Public Health* 93(6): 999–1006.

Johantgen, M., L. Fountain, G. Zangaro, R. Newhouse, J. Stanik-Hutt, and K. White. 2012. "Comparison of Labor and Delivery Care Provided by Certified Nurse-Midwives and Physicians: A Systematic Review, 1990 to 2008." *Women's Health Issues Off Publ Jacobs Inst Women's Health*. 22(1): e73–e81. doi:10.1016/j.whi.2011.06.005.

Malloy, M. H. 2010. "Infant Outcomes of Certified Nurse-Midwife Attended Home Births: United States 2000 to 2004." *J Perinatol Off J Calif Perinat Assoc*. 30(9): 622–627. doi:10.1038/jp.2010.12.

Schuiling, K. D., T. A. Sipe, and J. Fullerton. 2013. "Findings from the Analysis of the American College of Nurse-Midwives' Membership Surveys 2009–2011." *Journal of Midwifery and Women's Health* 58(4): 404–415.

Stapleton, S. R., C. Osborne, and J. Illuzzi. 2013. "Outcomes of Care in Birth Centers: Demonstration of a Durable Model." *J Midwifery Women's Health* 58(1): 3–14. doi:10.1111/jmwh.12003.

Yang, T., L. Attanasio, and K. Kozhimammil. 2016. "State Scope of Practice Laws, Nurse-Midwifery Workforce, and Childbirth Procedures and Outcomes." *Women's Health Issues* May/June.

In an effort to end that internecine warfare, and with a deep sociological awareness that oppressed groups often fight each other and should redirect those energies toward higher common goals, in 2011 all key midwifery organizations came together to form US MERA—United States Midwifery Education, Regulation and Association—and to work together within that group toward common goals, such as cooperation on research and legislative efforts (such as getting bills passed that legalize and license CPMs and CMs, and/or grant more autonomy to all licensed midwives) among others (see www.usmera.org). The formation of this association and the work of its members over the past few years represent "a massive shift of agreement toward a common pathway for meeting the ICM educational requirements" (Lisa Kane Low, personal correspondence, August 2016). In addition, this group's work has also led to ACOG's at least tacit support for midwives who meet the international definition (which, again, includes all CPMs who graduate from MEAC-accredited schools and are state-licensed; previously, ACOG supported only CNMs and CMs).

In addition, popular films like Ricki Lake's *The Business of Being Born* and Debra Pascali-Bonaro's *Orgasmic Birth* have brought midwifery much more into public awareness, though there still seems to be little popular understanding of the similarities and differences in the CNM, CM, and CPM certifications—as I noted at the beginning of this chapter, many consumers still elide them into just one category: "midwives." I hope this chapter will contribute to the broader development of such understanding and to a greater appreciation of the contributions midwives of all types make to the betterment of American birth and to the service of American women and families.

Questions for Thought and Discussion

1. What are the three types of midwifery certification in the US and what are the differences among them?
2. Why was the CM created and why has it not accomplished its intended purpose?
3. Where do CNMs and CPMs primarily attend births?
4. Why can't American midwives unify under one organization and have only one certification? What are the primary issues dividing them? Is there a possibility that might happen one day? What sort of progress is being made?

Recommended Films

Birth Story: Ina May Gaskin and the Farm Midwives: produced by Kate Roughan and Zachary Mortenson, 2012. This feature-length documentary tells the story of counterculture heroine Ina May Gaskin and her spirited friends, who began delivering each other's babies in 1970, on a caravan of hippie school buses, headed to a patch of rural Tennessee land. With Ina May as their leader, the women taught themselves midwifery from the ground up and, with their families, founded a communal, agricultural society called the Farm. They grew their own food, built their own houses, published their own books and, as word of their social experiment spread, created a model of care for women and babies that changed a generation's approach to childbirth. Available at: http://birthstorymovie.com/the-film/

It's My Baby, My Body, My Birth: With epidural and caesarean rates on the rise, we in the US increasingly assume birth requires medical and surgical procedures. The women in this film challenge this idea by sharing their life transforming birth experiences with midwives. www.ItsMyBodyMyBabyMyBirth.com

Mama Sherpas: From executive producers Ricki Lake and Abby Epstein (*The Business of Being Born*), this topical documentary, directed by Brigid Maher, examines a growing shift in the birthing industry: the rise of Caesarean sections. With C-section rates dangerously over 30% in America, midwives may be the solution. In recent years, the idea of a "collaborative care" practice where doctors and midwives manage women's care together has begun to gain traction. Research has demonstrated that collaborative care models produce better outcomes for mother and baby, including fewer C-sections. This moving and urgent film provides an intimate lens into how midwives across the country work within and better the hospital system, redefining how the US looks at the birthing process. http://www.themamasherpas.com/#watch-the-film

Orgasmic Birth: produced by Debra Pascali-Bonaro. http://www.orgasmicbirth.com/ (Also available under the title *Organic Birth*)

The Business of Being Born: produced by Ricki Lake and Abby Epstein. http://www.thebusinessofbeingborn.com/

Glossary of Acronyms Frequently Used in US Midwifery

ACME—Accreditation Commission for Midwifery Education, the ACNM sister organization responsible for evaluating and accrediting programs that graduate students eligible to become AMCB-certified CNMs and CMs.

ACNM—American College of Nurse-Midwives. Founded in 1955, the ACNM is the professional organization for CNMs and CMs.

AMCB—American Midwifery Certification Board, the ACNM sister organization responsible for testing and certifying CMs and CNMs.

CfM—Citizens for Midwifery, a consumer organization supporting the Midwives Model of Care™.

CM—Certified Midwife, a national certification granted by the AMCB.

CNM—Certified Nurse-Midwife, a national certification granted by the AMCB.

CPM—Certified Professional Midwife, a national certification granted by NARM.

DEM—direct-entry midwife (in the US, a professional midwife who enters midwifery without passing through nursing first). All CMs and CPMs are DEMs; that term is also used by many "plain" or unlicensed midwives.

DOR—ACNM's Division of Research, which is currently working on a major benchmarking project, or MANA's Division of Research. MANA's DOR compiles and analyzes data on the outcomes of midwifery care through the MANA Statistics Project. Upon formal request, they often allow other researchers access to these databases, which are quite extensive, with a total over 112,000 births properly and prospectively logged in as of 2017.

FAM—Foundation for the Advancement of Midwifery, a fund-raising organization that supports various midwifery-related projects and endeavors.

ICTC—International Center for Traditional Childbearing, an organization founded in 1991 by Shafia Monroe. ICTC is a nonprofit infant mortality prevention, breastfeeding support, and midwife training organization, comprised of women and men who want to improve birth outcomes and provide training opportunities in their communities, and most particularly fight for social justice in birth for both midwives and women of color.

LM—Licensed Midwife, a midwife who achieves state licensure. All CNMs/CMs are licensed; most CPMs whose practices are legal in their state are also LMs.

MANA—Midwives Alliance of North America, an organization founded in 1982 that welcomes all certified midwives as voting members yet mostly represents homebirth midwives.

MBC—Midwifery Bridge Certificate (see Appendix).

MEAC—Midwifery Education Accreditation Council, the MANA and NARM sister organization responsible for evaluating and accrediting direct-entry educational programs that graduate students eligible to become CPMs.

MMOC—Midwifery Model of Care, a woman-centered ideology held by many or most practicing midwives of all types that views birth as a normal, physiologic process that benefits much more from compassionate care than from medical interventions. (See Chapter 11.)

MMOC™—Midwives Model of Care, a definition trademarked by the Midwifery Task Force (a coalition of MANA members and consumers) in 2000.

NACPM—National Association of Certified Professional Midwives. This organization has set national standards for CPM practice and primarily works at the national level, lobbying to get CPMs inserted into national legislation that affects midwives and for insurance reimbursement.

NARM—North American Registry of Midwives, the body responsible for testing and certifying CPMs. This credential is only legally recognized in the US (in 30 states), although quite a number of CPMs do practice in other countries.

PEP—Portfolio Evaluation Process, an education evaluation process through which all aspiring CPMs who do not attend MEAC-accredited schools must pass to gain and then demonstrate the knowledge, skills, and competence they have gained through apprenticeship or other types of training.

RM—Registered Midwife (licensed in her state but called a Registered Midwife instead of a Licensed Midwife, as in Colorado and Canada).

SNM—student nurse-midwife

US MERA—United States Midwifery Education, Regulation and Association, a coalition of leaders of most of the above-mentioned organizations designed to coordinate legislative work, research efforts, and other issues among those organizations and avoid the internecine conflict that used to characterize their relationships. (See www.usmera.org and the Appendix below.)

Acknowledgements and Research Description

I wish to thank Judith Rooks CNM, former president of ACNM, Lisa Kane Low CNM, current ACNM president; Melissa Cheyney CPM, associate professor of Anthropology and chair of MANA's Division of Research; and Ida Darragh CPM, NARM board chair; and several anonymous reviewers for their excellent edits on this chapter and for the important references they provided. Funded by the Wenner-Gren Foundation for Anthropological Research Grants #6015 and #6247, between 1996 and 2000 I carried out research on "The Development of Direct-Entry Midwifery in North America: Politics and Professionalization." My research methodology involved attending international, national, and local midwifery and childbirth conferences, participation on one midwifery board and in a national coalition, and carrying out over 70 interviews with leaders and educators in nurse- and direct-entry midwifery, focusing on their motivations for developing two new direct-entry certifications, the practical and philosophical issues that divide them, and the legislative processes in several states. In addition, I interviewed 75 midwifery students (30 direct-entry and 45 nurse-midwifery) about their educational processes, seeking to understand the relative benefits and disadvantages of each. Some of the results of this research have been published in Davis-Floyd 1998b, 1999, 2002a,b, 2003a, 2004a,b, 2005, 2006; Benoit et al. 2001; the full results appear in Davis-Floyd and Johnson 2006. I wish to express my deep appreciation to Wenner-Gren for its financial support. I have continued to carry out research on American midwives to build on the solid base I have already established and to keep up with current events as they unfold.

APPENDIX

The Collaborative Work of US MERA

by Ida Darragh CPM

For those who wish to understand the full complexity and heroic accomplishments of the work of US MERA, here is a full description of its organization and recent work provided to me by Ida Darragh, NARM board chair:

The US MERA is a collective of organizations reviewing US Midwifery in light of the ICM (International Confederation of Midwives) international standards. US MERA's membership has consisted of 5 representatives from 7 organizations: ACNM, ACME, AMCB, NARM, MEAC, MANA, and NACPM, and, most recently, ICTC has joined this collective. (See Glossary above.) MERA means Midwifery Education, Regulation, and Association—these are the three pillars on which ICM is founded. So the groups that represented the CNM/CM and CPM credentials (professional organizations, school accreditation agencies, and certification agencies) met between 2013 and 2015 to evaluate the strengths and weaknesses of all credentials in light of the ICM standards, focusing their work on the issues surrounding education. [Editor's note: Again, two major issues prevent unity among these groups: disagreement over appropriate educational routes and differences in scope of practice.]

As in the past, the CNM/CM groups were strongly in support of formal, accredited education programs for all midwives. Also as in the past, the CPM groups were strongly supportive of NARM's Portfolio Evaluation Process (PEP), which includes the apprenticeship route, as well as the formal, accredited programs.

The ICM standards gave us a place to start the discussions, though the driving issue was reaching a compromise that would allow ACNM to support licensure for CPMs in states that did not yet have a licensure law. The language that was finally agreed on by all groups was support for licensure bills that would *require a MEAC education for CPMs certified after Jan 1, 2020,* but would allow CPMs certified before that date to qualify for licensure by obtaining the newly-created *Midwifery Bridge Certificate* (MBC), a certificate issued by NARM that a CPM can receive if she documents accredited continuing education in three categories: maternal emergencies, newborn emergencies, and a third category, which specifies content areas approved by the Professional Regulation Committee. About 35 CPMs received the MBC in 2015. (You can find the details of what is accepted on the NARM web page under Midwifery Bridge Certificate.) [The "bridge" is from preceptor verification (also called the Portfolio Evaluation Process or PEP) toward third-party verification (accredited CEUs)]. By the end of the process of developing the Bridge Certificate, all involved agreed that the PEP covered all necessary education for providing midwifery care to low-risk women during the childbearing year. The only thing it lacked was the "accredited" part of the education. The ACNM reps agreed (even suggested) that accredited CEUs could be the bridging from PEP towards a future when MEAC-accredited education would be the norm.

In March 2016, ACOG actually came out with a statement in support of the Midwifery Bridge Certificate—another huge step forward (see the box below).

Now, the focus is on creating educational programs similar to the PEP that will be Direct Assessment programs that can get MEAC-accredited. The first such program started in September 2016 at the Farm and is run by Carol Nelson and Sharon

ACOG Statement on the MERA Bridge Certificate

March 23, 2016

ACOG supports the International Confederation of Midwives (ICM) educational standards as the minimum education and licensure requirement for all midwives practicing in the US. ACOG recognizes that the US MERA Bridge Certificate is an attempt to elevate the training and education of midwives who lack accredited education and do not currently meet ICM criteria.

The US MERA Bridge Certificate at present is only intended to address the training and educational needs of CPMs in states that do not currently license these providers. ACOG strongly encourages all apprentice (PEP) trained CPMs to utilize this bridge certificate opportunity. Every CPM, no matter when they were credentialed or where they practice, should at least meet the educational and training standards required of midwives in other nations.

ACOG looks forward to working with ACNM and the other US MERA organizations. It is essential that we send a unified message to legislators, regulators, the public, and our patients that we support nothing less than high-quality maternity care.

Wells. They will apply for MEAC accreditation after their first year of having a class. It remains to be seen how different this is from a regular MEAC school since the latter are almost all distance education or hybrid programs.

The US MERA groups agreed to support licensure bills that contained these requirements for licensure in proposed bills, but were not intended to be applied in states that already had licensure. As of May 2017, three states have passed a licensure bill with the MERA language: Maine, Michigan, and South Dakota. We do expect more states to pass such bills in upcoming legislative sessions.

Note: NARM is not yet giving up the [apprenticeship-based] Portfolio Evaluation Process (PEP), which is still a route for licensure in 22 states. NARM is offering the Midwifery Bridge Certificate (MBC) as an add-on based on accredited continuing education.

The ACOG president was present for parts of the meetings, and at least one ACOG rep fully participated. They were encouraging of the process. ACOG would not officially sign on to the MERA proposal but informally agreed not to oppose bills that contained that language. That was huge progress. Now, ACOG has come out with their new Committee Opinion on Home Birth, which supports homebirth only if strict risk criteria are used (no VBAC, for example), only if there are integrated home-to-hospital transfer arrangements, and only if attended by CNMs, CMs or a midwife who has met the educational standards of ICM. These are all steps in the right direction if our goal is an integrated maternity system with increased access to midwifery care across all locations of birth. Yet, we remain in limbo.

The US MERA groups agreed to support licensure for CPMs meeting the new criteria, but ICM does not take a stand on any statements from any country, and does not evaluate any country's systems as being ICM-compliant. So, it is left to the states to determine if their licensure program meets ICM standards. If that language ("meets ICM educational standards") is used in a law, then it has the burden of proving that criteria given that ICM does not issue any evaluation of credentials. CPMs have to argue that the MERA language is sufficiently close to ICM to be acceptable; the ACNM has agreed to support that interpretation, and ACOG was in the background—wanting midwives to be licensed yet unable to mention the CPM or the US MERA statements. ACOG did eventually endorse licensure based on the US MERA statement in March 2013, which then enabled them to come out with the statement above in 2016.

Here's an example of the conundrum: ICM standards are for a three-year educational program following completion of secondary education. PEP has a two-year minimum and most MEAC schools are two-year programs. ICM has an outline of curriculum for three-year programs, where basic midwifery for childbearing mothers is covered very well in the first two years (and is met by all CPM routes) but the third year is advanced skills, such as diagnosis and treatment, abortions, and professional issues such as interpreting research, and evaluating public health issues like sanitation and literacy. Those third-year areas are really beyond what is required of CPMs and would not be allowed by a licensure law in most states anyway. [Editor's note: They would be legally interpreted in the US as "practicing medicine without a license."] The ICM standards also oppose linking midwifery to nursing, which the ACNM acknowledges they are not willing to accommodate. CNMs also do not perform abortions, treat malaria and tuberculosis, or perform deworming procedures. Even the ICM acknowledges that not all countries will be able to meet all of these standards, especially in scope of practice—the ICM wanted to include all possible roles of any midwife, as midwives may be the sole health-care providers in their communities.

So, we have ACOG publicly stating that they would only support a non-CNM/CM who met ICM standards, but obviously not knowing what those standards are. We have ACOG representatives supporting the MERA work but who are unwilling to publically state that support. And we have physicians lobbying legislatures to include requirements that licensed midwives meet ICM standards. And all the while, at least ACOG is going neutral on bills that contain the MERA language. The US MERA groups continue to meet on a more limited basis to look at future goals or additional projects. There will be some exciting upcoming legislative seasons. (Ida Darragh, NARM board chair, personal correspondence, Aug. 31, 2016.)

From Robbie: To give my readers the feel and flavor of what happens in those "exciting legislative sessions," I include here a recent (June 2017) email from Susan Jenkins, fearless leader of The Big Push for Midwives, an organization dedicated to legalizing CPMs in all 50 states:

A Short Report to the Community from The Big Push

The new Alabama bill has one especially remarkable feature: It calls for an independent Licensed Midwife Majority board with no physicians: 4 LM/CPMs, 1 CNM, 1 Nurse Practitioner, and 1 home birth consumer.

The Push States are on a roll, folks. New licensure bills in:

MICHIGAN (Dec 2016): No scope of practice restrictions, Licensed Midwifery Board

SOUTH DAKOTA (February 2017): No scope of practice restrictions, Licensed Midwifery Board

ALABAMA (May 2017): Completely independent, no-physicians Licensed Midwifery Board

CALIFORNIA: Defeated (by tabling at committee level) an ACOG-backed bill that would have brought all home birth under control of the state medical board.

With each of these new licensing laws, the state midwives' association and state consumer organization defeated continuing opposition from ACOG and/or the state medical society with an overwhelming floor vote in favor of the bill—"yea" votes in the 90s or 60s against single-digit "nays." We had good numbers in the CA committee vote to table also. We didn't just win—organized medicine lost. Lost big.

Our primary weapons: Persistent sustained relentless telephone calls and emails from consumers, their families, their friends, coupled with the smarts and hard work of state consumer and midwifery leadership.

And the spirits/good energy of Margaret Charles Smith [a famed and beloved Southern black "granny" "Grand" Midwife, now deceased] and all our other foremothers filling those chambers.

From: Susan M. Jenkins, The Sanchez Law Firm, P.C., 1155 F Street, N.W., Suite 1050, Washington, D.C. 20004, 866.686.1348 (office), 202.431.9040 (cell)

7

Intuition as Authoritative Knowledge in Midwifery and Homebirth

with Elizabeth Davis

Diagnostic technologies, from the most mundane and routine ultrasound to the most exotic embryo transplant have in common that they work toward the construction of the fetus as a separate being . . . a visible, audible presence among us, and they do that by doing two other things. They medicalize pregnancy, and they render invisible and inaudible, women.

The history of Western obstetrics is the history of technologies of separation. We've separated milk from breasts, mothers from babies, fetuses from pregnancies, sexuality from procreation, pregnancy from motherhood.

It is very very hard to conceptually put back together that which medicine has rendered asunder. . . . As I speak to different groups, from social scientists to birth practitioners, what I find is that I have a harder and harder time trying to make the meaning of connection, let alone the value of connection, understood.

— Barbara Katz Rothman, Plenary Address, Midwives' Alliance of North America Conference, New York City, November 1992.

This article is revised and updated from Davis-Floyd, Robbie and Elizabeth Davis. 1996. "Intuition as Authoritative Knowledge in Midwifery and Home Birth" in *The Social Production of Authoritative Knowledge about Childbirth,* a special issue of *Medical Anthropology Quarterly*, eds. Robbie Davis-Floyd and Carolyn Sargent, 10(2):237–269.

Both of us (Elizabeth and Robbie) were in the audience when sociologist Barbara Katz Rothman gave the speech from which the above quotes are excerpted. Her words, spoken to an audience of midwives who have no trouble at all understanding the value of connection, crystallized for these midwives their aloneness in the world of medicine—a world in which the subtle rewards of connection are often lost as the value of those technologies of separation is increasingly taken for granted. The warm exchange of breath and sweat, of touch and gaze, of body oils and emotions, that characterizes births in which there is an intimate connection between the mother and her caretaker, has given way in the US to the cool penetration of needles, the distant interpretation of lines on a graph. Building on Rothman's earlier work (1982, 1989), in *Birth as an American Rite of Passage* 2003 [1992], Davis-Floyd identified the "technocratic model" of birth as the core paradigm underlying contemporary obstetric practices, including diagnostic technologies. As Rothman points out, separation is a fundamental tenet of this paradigm, which she calls the "medical model." Other basic tenets, as we have seen in previous chapters in this volume, include the metaphorization of the female body as a defective machine and the working premise that birth will be "better" when this defective birthing machine is hooked up to other, more perfect diagnostic machines.

Under this model, authoritative knowledge—the knowledge on the basis of which decisions are made and actions are taken (Jordan 1993)—is vested in these machines and in those who know how to manipulate and interpret them. In Chapters 1 and 2, Robbie discussed these machines as symbols of our culture's "supervaluation" of technology over bodies and over nature. She analyzed obstetrical procedures, diagnostic and otherwise, as rituals that not only convey cultural core values to birthing women but also enhance the courage of birth practitioners by deconstructing birth into identifiable and (seemingly) controllable segments, then reconstructing it as a mechanistic process. She found that these ritual procedures enhance courage not only for obstetricians and nurses but also for the women themselves—being hooked up to some of the highest technologies society has invented gives many American women the feeling that they are being well taken care of, that they are safe. A reassuring cultural order is imposed on the otherwise frightening and potentially out-of-control chaos of nature (see Chapter 3).

Yet not all women are reassured by the technocratization of birth. There are some women in the United States who supervalue nature and their bodies over science and technology, who regard the technological deconstruction of birth as harmful and dangerous, who desire to experience the whole of birth—its rhythms, its juiciness, its intense sexuality, fluidity, ecstasy, and pain (see Chapter 3). Those women who most deeply trust birth place themselves quite consciously as far out of the reach of the technocratic model as they can get, choosing to give birth in the sanctity and safety of their own homes, and grounding themselves philosophically in a holistic model of birth. Like the midwives who attend them, these homebirth mothers have no trouble understanding the value of connection; indeed, connection is the most fundamental value undergirding their holistic paradigm (or their religious beliefs—as Klassen [2001] has shown, many deeply Christian homebirthers ground themselves in their connectedness to and faith in God).

There is increasing evidence that midwife-assisted homebirth is as safe as, and for some outcomes, safer than, hospital birth (Janssen et al. 2002; Janssen et al. 2009; Janssen, Henderson, and Vedam 2009; Johnson and Daviss 2005; Miller and Skinner 2012; Hutton, Reitsma, and Kaufman 2009; de Jonge et al. 2009; Cheyney et al. 2014a, b; Cheyney et al. 2015), but this evidence is little known and not at all acknowledged in the wider culture, which still assumes the authority of the technomedical tenet that hospital birth is far superior to birth at home. Thus, as health care practitioners, all midwives—even those who attend women in their homes—are under tremendous cultural pressure to "do birth according to medical standards," as one midwife put it.

But "doing birth according to medical standards" will in some cases mean using interventions and/or transporting the woman to the hospital, despite the midwife's alternative judgment. Midwives must attempt to meet these cultural imperatives. Such attempts place many midwives in conflict with their own holistic paradigm and the patience and trust in birth and the female body that it charters. Contemporary midwives cannot fail to be aware of this dilemma—it is a defining theme of their practices and their lives, ensuring that for them, every homebirth that is not textbook-perfect will pose ethical, moral, and legal dilemmas that might end them up in a courtroom in danger of losing the right to practice. The level of tension between the technocratic and holistic paradigms with which homebirth midwives must constantly cope makes their occasional willingness to rely solely on *intuition*—honored by the holistic model and condemned by the technocratic model—a strong marker of their commitment to holism and its underlying principle of connection.

The purpose of this chapter is to call attention to midwives' use of intuition as a salient source of authoritative knowledge. Our intention is not to refine the concept of intuition, but simply to utilize Brigitte Jordan's (1993) formulation of the notion of authoritative knowledge as a theoretical tool to help us understand the role that intuition plays for contemporary midwives. To begin, we will explore some theoretical perspectives on the nature of intuition.

On the Nature of Intuition: Theoretical Perspectives

I think, because we're in a culture that doesn't respect intuition, and has a very narrow definition of knowledge, we can get caught into the trap of that narrowness. Intuition is another kind of knowledge deeply embodied. It's not up there in the stars. It is knowing, just as much as intellectual knowing. It's not fluff, which is what the culture tries to do to it.

— Judy Luce, homebirth midwife

"Intuition" is defined by the *American Heritage Dictionary* as "the act or faculty of knowing or sensing without the use of rational processes; immediate cognition." One of the best studies of the topic is by Tony Bastick (1982) in which he isolated a number of characteristics of intuition, including confidence in the process of intuition, the sense of certainty of the truth of insights, the suddenness and immediacy of awareness of knowing, the association of affect with insight, the nonanalytic (nonrational, nonlogical) and gestaltic nature of the experience, the empathic aspect of intuition, the "preverbal" and frequently ineffable nature of the knowledge, the ineluctable relationship between intuition and creativity, and the possibility that an insight may prove to be factually incorrect.

In *Women's Intuition* (1989), Elizabeth Davis points out that, regarding the acquisition of information, Western society gives authoritative status only to the highly linear modes of inductive and deductive reasoning. Yet it is well established that "there is no creativity in science, indeed, in any domain of creative activity, that does not entail intuition" (Laughlin 1997:6; see also Bastick 1982; Hayward 1984:29–33; Jung 1971; Poincare 1913; Slaatte 1983; Vaughn 1979; Weil 1972; Westcott 1968). Why then is intuition so devalued in the West?

As a number of social scientists (Martin 1987; Merchant 1983; Rothman 1982) have pointed out, mechanistic metaphors for the earth, the universe, and the body have gained increasing cultural prominence since the time of Descartes. Conscious deductive reasoning, which can be logically explained and replicated, is the most machine-like form of human thought. Thus, ratiocinative ("to ratiocinate" means "to reason methodically and logically") processes are reified in the West and are often couched in terms of normative rules (Rubinstein et al. 1984:34; Beth and Piaget 1966). Intuition, in contrast, refers to our experience of the results of deep cognitive processes that occur without conscious awareness and cannot be logically explained or reproduced. Laughlin (1992, 1997) postulates that intuition is *neurognostic*—inherent to the basic structure of the human central nervous system—which would account for the panhuman attributes of the experience of intuitive insight. He suggests that language and its concomitant ratiocinative conceptual structures did not evolve to express the entire human cognitive system and its operations but only those relevant to social adaptation. The kind of knowledge that can be expressed by the human brain's linguistic and conceptual structures is superficial in relation to the deeper neurocognitive processes "upon which knowledge in its broader creative sense depends" (Laughlin 1997:17).

Neurophysiological research on the complementary functions of the two brain hemispheres has shed some light on the process of intuition. The left hemisphere primarily mediates language production, analytic thought, and lineal and causal sequencing of events, whereas the right hemisphere primarily mediates the production of images, gestaltic or holistic thought, and spatiotemporal patterning (Bryden 1982; Ley 1983; Sperry 1974, 1982). Simplifying a bit, one could say that the left lobe distinguishes parts of wholes, making analytic thought and linguistic communication possible, while the right lobe makes gestaltic perception possible—and difficult to communicate or analyze in our Western linguistic system. (See the table below, from Davis-Floyd and Laughlin 2016:34.)

Some researchers have used these findings to suggest that we humans have two modes of consciousness, one corresponding to what we call "reason," associated with left-lobe functioning, and another called "intuition," associated with right-lobe functioning (Lee 1976). As Laughlin (1997:9) points out, some anthropological theorists have gone to the extreme of suggesting two different types of culture defined by these two ways of knowing. For example, Warren TenHouten (1978–79) used the labels "propositional" and "compositional" and argued that these two ways of knowing lie on a continuum with a third mode, the "dialectical" in the middle as an integration of left and right lobe cognition. In 1941, Sorokin suggested that all societies oscillate over time like a pendulum between two extreme poles, one charac-

The Two Sides of the Human Brain (Frontal Cortex)*

Left hemisphere functions	Right hemisphere functions
analytic—dissects, segregates,	synthetic—receives the gestalt, the whole
categorizes, evaluates; either/or logic, digital thinking	poetic, metaphoric, analogic
emphasizes differences, discontinuities	stresses similarities, relationships
works things through	creates A-HA! experiences
verbal	musical, pictorial, general semantics
speech	gestures, tone of voice
temporal (watches clock)	spatial
linear	holistic
intellectual, rational	emotional
individual more likely to be conscious of its functions	individual less likely to be conscious of its functions

*Please note: This table is oversimplified, because the whole brain operates in all brain functions, yet it is still generally useful in terms of brain hemispheric predominance. For an example of how this list can be useful, note that people often don't say in words what they really mean; to get at their actual meaning, it is more helpful to pay attention to gestures and tone of voice (e.g., cheerful loving words spoken in a sarcastic tone); these are much more reflective of what the person actually means.

terized by rational knowledge and materialistic values, and the other by intuitive knowledge and spiritual values. Sorokin's suggestion is paralleled in popular writings by Rianne Eisler's (1988) distinction between "dominator" and "partnership" cultures, and Daniel Quinn's (1993) between "Takers" and "Leavers." These distinctions are also paralleled by the differences between contemporary American homebirth midwifery and the technocratic society in whose midst midwifery exists and struggles to flourish. The technocracy is largely hierarchical, male-dominated, technology-oriented, and based on left-brained principles of separation and discrimination, while homebirth midwifery is primarily egalitarian, nature- and female-oriented, and based on right-brained principles of holism and connection.

However, such apparently clear-cut dichotomies often mislead. It is important to remember that, in spite of hemispheric dominances, the whole brain is involved in all brain functions. Sharp functional division between the hemispheres occurs only in subjects whose brains have been physically split or damaged, either by injury or by surgery (Sprenger and Deutsch 1981). In the normal, healthy brain, similarity and replication of function are much more common (Davis-Floyd and Laughlin 2016). Laughlin suggests that intuition is "mediated by neural networks in both lobes, not merely in the right lobe" (1997:11), calling the neurocognitive processes that produce intuition "transcendental" in part to stress their cross-hemisphere, whole brain functioning. The corpus callosum, which plays a major role in conveying information between hemispheres, may be most significant in the genesis of intuition. In *Women's Intuition*, Davis (1989) postulates that interhemispheric coherence linked to transcendent states (Goldberg 1983) and intuitive connections may occur more readily in women than in men, since it appears that the corpus callosum in the female brain is significantly larger. It can be argued, however, that this part of the brain can be deliberately developed in either sex, and as such, any gendering of intuitive ways of knowing must also be understood as a product of socialization and acculturation.

As noted above, science, for all its supervaluation of left-brained deductive reasoning, could never have proceeded without the creativity of intuition; concomitantly, no intuition-oriented culture could survive without heavy reliance on ratiocination. Likewise, even the most technocratic of physicians can find themselves following their intuition instead of their reason (Fox 1957, 1980), and even the most holistic of midwives, in this postmodern era, is likely to have attained a high level of competence in using the technocratic tools of birth, and to be able to explain and defend her actions in scientific, linear, and logical terms. The praxis of postmodern midwifery entails, in many ways, the careful exercise of inductive and deductive reasoning even as it continues to rely for its primary ethos on the enactment of bodily and psychic connection (see Chapter 9).

Background and Context: Midwifery as Radical Cultural Critique

The fact that the legal system so completely supports the praxis of technobirth has forced those midwifery practitioners who take the risk of opposing it to become hyper-educated in obstetrics so that they can both defend themselves against legal persecution by the medical establishment and work to change the laws that keep them legally marginal. In response to such pressures, and in service to the increasing numbers of urban middle- and working-class women who request their services (Janssen, Henderson, and Vedam 2009; MacDorman, Menacker, and Declerq 2010), as we saw in Chapter 6, midwives in the US originally known as "lay" have expanded from their original base of traditional practitioners serving specific ethnic groups in bounded communities (see for example Susie 1988) to full participation in the postmodern world. In the Third World, as the viability of indigenous systems of birth knowledge is everywhere challenged by imported biomedical systems, midwives are emerging as articulate defenders of traditional ways, as well as creative inventors of systems of mutual accommodation (for example, see Barclay 2009 on how Samoan midwives have managed to integrate home and hospital birthing systems). This phenomenon, which Davis-Floyd has labeled *postmodern midwifery*—midwives who are educated, articulate, organized, political, and highly conscious of both their cultural uniqueness and their global importance—is not limited to the US but is increasingly emergent all over the world (see Chapter 8).

Robbie's juxtaposition of "postmodern" (a charged word in the anthropological lexicon) with "midwifery" is far from casual. With that juxtaposition, she is trying to make salient the qualities emergent in the praxis (a term anthropologists use to encompass both practice and the sociocultural context within which it is embedded), the discourse, and the political engagement of a certain kind of contemporary midwife. George Marcus has stressed that the power of the postmodern intervention in anthropology has inhered in its "radical critique" (1993:6) of unexamined conventions and monological assumptions, both ethnographic and cultural. As Linda Singer points out in "Feminism and Postmodernism," in feminist writings this radical critique "recurs with variations."

> [As] an explicit discursive strategy of challenging the terms, conventions, and symbols of hegemonic authority in ways that foreground the explicitly transgressive character of this enterprise . . . postmodern discourse disrupt[s] the project of closure by consensus, by insisting on exposing how differences inscribe themselves, even when they are explicitly refused or denied. The voice of rationality is shown to be riddled with contradictions it cannot exclude. (1992:469–470)

This surely is an apt and accurate description of midwifery practice as described in this chapter. We will see how midwives, in their intentionally transgressive reliance on intuition, quite regularly expose the contradictions that the voice of rationality proves, in the domain of birth, to be unable to exclude. As we shall see, the transgressive nature of postmodern midwifery is further displayed in the fluidity with which the midwives interviewed for this study move between the biomedical and midwifery domains, appropriating the authoritative lexicon and the whiz-bang technologies of biomedicine to the holistic philosophy and "of service to women" ethos of homebirth midwifery. These same midwives, and others like them, have become adept at challenging the terms, conventions, and symbols of hegemonic authority in the courts, in the press, in state and national legislatures, and through the politics generated by the actions and interactions of their national organizations. Through such ongoing activities, as well as in countless aspects of the daily discourse and praxis of midwifery, these midwives self-consciously engage in the most radical of cultural critiques.

Methods and Collaboration: How an Anthropologist and a Midwife Came to Co-Create This Study

This chapter is based on interview data obtained from 23 white middle-class American midwives about the role that intuition plays in their behavior at births. Seventeen of these midwives were empirically trained and primarily attended homebirths; by 2017 all of those who were still in practice had become Certified Professional Midwives (CPMs); at the time of our study (1992–1993), that certification, which was created in 1994, did not yet exist (see Chapter 6). Six were certified nurse-midwives (CNMs). Most interviewees were experienced midwives with three to sixteen years in practice; three had been in practice less than a year. Three of the CNMs attended births both at home and in the hospital; the other two were hospital-based. All of the midwives were attendees at the 1992 conference of the Midwives Alliance of North America (MANA) in New York or the 1993 MANA conference in San Francisco; most interviews were conducted at these two conferences, with others conducted at what was then called the Seattle Midwifery School (now the midwifery program at Bastyr University). While we can make no definitive claims as to the representative nature of our interview sample, we can affirm from many years of interaction with midwives that the attitudes, beliefs, and experiences of our interviewees are typical for midwives who practice humanistically and holistically under "the midwifery model of care" (see Chapter 11) regardless of setting (home, hospital, birth center).

Our interviews, which were tape-recorded, were generally from one-half to one hour in length; all of them were conducted by Davis-Floyd, who began by interviewing midwives who were recommended to her as having "good stories" to tell. Some of the interviews ended up taking the form of story-telling sessions formed in clusters in hotel hallways, as midwives walking by felt moved to join the session and recount their own experiences. Each one was asked to tell as much as she wished about incidents surrounding birth in which intuition had played a role. Robbie's goal was to elicit as many "intuition stories" from the midwives as she could, to begin to gain a sense of whether, and if so, how much or in what instances these midwives relied on intuition, of the results in actual births of their acceptance or rejection of intuitive messages, and of their feelings about the value and usefulness of intuition as a diagnostic tool and guide to action—in other words, as a form of authoritative knowledge.

An additional 20 stories were gathered at a tape-recorded workshop on intuition called "Spinning Tales, Weaving Hope" that Elizabeth Davis led at the 1993 MANA conference in San Francisco, during which all the midwives present were asked to share any experiences with intuition they felt were important. While we cannot be sure what role this workshop and the interviews we conducted played in these midwives' opinions and ideas about intuition, the mere fact that we, as authoritative figures, were particularly focused on intuition no doubt helped to validate or to enhance the idea of intuition as a legitimate source of authoritative knowledge in the minds of our interviewees. This in fact was explicitly intended by Elizabeth, who designed her workshop for just that purpose; in Robbie's case, it was an inevitable by-product of the interview process—yet another illustration of the essential connectedness of the anthropologist to her subjects of "study," and of the intense subjectivity of the anthropological endeavor (Clifford and Marcus 1986; Marcus and Fischer 1986).

That subjectivity was also much in evidence during the process of data analysis. As anyone who works with interview data knows, the process by which one arrives at an interpretation of those data is difficult to describe. Asked to do just that by a reviewer for the *Medical Anthropology Quarterly*, the journal in which this essay was originally published, we confronted a hard-to-delineate "fuzziness" in that process. When one interviews from a predesigned list of questions, one can compare the answers to a certain question or set of questions across the database. In this case, however, we were not working from such a list, but rather asking for stories and listening to them as they unfolded. We transcribed the tapes, read the transcriptions over and over, and discussed them at length, until salient themes and patterns began to emerge that shed light on our central organizing question: *To what extent and under what circumstances do midwives utilize intuition as a source of authoritative knowledge for decision making during birth?*

Our collaboration emerged gradually. In 1992, Elizabeth Davis was one of Davis-Floyd's (no relation) first interviewees for this study. One year later, we agreed to coauthor this article, which Robbie has now revised and updated as a chapter for this book. We merged in this endeavor our unique perspectives. Robbie Davis-Floyd is a cultural/medical anthropologist who has applied symbolic, cognitive, and feminist perspectives to the study of childbirth, midwifery, and obstetrics. For over 33 years, she has been conducting research on women's experiences of pregnancy and childbirth (1987a, 2003 [1992], 1994), on the beliefs, attitudes, and training of obstetricians (Davis-Floyd 1987b; Davis-Floyd and St. John 1998; Chapter 5, this volume), on the ritual and symbolic dimensions of hospital and homebirth (2003 [1992]; Davis-Floyd and Laughlin 2016), and on the politics, educational processes, and ideologies of contemporary midwives, both traditional and professional (Davis-Floyd 2001a, b, 2003, 2004a, b, 2005, 2006, 2010; Davis-Floyd and Johnson 2006). Elizabeth Davis is an independent midwife who has attended over 300 births as primary caregiver; 90% of them took place at home. Internationally known for her work on women's sexuality and reproductive rights for more than 35 years, she has authored a number of books on birth and related topics, most notably the midwifery textbook *Heart and Hands,* now in its 5th edition (2012), *Orgasmic Birth* (with Debra Pascali-Bonaro 2010), *The Rhythms of Women's Desire* (2013), *The Women's Wheel of Life* (with Carol Leonard, 2012), *Women's Sexual Cycles* (1994), *Woman, Sex, and Desire* (1995), *Women's Intuition* (1989), and *Energetic Pregnancy* (1987). She initiated the development of midwifery certification in California and was instrumental in getting legislation passed to decriminalize direct-entry midwifery in that state. She is a past chair of the Midwives Alliance of North America (MANA) Education Committee, and a past president of the Midwifery Education Accreditation Council (MEAC), a national accrediting body for direct-entry midwifery education (see Chapter 6). She is currently codirector of the MEAC-accredited National Midwifery Institute, Inc., lead instructor of the Heart and Hands Midwifery Intensives course work, and a frequent lecturer at childbirth and midwifery conferences around the world (see www.elizabethdavis.com).

Midwives and Intuition

Connection as a Prerequisite

The first thing that jumped out at us from our interview data was the enormous value midwives place on "connection." Connection, as these midwives experience it in homebirth, means not only physical but also emotional, intellectual, and psychic links. It is not merely two-way, as with the connectedness of midwife to mother, or mother to child.[1] If we were to dia-

[1] Breastfeeding constitutes a good example of the pragmatic ramifications of insisting on the value of connection. Ninety-eight percent of American women give birth in hospitals; around 50% of them breastfeed their babies during the early months of life (Merewood et al. 2005). Of the 1.36% of women who give birth at home or in freestanding birth centers—in other words, in accordance with the connection-based holistic model of birth—close to 100% choose to breastfeed.

gram it, we might draw something like a web, with strands connecting mother, child, father, and midwives, each to the other.[2] If, further, we were to look inside each individual, we might see other strands of the web connecting each individual to the deepest essence of herself. Our interviewees insisted that the degree of connection they are able to maintain with mother and child depends on the degree of connection they maintain to the flow of their own thoughts and feelings. So basic is the importance of this internal connectedness that many of them actively seek it during and even before birth. As Elizabeth explained during her interview with Robbie, "Sometimes, especially when I've been doing a lot, it's really hard for me to clear myself and arrive at the birth open. So before I leave, I lie down and just try to unwind and unfold my concerns of the day and open to myself, so that I can also be open to the woman and her birth."

This effort to "be open" to oneself and to the woman and her birth is a common theme among homebirth midwives. The connectedness it facilitates extends not only to the psyche and emotions but also to physical sensation and experience. Consider the following quote from a Canadian midwife:

> In our collective practice, one of the things that we became really aware of over time was that if one of the midwives at a birth had diarrhea [it was a message that we should] look at things a lot closer. Inevitably in those births something came up. . . .
>
> Q. How would you explain that? Why would a midwife get diarrhea if something's wrong with the birth—what's the connection?
>
> I think you're intuitively picking up that something isn't quite right here. It's coming out in the body—it hasn't gone into the head yet.

The physicality of this knowing of which she speaks is reinforced in this description by a California midwife:

> My scientific self believes that everything happens inside my skull, in my brain. [And I have intellectually learned many skills, many techniques.] But my physical experience is that [in dangerous situations in

[2] The importance of the web metaphor to the members of MANA as an expression of their lived experience was demonstrated during the closing ceremonies of the 1993 San Francisco conference. Four hundred and fifty midwives formed a giant circle around the edges of an otherwise-empty ballroom. They passed balls of yarn in many colors around the circle; each participant looped each color of yarn that came to her around her wrist, until all were physically connected. Then they tossed many more balls of yarn across the floor to each other, tying those around their wrists also, until all that yarn formed a giant rainbow-hued web that filled the ballroom floor, linking everyone to everyone through myriad connections. Spontaneously lifting the giant web into the air by lifting their arms, the midwives quickly discovered that, if one person moved her arm, the whole web would move in response. And if a ball of yarn got stuck in the middle of the floor, at least 30 people had to move in synchrony for one person to retrieve it. This of course was a perfect ritual and symbolic enactment of the high value these midwives place on human interconnectedness.

> which my mind isn't sure what to do, which technique would be the very best]—say, the baby's head comes out, but it won't rotate, and the shoulders are stuck—a cone of power comes straight down the width of my head, through my body, and out through my hands. And my hands begin to do a maneuver, and my mouth begins to speak and I tell the woman to turn over [on her hands and knees], or I reach up and grab hold of the baby's butt and draw the baby down, or I do whatever I do—but I didn't know what I was going to do before that moment—and that's midwife intuition. [Maggie Bennett][3]

From whence does this "cone of power" originate? While both Maggie and the Canadian midwife quoted above describe intuition as intensely physical, Maggie's "cone of power" adds a spiritual dimension as well. Asking our interviewees where intuition is located for them, we received the following responses: "All through the body"; "It's cellular"; "It's in my stomach"; "It's inner knowledge—you don't know where it comes from"; "Your heart, your dreams"; "Your connection to the universe"; "My higher self"; "My heart, my chest, my throat"; "I'm very auditory—I hear it as a voice coming from deep inside." We can conclude that for our interviewees, intuition seems to involve the body, psyche, and spirit, but not the rational mind.

The midwives say that they experience the kind of openness described by Maggie and Elizabeth, and the connectedness it facilitates, as essential to receiving intuitive messages. If they are closed—"shut down," "disconnected"—they cannot hear that inner voice, and must rely on their extensive intellectual knowledge and accumulated expertise. While they see nothing wrong with this reliance, they do seem to regard it as a qualitatively different type of care, as will be evidenced in the following section.

Learning to Trust

In formal interviews and casual conversations, we heard midwives express strong familiarity with biomedical diagnostic technologies. Their in-group jargon is filled with technomedical terms, their midwifery bags bulge with technologies (see chapter Appendix), and their homebirth charts look quite hospital-like, with maternal temperature and blood pressure and fetal heart tones duly recorded at proper intervals. Yet these same midwives who are so competent at using the jargon and the diagnostic tools of technocratic medicine often perceive the information thus obtained as a highly adulterated blessing, perhaps a source of as many problems as it solves. As Elizabeth explained:

> What I see going on in a lot of midwifery training programs is the idea that here's this body of knowledge, and one needs to be schooled, and one needs to be tested—the idea that the student is empty and waiting to

[3] Interviewees Maggie Bennett, Jeannette Breen, Elizabeth Davis, and Judy Luce insisted on being identified by their own names, in keeping with their strong beliefs in the value of their work and of their intuitive experiences. All other names following quotations are pseudonyms.

> be filled, and the knowledge is there, and after you stuff it in, then the student is "qualified." But in midwifery, no amount of that is ever going to compensate for a lack of self-confidence or an ability to blend critical thinking with personal responsibility. What makes a really good midwife, I think, are those inner-based qualities of analysis and discernment, the emotions that she stays in touch with because she does not divorce her *self* from the process of learning, so that the feelings of self-respect, and self-love, and self-trust blend to make her humane and to keep her connected. *I think in birth, if you're not part of the process, you're a threat to the process.*

The other midwives we interviewed were in complete agreement with Elizabeth. For all of them, being part of the process of birth, being connected, constituted the primary ingredient of their success—an ingredient far and away more significant than their albeit considerable technical diagnostic skills. Jeannette Breen even went so far as to say:

> Assisting women at birth—that's all it is, is intuition. I listen to the baby's heartbeat, because, you know, I listen to the baby's heartbeat, but I don't really care about it, because I have this inner knowing that everything's fine.
>
> Q. Do you also know when everything isn't fine?
>
> Sure you know, there's an energy there.
>
> Q. Has there ever been a time when the stethoscope told you one thing but your intuition another?
>
> No. If I detect a problem with the baby's heartbeat, there have already been signs that I'm suspecting there may be a problem. The heartbeat almost never tells me anything, except it looks nice on a piece of paper to document it. I do that for the lawyers.

Donna and Fran: Ignoring vs. Listening to That Small Inner Voice

It is a working hypothesis of ours that the more intensely midwives are trained in didactic models of medical care based on ratiocinative processes, the less they will trust in and rely on their intuition. Since our interviews focused on midwives who demonstrated their commitment to holism by attending MANA conferences, we have been unable to evaluate the evidence for this hypothesis. To do so, we would have to interview equal numbers of more medically-oriented CNMs. All of our interviewees report that learning to trust their intuition is an ongoing process. Our data do however indicate some differences in the ways that more medically trained CNMs and empirically trained midwives (who at the time learned their skills through the one-on-one interaction of apprenticeship) experience this process. The CNMs seem to begin by regarding intuition with mistrust, then move into trust through lived experience. The empirically trained midwives seem to begin by trusting intuition, and move into confirmation of that trust through lived experience. Consider the following story told to Robbie by Donna Hartmann, a hospital-based CNM from the Midwest about her first salient experience with intuition at birth:

> Last year I [was] seeing a Laotian Hmong woman. She came when she was about four months pregnant from a refugee camp. The very first time I met her I felt like there was something that was not right, but, although I kept looking, I couldn't find anything, ever. . . . Well I happened to be on call the night she was in labor, and her interpreter called me and told me she was going into the hospital and I asked the interpreter if she was coming and the interpreter said no, and—I had had this feeling all along, this voice that was telling me something bad was going to happen, and I thought, it's a mistake for the interpreter not to come, but I didn't say anything—I respected their plan.
>
> And the woman got to the hospital and she was complete with a bag of water that was bulging and a high presenting part. And the nurse said to me, "I think she should go to the high-risk birth center," and I knew that this woman would not be protected—I knew there'd be residents—and so I pushed aside the part that had been telling me something was wrong, and admitted her to the alternative birth center. And when I got there, about five minutes after she arrived up there, she was pushing already, and I [started to check her] and the bag of water broke with her next contraction, and my whole hand filled with umbilical cord.
>
> She'd been in labor all day at home, and I don't know how long the cord was prolapsed, but as soon as I found it we tried to get her to push through, but she wouldn't push, so I pushed the baby's head up and we did a cesarean section, and we got the baby out pretty fast but the baby has only lower brain stem function. Even though we did things right, we did things fast, it was a terrible outcome. And I think, had I listened to that voice, [the translator would have been there and could have convinced her to push] or she would at least have been admitted to a unit where things could have been done faster, and I don't know if there would have been a better outcome or not, but it's the strongest message of intuition I've ever had and from it I learned a lot about listening. I had never been raised to believe in the inner voice, but now I listen, when I slow down enough to hear those things.

Donna Hartmann's difficulties with learning to listen to her inner voice are echoed in Fran's story:

> I went to nursing school, and before I finished my CNM I attended a number of homebirths with a midwife who was not a nurse and watched her make decisions based on intuition and just connection with the client. The nurse-midwifery education that I had didn't teach us that—it was very linear and very objective and taught us to make decisions based on very objective and very specific criteria. In the last few years I've had

> some very high-risk births, very scary outcomes and have felt in my heart, in my chest, in my throat that things were going to be okay, and have gone against my physician backup and said, "Let's keep going for just a little while," and ended up with lovely babies, even with lots of meconium[4] and with strong decelerations.[5]
>
> And quite recently I was in a situation where I had all the objective criteria for a really nice birth. The strip [electronic fetal monitor printout] didn't look very bad and we had no meconium. But the whole time my heart and chest were telling me "Things are not going right." And I was trying to get my physician backup to intervene and he was saying, "Based on these objective criteria, things are going to be OK" and they were not. . . . the baby was born with Apgars of 2 and 2.[6] I think we need to listen to our intuition and we need to keep apprenticeships so that we can watch each other and talk to each other during these decisions. If you can say to other midwives you're working with, "I'm having a bad feeling about this," even though everything else—all the objective criteria—look good, you need to trust those feelings. That's what I've learned.

Elizabeth's Story: Acting on Intuition "Just in Case"

Recounting her early years of homebirth midwifery practice, Elizabeth, who was empirically trained, introduced the following story by saying, "This is the experience that first got me interested in the role of intuition in birth." In contrast to the two CNMs quoted above, her first reaction to a strong intuitive experience was not to resist or ignore, but to act upon it:

> I had received a call that someone was in labor and [I lay down to unwind and open myself], and I heard this voice—I'm pretty auditory, and that's one of the ways my intuition shows up—and the voice said, "She's going to have a partial [placental] separation." I immediately fought back the voice—I think a lot of us, when we get intuitive messages, will argue back with our rational minds and refute them—we're schizo enough to do that . . . and that's what I did. I went over her history in my mind, and there was nothing that would indicate any risk for post-

[4] Meconium is the baby's first bowel movement. If present in the amniotic fluid, it is sometimes associated with fetal distress, which is usually also indicated by fetal heart patterns. It is generally recognized, even in most hospitals, that thin or light meconium staining during labor is not problematic, especially when the heart rate patterns fall within a normal range. Heavy, thick, and chunky meconium in the amniotic fluid is usually indicative of fetal distress.

[5] Decelerations of the fetal heart rate, as recorded on the electronic fetal monitor, are sometimes indicative of fetal distress.

[6] The Apgar score provides a standardized means by which birth attendants can assess the baby's condition at birth. Signs rated at two points each on a preprinted chart are skin color, muscle tone, breathing attempts, heartbeat, and response to stimulus, such as a touch or pinprick. Babies are rated twice, at one minute after birth and again at five minutes, because many babies, especially anesthetized ones, take some time to turn pink and begin full breathing on their own. Ten is the highest obtainable score. Babies with Apgars of 2 and 2 (2 at one minute, and still 2 at five minutes) are severely distressed.

partum bleeding. And the voice said, "No, sorry, this is going to happen." Then I responded with great confidence and said, "Well that's OK, because I've handled this before—I've done manual removals." But after that it came back, "No, you've never done this. You've never had to go this far up and you've never had this much bleeding." I was really scared, but I thought, "Well, this is my fear, and I'm just projecting, God only knows why."

But, I told my partner about it, and at the birth I drew up a syringe of pitocin in advance, and pushed fluids by mouth, and the kinds of things that I would do if I anticipated a potential problem with bleeding.

So she gives birth to this gorgeous little girl, the labor was uneventful, nothing strange, and she's holding her baby, and this bleeding starts. I follow up the cord to see where the placenta is and suddenly there's so much blood, and my hand is continuing from that point of exploration on up inside the uterus—I'm on automatic pilot, doing this manual removal as it was foreshown. And my partner is injecting the syringe of pitocin, and everything worked out great, I think because of the immediacy of the response and the complete lack of double guessing myself. Just going ahead and doing what was necessary without wasting time really kept her blood loss to a minimum, even though it was considerable. We didn't have to transport, she didn't have to be transfused, she didn't go into shock, and that was amazing to me.

Reason vs. Intuition: How Do You Know an Intuition Is Real?

Bastick's (1982) comprehensive list of the qualities of intuition (see above) includes the possibility that an intuition may be incorrect. With this most of the midwives in our study would disagree, as they tend to define intuition per se as inherently accurate (see also Vaughn 1979). Many of them told us that the trick, each time the inner voice speaks, is how to know whether or not it is a "real" intuition, and the struggle is to learn the difference between the inner doubt and debate that accompanies ratiocinative thinking, and the true voice of intuition. Their unwillingness to assume that an intuition can be wrong, we find, comes from their consensual belief that intuition finds its source in the spiritual realm or their own "higher selves," which by definition cannot be wrong, or from the deepest recesses of their bodies, which, according to the holistic model, are essentially energy fields operating in connection with all other energy fields, and therefore cannot be wrong either.

In contrast, reason/ratiocination, which is site-specific to the neocortex, *can* be wrong, and often is so. Thus, if a midwife has what she thinks may be an intuition, but it turns out to be wrong, she is likely to conclude that it must not have been an intuition in the first place, but a product of her "rational mind." This is not to say that midwives devalue reason and ratiocination. They tend to be comfortable with their ratiocinative abilities and keenly aware that these are culturally supervalued. The voice of reason is loud and aggressive; the harder task, as the midwives see it, is to identify and heed the truths spoken by the still, soft, and culturally devalued inner voice. The worth of this enterprise is attested to by the outstanding safety record that contemporary homebirth midwives are achieving—a record that compares most favorably with the interventionist, expensive, and often iatrogenic "active management" of labor and birth in many hospitals. The midwives we interviewed for this study reported they averaged a 90% or higher success rate for the home- or birth-center births they have attended, the vast majority of which took place without drugs or other technological interventions. Out of every 100 clients, they transferred 8–10 to the hospital during labor; fewer than 4% ended up with cesareans; and their perinatal mortality rates averaged around 2/1,000. These statistics correspond almost exactly with those reported in much larger formal studies (Johnson and Daviss 2005; Cheyney et al. 2014a, b), and contrast with the extremely high percentage of women in the hospital who receive drugs during labor (over 90%), the near-universal technological interventions in hospital birth, the national cesarean rate of 23% in 1996 when this research was first published and 32% in 2016, and hospital perinatal mortality rates of 7–9/1,000 (Janssen et al. 2009; de Jonge et al. 2009).

Maggie's Story: A Case Study in Reliance on Intuition

Although all these midwives know "the rules," the protocols of standard midwifery practice, they often circumvent or ignore them completely in the actual doing of birth. Clearly they do not consider such protocols authoritative per se. Brigitte Jordan (1993) has said that authoritative knowledge is interactionally displayed knowledge on the basis of which decisions are made and actions taken. How far into actions and interaction can intuition take a midwife? Given the external diagnostic technologies at her command, including those of the hospital to which she can transport her client, how authoritative can she consider that inner voice to be? What happens when something that voice tells her conflicts with more culturally accepted external parameters of normal, with standard protocol? We take as a case study a birth attended by midwife Maggie Bennett (who was president of the California Midwives' Association at the time of this study), which took her far beyond medically accepted standards, right out onto the ragged edge of intuition and trust:

> [Once I had a client named Jane]—it was her third pregnancy and she was 39. Her first pregnancy . . . was complicated and that child had some physiological problems. Her second labor began prematurely, and she was delivered by cesarean section—the baby was six weeks premature and had cerebral palsy. Her father is an obstetrician. So she came to me feeling that hospitals and doctors offered her nothing as far as safety. She was also a VBAC [vaginal birth after cesarean] at a time when VBACs were new to me, and she also had a vertical scar, exterior and interior—a no-no.

Maggie has so far listed no less than five factors that, from a medical point of view, would define this woman as far too high-risk for any midwife to take on for a homebirth: two previous problematic births, both with pathological outcomes, a father who is an obstetrician (a strong indicator for a medically-oriented daughter and a potential threat to the midwife's ability to continue to practice), and a woman who wants to give birth vaginally at home, but who happens to have the kind of scar, on both her abdomen and her uterus, that is most likely to rupture during a subsequent labor. But, Maggie continues:

> What she did have going for her was God. She was a born-again Christian, and believed that this was of God's design, and so she had a lot of power from that source. So the first thing that happened was that we got close to term—37, 38 weeks, and her baby was breech. And we kept waiting for it to turn on its own, and we did crawling and slant-boarding[7] and all sorts of things, but the baby didn't turn. So we decided that the baby had to be turned. And the baby was really hard to turn, and it didn't go easily, and at one point I felt that we should stop, because it was just too difficult. But then I had this intuition that the baby could go head down, but that *I* was blocking the process.
>
> One of the things that was happening was that the woman wanted to have a beer [to help her relax] and I wouldn't let her do that because I wanted her 100% present and in her body, and I wasn't willing to let her check out while I did this procedure on her. I just wouldn't allow it. [But then she began making these statements that semiequated me with the devil, and finally I realized that my refusal was causing a lot of unpleasant tension between us.]
>
> And so I let go of my beliefs about the alcohol, and I called her husband and said, "You need to pray." I had to let go of my being righteous about my own belief system—I am not a Christian—and about religion and about alcohol, and let this woman be in her body the way she had to be in her body, and be in her beliefs the way she had to be in her beliefs. And if that meant that I had to bow my head and pray, then that's what I had to do—so it was as much about me as it was about her.
>
> So she had a glass of wine and a half a beer, and I had a half a beer, and my partner had a half a beer, and we mellowed out a whole bunch, and she lay down on the slant board again, and the baby just went around. So again, it was the intuition about knowing that the baby wanted to turn around, and looking at what everybody had been doing that was stopping that from happening.

[7] "Slant-boarding" is a midwifery technique that often proves effective in getting breech babies to turn before delivery. The mother must get her head lower than her pelvis. A bean bag chair can be used, or an ironing board (or door) can be placed against a sofa or heavy chair at a 45-degree angle; the pregnant woman lies on her back, head down on the board with her feet pointing upwards for 15 to 20 minutes, two or three times a day. During this time she is encouraged to relax and to visualize the baby turning. (For other such techniques, see Kitzinger 1991:98.)

In her willingness to compromise her own religious and health beliefs to facilitate the turning of the baby and to maintain connectedness with the mother, Maggie demonstrates the malleability of the midwife, her willingness to go the distance with the mother on the mother's terms. Maggie as practitioner-in-charge could have retained her authority to deny the woman alcohol by insisting on the authority of her "knowledge" that alcohol would be harmful. Instead, she gave up that claim altogether, gladly surrendering authority to what she saw as the higher good of connectedness and trust. (We should mention here that having the mother—and sometimes the midwife—drink a beer before an external version [the manual turning of the baby in the uterus] for relaxation is a common practice of traditional midwives throughout Latin America; breech babies often won't turn if the mother or the midwife is tense. See Chapter 8, p. 235.)

Yet another opportunity to give up authority quickly arose: hospital guidelines and many midwifery protocols state that babies must be born within 24 hours of the rupture of the membranes, as the danger of infection of the baby rises significantly thereafter. This rule of thumb has sent many would-be homebirth mothers to the hospital and has resulted in many cesareans, as it is very common for labor and birth to take far longer than 24 hours. Indeed, as midwives know, normal labors can take up to five or six days as the uterus tones and prepares during the latent phase (up to 5 cm; active labor is defined as beginning at 6 cm). During that time, if left unpenetrated, ruptured amniotic sacs will often reseal). But a cesarean was not to be Jane's outcome. Maggie continued:

> So she goes into labor four days later, but she doesn't just do it normally—she has premature rupture of the membranes for 24 hours, 72 hours, four days she has premature rupture of the membranes, and you better believe that intuition played a role every single day, because I had to reexamine where we were going with it all the way along. But the answer was always the same—her waters were clear, she had no temperature, and she still had God. She was filled with her faith in God that that baby was safe. And I was able to participate in that faith.
>
> So on the fourth day [after her membranes ruptured], after she is finally in labor, her backup doctor called to check on her, and someone told him that she was in labor and was out walking with her husband. . . . So now the *doctor* knows that she's in labor. And remember that I told you that her father was an obstetrician in a town about four hours away? Well *he* calls up and finds out that she's in labor, and then he starts calling every three hours. And he starts to say, "What's going on there? That baby should have been born by now."
>
> So I have a woman who's four days with ruptured membranes, who's been in labor for about 18 hours with contractions about five minutes apart. . . . And while I was out for a few minutes picking up food for everybody,[8] I ran into her backup doctor at the restaurant and he said to me, "I

> just want to know is the baby coming out above or below?" and I said—this was an intuition, come to think of it—"The baby's coming out normally."[9]

The pressure builds. Maggie is attending a woman with significant risk factors from past and now this present birth; two physicians are aware that she is in labor and are trying to monitor the situation from afar. Every midwife knows how fraught with personal peril such a situation is, and that there is also peril for the mother, as the tension induced by such pressure can easily stop or slow labor. Maggie's response at this point to "all this energy, this highly political birth," is that of guardian and protector of the natural process: she pulls the plug on the telephone (this was before the age of cell phones). She said:

> I think that every time a midwife goes to the edge, it is the intuition that everything is all right that takes her there. I had to keep examining with this woman whether or not it was all right for us to continue, and every single time was an internal process about—we have these signs, and this is not the rules, but I *know* the baby's all right, and I *know* that the mother is all right, so we can go on from this point.
>
> So eventually, she begins to push the baby out, and the waters broke [again—the bag had resealed] just as she began to push and there was slight meconium staining. And she begins to have a slight temperature, like maybe 99, but this is all right [according to protocols] because she has begun to push.
>
> Guess what? She doesn't push the baby out in one hour, she doesn't push the baby out in two hours, not even in three hours. She takes a rest at four hours.[10] She finally gets that baby out in five hours . . . squatting . . . little by little by little by little. . . . And the baby actually breathes spontaneously and has Apgars of 7 and 8.
>
> So in the end, in retrospect, it was just a challenged birth—a challenged pregnancy, a problem in late pregnancy, a challenged labor all the way along. And I couldn't have done that birth if I had followed *my own* protocols. And there was a point where I had to say, "I am called mid-

[8] Hospital labors are usually artificially speeded up with drugs, episiotomies, forceps, or cesarean section. Homebirth labors, which are allowed to take their natural course, tend to take far more time than hospital births do. During a long labor, it is essential for a mother (and indeed, her birth attendants) to keep up their strength by eating and drinking plenty of nutritious food and fluids. Homebirth midwives recognize that contractions that have been going on for 18 hours and are still 5 minutes apart mean that the mother is still in "early labor"—"active labor" has not yet kicked in—and there is plenty of time for the midwife to go out for food.

[9] Note Maggie's refusal to adopt the physician's technomedical discourse here—a discourse that simultaneously reduces the differences between cesarean and vaginal birth to a matter of geography and subtly expresses the value that this culture consistently places on "above" in relation to "below."

[10] Hospital practitioners generally allow one, and a maximum of two, hours for pushing, after which a cesarean will usually be performed. Homebirth midwives accept a wide range of pushing stages, but more than four hours of pushing is rather unusual, even at home.

> wife, and I am in here for whatever happens, because I have to let go. I have to absolutely let go of my desire to control this, because I can't."

Some perspective on the value Maggie places here on letting go of control is provided by an earlier study carried out by Robbie on differences between home- and hospital birthers (Chapter 3, this volume). She found that the hospital birthers placed high value on control, while the homebirthers felt that giving up control was far more valuable in birth and in life than trying to maintain it—a philosophical position they arrived at through lived experience. As Liza explained it:

> I was brought up in the mainstream, and I used to knock myself out trying to control everything. Then I got sick, and I realized that I actually can't control anything or anyone. As soon as I let go of trying, and just began to surrender to what is, everything in my life started to work. I got well, I got married, I had a baby.
>
> And if the lesson needed reinforcing, labor did it. That is a force beyond control, a powerful wave that will drown you if you fight it. Better then to dive into it, to relax, let it carry you. Whenever I tried to control my labor or myself during labor, I was in agony. But when I let go and surrendered to the waves, they carried me.
>
> And honestly, contractions only last around 45 seconds, and then you get a break. I think anyone can handle 45 seconds of pain, especially if you stay focused in the moment, on relaxing into this contraction, and then the next, without constantly asking, "How much longer do I have to go?" Because if the answer is hours and hours, you can get really discouraged. But if you just dive into one contraction at a time, and just stay right there in that moment, again, the waves will carry you. [Originally quoted in Davis-Floyd 1994:1133; see also Chapter 3.]

Maggie reinforces this philosophical position on the value of surrender at the same time as she indicates how difficult it is to maintain this view in a society that supervalues control in most aspects of life:

> You know, I would never have the audacity to go to a birth and think that I could control everything that happened, for either the safety or the outcome. Sooner or later, I, along with the mother, have to give up the control. You would think after 17 years [of attending births] I would know that, but I have to relearn that at almost every birth, over and over again.

We asked Maggie, "How do you feel about staying the course with that birth?" and she responded, "I feel that it was a great gift, a great learning, and I am so incredibly inspired by the woman, and the goddess that she is (she would hate me for saying that)—that I was able to witness that miracle."

In calling this woman a "goddess," Maggie expresses an attitude toward women that is held by many midwives who tend to see the birthing woman as a powerful creatrix—a birth- and lifegiver. Such midwives espouse the principles of ecofeminism, which link the fate of the planet, metaphorized as Gaia, the Mother Goddess, to the cultural treatment of the female body (see, for examples, Diamond and Orenstein 1990; Starhawk 1988, 1989, 1993; Diamond 1994; Hill 1998). Much as they interpret intuition as both spiritual and embodied, they honor the Goddess as a spiritual reality embodied in the earth and its energy field, and as a metaphor of and for women's creative power, of which birth is but one expression. As Maggie points out above, to serve the Goddess is to learn to give up one's desire for control, to surrender to the ebb and flow of Her inscrutable rhythms.

Spirituality is a strong component of independent midwifery, but there is a great deal of variation in their spiritual orientations. While many home-birth midwives actively celebrate the Goddess or are quite comfortable with the Goddess-as-metaphor, some have a strongly Christian orientation toward birth. Christian midwives tend to interpret birth not so much as a manifesta-

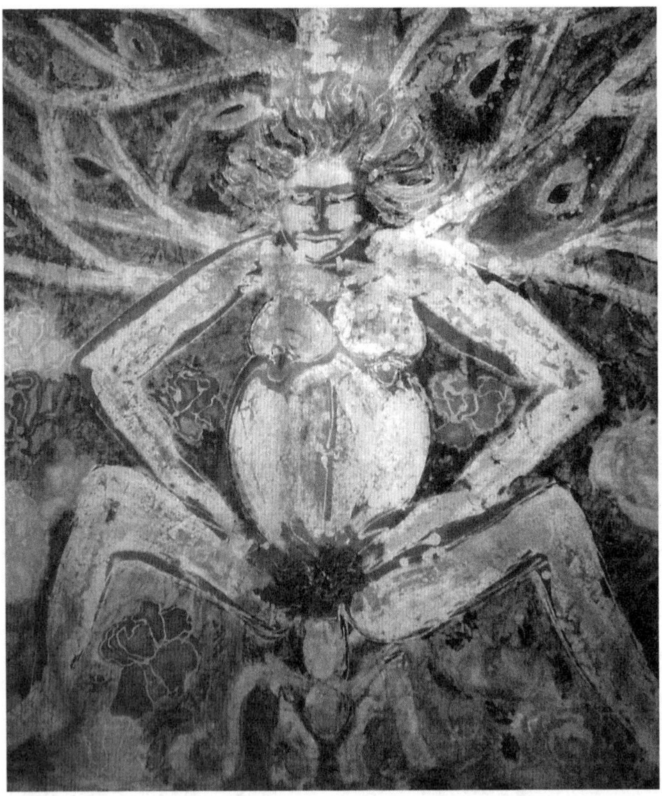

Woman as Goddess and Earth Mother, placenta as Tree of Life. A holistic as well as ecofeminist view of birth presented in a batik by the late Sheila Kitzinger. Photo taken in Sheila's home.

tion of the woman's own personal power but of God's power flowing through the birthing woman. This is the view held by Maggie's client Jane, and the reason why Jane would not appreciate Maggie's calling her a Goddess, which for Maggie is the highest compliment she can give to express her appreciation for Jane's profound inner connectedness and strength.

At this point in Maggie's recounting of this birth, the question of protocols and external diagnostic technologies again came up. The high authority that Maggie placed on her inner knowing during this birth was clearly demonstrated when she said she had never made a decision based on anything that was written on Jane's chart—her blood pressure, urinalysis, information about rate of dilation and progression of labor, and so forth—because, as she put it, "it wouldn't be neat, it wouldn't add up, it wouldn't follow any kind of progression that was any kind of normal anything." I asked: "So why didn't you make an effort to make this labor conform to normal by transporting her?" and Maggie answered:

> Because every time I [checked with Jane, she would tell me that she was fine and that she knew the baby was fine]. And every time I looked at her, and every time I looked inside myself, and every time I saw that—whatever it is—the place where the baby was—the baby was safe. . . . Inside my head I saw the baby safe—and this is my own metaphor, I realize, but I saw the baby surrounded by sparkling light, kind of like glittery flecks of amniotic fluid.
>
> Q. So your inner vision of the baby corresponded with the mother's?
>
> Yes.

This correspondence of Maggie's inner vision with the mother's is a prime example of the kind of connectedness that midwives see as essential for the emergence and the credibility of intuition. Our other interviewees generally agreed on the persuasive power of such correspondence of intuitions. They also agreed that, in the rare instances in which the mother and the midwife have conflicting intuitions about a potential problem during labor, they are clearly not connected. In such a situation, they feel that transport is essential, as this "total lack of synergy" seriously impedes their ability to provide safe and empathic—i.e., connected—care.

Maggie and I explored in further conversation the mystery of why, in some cases, she will urge a woman to transport in the face of a minimum of indicators, while in a case like Jane's she would stay home in the face of a maximum of indicators for transport. We asked her, "Is that a matter of intuition for you every time?" She replied:

> Yes. You see, I don't know about where it all goes together, because I keep charts, and I do signs, and I check dilation, I look at the color of the amniotic fluid, I take blood pressure—I do those kinds of clinical things. . . . But . . . one month I realized that I had been to five births

> within a month, and only one of them fit within protocols. And I had to look at myself and say, I think of myself as a conservative midwife, but what's wrong here if four out of five births are out of protocol, am I a radical midwife, am I a dangerous midwife—what's going on here?
>
> And I really had to evaluate, and look at my charts with somebody else, before I could come up with a picture of me as a midwife, and what I resolved for *me* is that *where birth is not normal, part of a midwife's job is to return it to normal*. For example, in the case of a VBAC, which is regarded medically as high risk and almost universally by midwives as not high risk, what we're doing in that case is returning birth to normal. And when we go four, five, six hours of pushing, we are also returning birth to normal, a normal that says if the woman pushes for three hours and she's exhausted, then she can take a rest, and maybe in a couple of hours, she'll get her strength up, and then she'll be able to push again—she *will* get her baby out. When we do things like that, we're returning birth to normal.

Rather than de- and reconstructing labor to fit abstract and narrowly drawn technocratic parameters of normal—a process that often results in major surgery as the final reconstructive step—what Maggie and her sister midwives do is to continually redraw the parameters, processually expanding their definitions of normal to encompass the range of behaviors and signs actually exhibited by pregnant women as they labor and birth. In short, these midwives are willing to expand protocol parameters to reflect the realities of individual labors, rather than reshaping labor to fit protocol parameters. They see a labor that is unlike other labors not as a dysfunction to be mechanistically normalized according to the standardized technomedical system of authoritative knowledge, but as a meaningful expression of the birthing woman's uniqueness, to be understood on its own terms.

Normalizing Uniqueness

This midwifery *normalization of uniqueness* must be understood in the context of the technomedical standardization of care and pathologization of uniqueness. The technocratic model of birth defines as "normal" only those births that fall within specific parameters—12 hours for active labor, cervical dilation of one centimeter per hour, steady fetal heart tones, etcetera. Labors that take too little or too much time, cervixes that remain "stuck" at four centimeters for hours on end (again, this is simply the latent phase of labor, which can take days), heart tones that speed up or slow down, meconium in the amniotic fluid—all are defined as dysfunctional "deviations from the norm." Aware of technomedical parameters, midwives must constantly weigh their trust in and acceptance of women's individual rhythms against the consequences of straying too far outside the medical protocols that are regarded as authoritative in the courts.

Judy's Story: Letting Go

As in Maggie Bennett's story above, this tension between the techno-medical pathologization and the midwifery normalization of uniqueness is reflected in the following story told by Vermont midwife Judy Luce:

> A woman came to me . . . she was 39 and pregnant with her third child. The first child had been born by cesarean after 37 hours of labor. [The child had a severe genetic defect, and died at the age of three.] And within eight months of that her second child was born, prematurely—a vaginal birth but 31 hours of labor, four hours of pushing, and a forceps delivery for a six-pound ten-ounce baby. So she's due at the end of September, and wants to have a homebirth. She is an artist, she does huge oil paintings, brilliant . . . incredible intensity, vibrant colors, and she did a whole series that tell stories of her first child's birth, of the sickness, the dying, the death, and the grieving. Just a whole series which was so amazing and intense. So, the weight—the birth felt very *heavy* to me. There was a lot staked, not just on having another child, but also on what the birth was going to mean, and you know, the due date came and went and lots of early labor, but nothing happening. You know, it would begin—all-night backaches—but never really taking off . . .
>
> Finally she called and said "My water just broke, and it's really—it has brown meconium in it." So I go dashing over there again, and you know, the pad, her underpants, the floor, it's thick brown. And it's not thin—there's nothing thin about this. I listened to the baby through a couple of contractions, and the baby was wonderful, real reactive. . . . And I felt deeply, intuitively, that this baby was fine, but there was a weight around the whole birth. . . . If she had the baby in an hour, I could stay and deal with this, but [she was only two-to-three centimeters dilated, and] what am I going to do if it's 20 or 30 hours of labor, like the first two times? And how do you defend yourself in court, if the baby aspirates meconium [gets its own poop into its lungs], when you'd have to say, 20 hours ago, I knew this was here?
>
> [So I call my physician backup, and then I talk the couple into going to the hospital.] And the mother felt too grungy to go to the hospital without a bath, so she got in the shower at about 6:08, and I go in, and she's standing there, trying to get out, holding her stomach and going "Unnnhhhhhh" [a common sound women make when they push]. So I get her in the bedroom and check her, and the baby's head is just coming into my hand. And at 6:28 she had an eight-pound baby girl, beautiful birth, no tearing. The baby was clear as a bell, but every bit of the fluid was just filled with meconium—you could just stir it around.
>
> Afterwards, she said to me that when she got in the shower, out of this place she couldn't even touch, this immense grief came up and she cried,

> she just sobbed. Her husband said, "What's the matter?" and she said, "I just need to cry." And she opened, you know. That sobbing—everything opened. And that baby was born. And I think it's about holding on to the integrity of what you're feeling. It's not because you're *right*—there was a dance that went on between us about that decision making, and that space was big enough for that birth to happen. It was just immensely powerful.

Knowing that "there are no guarantees, even with intuition," Judy had been planning, "with grief," as she put it, to take the mother to the hospital in accordance with medical protocols, a decision to which the mother herself had acquiesced. Both of them apparently felt that the mutuality of the decision-making process left room enough, space enough, for the birth to happen at home after all. It was not a question of imposing authority, or even, in this particular case, of anyone holding the key to a particular kind of knowledge that either of them considered authoritative. They both knew that technomedical protocols indicated immediate transport in the case of thick meconium in the amniotic fluid, as the baby is in danger of aspirating the meconium. The midwife also knew, however, that majority of babies born with meconium have no problem with it.[11]

So, even though the midwife decided on transport, she was not anxious or nervous, but relaxed—her intuition told her the baby was fine, and her reason told her there was no cause for undue alarm, as even with meconium, the baby might be better off at home. The midwife's relaxed and accepting attitude allowed the woman the time and space to take the shower and thus to experience the emotional release she needed to be able to open up and give birth. Together, even as they both surrendered to the authoritative technomedical protocols that indicated transport, they still managed to hold a consensual space of connection in which the birth could happen at home—the "decision-making dance," as the midwife called it. In the eyes of midwives, birth has been made abnormal by technocratic medicine. As Judy's story illustrates, the give-and-take of this "dance" is instrumental in midwives' ongoing efforts to normalize uniqueness in birth.[12]

Brigitte Jordan speaks of authoritative knowledge as grounded in a community of practice, adding that within that community "authoritative

[11] As Melissa Cheyney (personal correspondence, 2017) notes, "We know now that meconium aspiration occurs in utero, not after birth. So it is only an issue when the baby is in primary or secondary apnea in utero and they reflexively begin gasping. This is why we don't put suction on the perineum anymore, as this would be too late."

[12] As one anonymous reviewer aptly pointed out, the words "normal" and "abnormal" may not even be appropriate when talking about birth from the standpoint of intuitive knowing, as the concept "normal" "has long been grounded in a worldview that is based on ratiocinative reasoning and the averaging of all experiences into one standardized experience. . . . Foucault's concept of 'normalization' might be an interesting springboard here." Space does not allow us to further address the issue of midwives' efforts to normalize uniqueness vs. medicine's efforts to pathologize it as "deviance," but it is an issue deserving of scholarly probing, and we call attention to it here in the hopes of stimulating further research and analysis.

knowledge is persuasive because it seems natural, reasonable, and consensually constructed. For the same reason, it also carries the possibility of powerful sanctions, ranging from exclusions from the social group to physical coerciveness" (1992:3). Certainly this is true of the authoritative knowledge of the technomedical community. But midwives who act on intuition do so in *opposition* to the cultural consensus on what constitutes authoritative knowledge in birth. Their protocols are their link to that larger biomedical system of authoritative knowledge; like physicians in the hospital, the farther they stray from those parameters, the more they place themselves at risk of the powerful sanctions of which Jordan speaks.

Yet within the midwifery community, intuition does count as authoritative knowledge—to quote Jordan again, "The knowledge that *participants agree* counts in a given situation, that they see as consequential, on the basis of which they make decisions and provide justifications for courses of action" (1992:3; emphasis in original). When Maggie shared her records with other midwives for peer review and evaluation, she was greeted with reassurance and acceptance; in spite of its devaluation, or simply non-recognition by the larger culture, these midwives, too, valued intuition as authoritative.

Jordan points out that "to legitimize one kind of knowing devalues, often totally dismisses, all other ways of knowing, [so that] those who espouse alternative knowledge systems are often seen as backward, ignorant, or naive troublemakers" (1992:2). Her words capture in a nutshell what the larger technomedical culture has done, in this country and many others, to the alternative knowledge systems of midwifery. Hanging out on the ragged edge, far outside of the safety net of cultural consensus, these women of tremendous hearts find their courage not in the normalizing performance of standardized routines, but in their connectedness to the women and babies they attend. As Maggie put it, "Mothers and midwives mirror one another. I know that I get all of my courage from the mother. And I bounce it back to her, and she gets her courage from me. . . . It's a dance—the woman has to trust her midwife, and the midwife has to trust her woman for that bouncing back."

Conclusion: The "Connective Dance"

We value the essential mystery of birth.

We value pregnancy and birth as natural, physiologic and holistic processes that technology will never supplant.

We value the integrity of a woman's body, the inherent rhythm of each woman's labor and the right of each mother and baby to be supported in their efforts to achieve a natural, spontaneous vaginal birth.

We value birth as a personal, intimate, internal, sexual and social experience to be shared in the environment and with the attendants a woman chooses.

> *We value the wisdom of midwifery, an expertise that incorporates theoretical and embodied knowledge, clinical skills, deep listening, intuitive judgment, spiritual awareness and personal experience.*
>
> *We value a mother's intuitive knowledge and innate ability to nurture herself, her unborn baby and her newborn baby.*
>
> *We value our relationship to a process that is larger than ourselves, recognizing that birth is something we can seek to learn from and to know, but cannot control.*
>
> — Excerpts from the MANA Statement of Values and Ethics, 2012

In this chapter, we have sought to examine the phenomenon of midwives' occasional willingness to rely on intuition as a primary source of authoritative knowledge in a society that grants conceptual and legal legitimacy only to ratiocination. We have seen that the trust these midwives place in inner knowing is a seamless part of their overall philosophy, as expressed in the "MANA Statement of Values and Ethics" excerpts quoted above, and as exemplified in the stories they tell about their individual experiences with intuition and birth. In contrast to the technocratic model, which charters an ever-expanding plethora of separation-based diagnostic and remedial technologies, this holistic midwifery philosophy supervalues inter- and intrapersonal connection and charters a range of behaviors expressive of that connective "dance."

Intuition, in these midwives' view, emerges out of their own inner connectedness to the deepest bodily and spiritual aspects of their being, as well as out of their physical and psychic connections to the mother and the child. The trustworthiness of intuition is intrinsically related to its emergence from that matrix of physical, emotional, and spiritual connection—a matrix that gives intuition more power and credibility, in these midwives' views, than the information that arises from the technologies of separation. That midwives nevertheless carry with them and freely utilize such technologies demonstrates not only that they also value ratiocination, but also that they are becoming experts at balancing the protocols and demands of technologically obtained information with their intuitive acceptance of women's uniqueness during labor and birth. We submit that their deep, connective, woman-to-woman webs, woven so lovingly in a society that grants those connections no authority of knowledge and precious little conceptual reality, hold rich potential for restoring the balance of intimacy to the multiple alienations of technocratic life.

Questions for Thought and Discussion

1. Why is intuition so important a source of knowledge for midwives?
2. Is intuition always correct? How do midwives know how to distinguish intuition from fear?
3. In what ways do midwives rely on intuition as authoritative knowledge during birth?

4. What do you think about the intuition stories you read here? Do they make you feel more, or less, confident in midwives' abilities to attend births?
5. Does reason/ratiocination play a role in midwives' decisions about birth care, or do they rely solely on intuition?

Recommended Film

Orgasmic Birth: produced by Debra Pascali-Bonaro. http://www.orgasmicbirth.com/ (Also available under the title *Organic Birth*)

Acknowledgments

We wish to thank anthropologists Carolyn Sargent, Ann Millard, Gay Becker, and midwives Judy Luce, Karen Erlich, Penfield Chester, Anne Frye, Marimikel Potter, and Sharon Wells for their excellent editorial assistance, four anonymous reviewers for their useful suggestions, and our midwife-interviewees for giving so generously of their time and experience. Robbie also expresses her appreciation to her wonderful student-intern Christina Weis for help updating the references in this chapter.

APPENDIX

Items that a Typical American Homebirth Midwife Carries with Her to a Homebirth

- a cell phone
- a computer or tablet for electronic charting (a recent technological improvement that midwives love because they always have access to these charts, as does the mother)
- a blood pressure cuff
- a stethoscope
- a fetoscope and/or a Doppler—a handheld ultrasound fetal heartbeat monitor
- sterile gauze
- antiseptics—alcohol, peroxide, Betadine, or Hibiclens
- alcohol prep pads
- flashlights
- urinalysis strips (to test for glucose, ketones, pH, blood, and protein)
- nitrazine paper (to test for leaks in the amniotic sac)
- urinary catheter kits
- sterile KY gel

- a variety of herbs, tinctures, and homeopathic remedies, including rescue remedy (for severe stress), arnica (for skin swelling and trauma), black cohosh or colophyllum (homeopathic blue cohosh) (for enhancing contractions), evening primrose oil (for assisting cervical dilation), spirits of peppermint (for assisting bladder function—often can be used instead of a catheter), angelica (for assisting placental expulsion), shepherd's purse (for preventing postpartum hemorrhage), herbs for afterpains, and valerian (for relaxation)
- olive oil for perineal massage (less and less frequently used as evidence has shown that simple perineal support is sufficient)
- a birthing stool
- an amni-hook for breaking the waters if they are still intact when the baby crowns
- waterproof pads and sheets
- an oxygen tank, mask for the mother, and infant resuscitation bag and mask (rarely used)
- special scissors for cutting an episiotomy (rarely used)
- syringes and drugs (injectable pitocin, Cytotec to stop a postpartum hemorrhage)
- IV lines and fluids
- instruments and sutures for repairing vaginal tears
- sheets to create a sterile barrier field while suturing
- a small lamp (for visibility during suturing)
- a local anesthetic (xylocaine or lidocaine) for numbing the skin during suturing
- a heating pad to assist in warming the baby
- a bulb syringe (for suctioning the baby's airways—rarely used anymore as airway suctioning has been shown to be unnecessary most of the time), and DeLee or Res-q-vac Suction Catheters (for sucking amniotic fluid out of the deeper respiratory passages of the newborn—rarely used)
- assorted hemostats and clamps
- special scissors for cutting the cord (current recommendations are to keep the cord dry and not put anything on it)
- scales for weighing the baby and a tape measure
- injectable or oral vitamin K
- erythromycin ointment (to place in the baby's eyes to prevent blindness from venereal disease—a requirement in most states)
- footprint pads in multi-colors (for taking the baby's footprint for the birth certificate)
- sitzbath herbs (for soothing the woman's vaginal area postpartum)
- red-top sterile vacuum tubes (for collecting umbilical cord blood for testing)
- a file full of papers for charting, preparing the birth certificate, etc.

Most midwives carry enough supplies with them at any one time to attend two or three births in a row without having to repack. Some midwives also carry:

- physician-prescribed antibiotics and Phenergan suppositories for stopping violent vomiting

- a laryngeal mask airway to create an airway in preparation for transport
- a pulse oximeter for checking babies' oxygen levels and screening for critical congenital heart defects
- breast shields (for cracked nipples) and breast shells (for helping the nipples to become more prominent so the baby can more easily latch on to the breast)
- a newborn screening kit (this kit consists of a lancet and a specially treated piece of paper, on which the midwife places samples of the baby's blood to be sent to the health department and checked for metabolic disorders)

[The above information was gleaned from a questionnaire handed out to 30 and returned by 25 homebirth midwives, all of whom were members of MANA back in 1995, and has been updated (August 2016) by Debbie Pulley CPM.]

8

Daughter of Time[1]

The Postmodern Midwife

with Etsuko Matsuoka, Holly Horan, Bonnie Ruder, and Courtney L. Everson

The Transnational Nature of Midwifery Knowledge: A Contemporary Exemplar

One bright winter's day in Oslo, Norway, in September of 2007, three of us who were speakers at the Midwifery Today conference being held in that fair city went to explore its amazing outdoor ethnographic museum, which contains homes and other buildings from many centuries that have been moved there and reconstructed. Turning a corner, we were overjoyed to see a lovely garden with a sign informing us that it contained every species of plant ever used by healers of all types from all historical periods and continents. Exclaiming in delight, my companions Elizabeth Davis, an American homebirth midwife (coauthor of Chapter 7), and Angelina Martinez Miranda,

[1] The title for this article, "Daughter of Time," originated in a song written in 1977 by American midwife Mary Offerman. The label expresses a hope that women today will be empowered to recuperate knowledges and skills maintained by women in the past, revitalize them for the present, and preserve them for the future. The phrase was further cemented in American midwifery lore in the early 1980s through a film about nurse-midwives called *Daughters of Time* (Durrin 1982—I have the date but can find no information about how to obtain the film) and through Barbara Katz Rothman's (1998) article by that title.

The original version of this chapter appeared as an article in *MIDIRS Midwifery Digest* 15(1): 32–39, 2005. This version has been greatly updated and expanded.

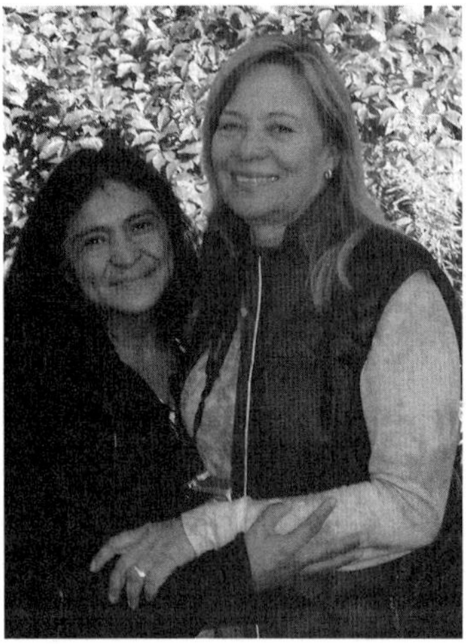

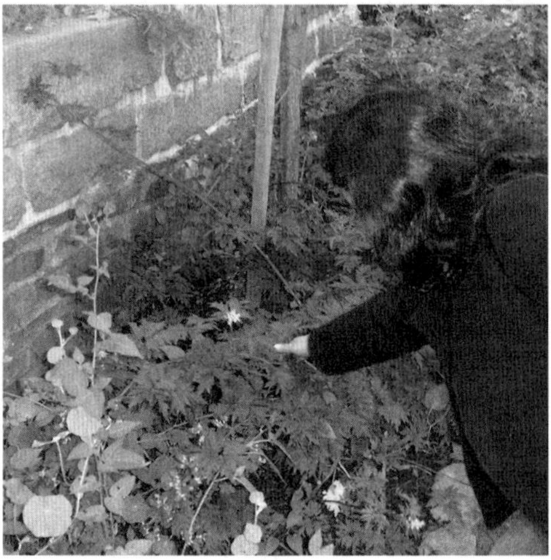

[left] Angelina Martinez Miranda and Elizabeth Davis, two thoroughly postmodern midwives—one traditional, the other professional, in the Botanical Garden at Norway's outdoor ethnographic museum. [right] Angelina caressing the plants and discussing their uses with Elizabeth, with myself as translator.

a Mexican partera tradicional (traditional midwife), knelt down to caress the plants and detail their uses. To my fascination, although they had different names for each plant, both of these midwives from disparate backgrounds and countries used each plant in exactly the same ways for exactly the same things. And there began for me a deeper, more visceral understanding of the transnational and transcultural nature of postmodern midwifery knowledge.

For past millennia, midwives have served women in childbirth. In premodern times, midwives were usually the only birth attendants. With the Industrial Revolution and the arrival of modernism, male physicians either replaced midwives or superseded them in the modernist medical hierarchy, leaving them with plenty of women to attend but with relatively little autonomy. As the new millennium dawns on a growing worldwide biomedical hegemony over birth, midwives—the daughters of time and tradition—find themselves negotiating their identities, searching for appropriate roles, and developing new rationales for their continued existence.

Back to the Future: Premodern, Modern, and Postmodern

In order to understand my use of the term "postmodern" in relation to midwives, we must first take a brief glimpse at the terms "modern" and "premodern" because all three terms create both an historical and a futuristic spectrum. "Modernity" as I see it is a narrow canal through which the vast majority of contemporary cultures have passed or are passing. The process of modernization began in various parts of the world at different times; first in the industrializing countries of the North, and more slowly in the colonized and exploited countries of the South. So anthropologists consider "modernism" or "modernity" not to be a particular point in time but rather a univariate (single-pointed, single-minded, unvarying) orientation toward "progress," defined in terms of Westernized forms of education, technologization, infrastructural development (railways, highways, waterways, airways, and electronic systems, etc.), factory production, economic growth, and the development of the global marketplace. This univariate orientation identifies a single point in a given area toward which development should be progressing: in economics, that single point is capitalism; in health care, it is Western biomedicine. Thus in modernizing societies traditional systems of healing, including midwifery, have become increasingly regarded by members of the growing middle and upper classes as "premodern vestiges" of a more backward time that must necessarily vanish as modernization/biomedicalization progresses. I use the term "premodern" simply to mean all that was before "modernization." A steadily decreasing number of cultures around the world still live in a relatively "premodern" state; almost all of them are subject to the pressures of modernization.

Modernity's Progression toward Univariate Points

- In economics, capitalism
- In national development, the building of infrastructures: water, sewage, electricity, telephones, and transportation systems (water-, air-, rail-, and highways)
- In production, the elimination of the small in favor of the large: industrial agriculture and the factory production of goods
- In education, university
- In health care, biomedicine

Yet around the world, the univariate orientation of modernization is increasingly contested. Postmodern thinking widens the narrow canal of modernization beyond uncritical acceptance of modernization as good, noting the enormous environmental, social, and cultural damage modernization entails, and seeking to generate more polymorphous societies in which multiple knowledge and belief systems can coexist and complement each other. In postmodern societies and groups, conservation and preservation of the envi-

Some of the Many Costs of Modernity

- The colonization of most of the world by a few Western capitalist and industrial countries
- The ongoing elimination of subsistence agriculture and indigenous cultures
- Massive worldwide pollution of the environment and its concomitant health costs to people and the planet
- The supervaluation of "the modern" and the devaluation of indigenous cultures and knowledge systems

ronment and of indigenous or traditional languages, cosmologies, health care, and economic systems take on particular urgency and importance, and such endeavors are sometimes considered to be more important than expanding the reach of industrialization, capitalism, and biomedicine. Postmodernism as I define it here in effect means going "back to the future" to scoop up the many good things that remain from the premodern world to bring them with us to replace univariate modernism with a more expansive, multimodal global society.

Postmodern efforts at conservation are fueled both by global organizations and by myriad local grassroots social movements. In the cultural arena of childbirth, for example, as some governments and development planners urge the elimination of traditional birthways and the traditional midwives who practice them (usually called "traditional birth attendants" [TBAs] in government and development agency lexicons), other international workers seek to conserve them. Many indigenous women who have tried out government-funded hospitals and clinics subsequently reject them because of the impersonal, dehumanizing care they receive there, and deliberately return to TBAs/traditional midwives for out-of-hospital birth. In some regions, professional midwives trained in a modernist ideology of biomedical superiority act, in fact, superior, while other professional and traditional midwives are displaying a variety of creative and highly relativistic responses to biomedical encroachment and constraints.

My familiarity with midwives and midwifery systems in many countries leads me to see the midwife/TBA distinction not as a dichotomy but as a continuum, so I prefer the labels "professional midwives" (to indicate those who have had professional training) and "traditional midwives," to indicate those who practice within the traditions of their communities, without professional degrees or certifications, but who are recognized as midwives within those communities.

Informed Relativism: The Characteristics of the Postmodern Midwife

Around the world we are witnessing the emergence of a phenomenon that I call *postmodern midwifery*—a term aimed at capturing those aspects of contemporary midwifery practice that fall outside easy distinctions between traditional birthways, professional midwifery, and modern biomedicine. With this term, I am trying to highlight the qualities that emerge from the praxis, the discourse, and the political engagement of a certain kind of contemporary midwife—one who often constructs a radical critique of unexamined conventions and univariate assumptions. Postmodern midwives as I define them are relativistic, articulate, organized, political, and highly conscious of both their cultural uniqueness and their global importance. By "postmodern midwife," I specifically do not mean midwives who accept without criticism either their own folk system or that of biomedicine, but rather midwives who fully understand these in a relative way, as different ways of knowing about birth, discrepant systems that often conflict but can be complementary.

Postmodern midwives are scientifically informed: they know the limitations and strengths of the biomedical system and of their own, and can move fluidly between them. These midwives play with the paradigms, working to ensure that the uniquely woman-centered dimensions of midwifery are not subsumed by biomedicine. They are shape-shifters, knowing how to subvert the medical system while appearing to comply with it, bridge-builders, making alliances with biomedicine, development agencies, governments, and consumers where possible, and networkers, attending conferences and meetings and making connections with other midwives in other parts of the world. Such networking increases their ability to translate between systems, and to gain consciousness of midwifery as a worldwide movement. These transnational interlinkages among midwives work to create a global culture of midwifery as well as to preserve, carry forward, and teach to others the best of one's own cultural traditions around birth.

Lacking or actively rejecting a sense of structural inferiority to biomedicine, the postmodern midwife is free to observe the benefits of traditional midwifery practices common in many cultures, such as massage, external version (turning the baby in utero to the head-down position best for birth), eating and drinking during labor, birthing in upright positions, birthing at home, and uninterrupted contact between mother and baby. A comparison with what takes place in the hospital and what can be learned from scientific evidence results in the conclusion that there is value in the midwifery approach that biomedicine does not recognize. The postmodern midwife then develops a sense of mission around preserving that approach in the face of biomedical encroachment, and an understanding that *for midwives, the professional is always political*: midwives and their colleagues must have an organized political voice if they are to survive. So postmodern midwives work to build organizations in their communities to create unified voices, join national and international midwifery organizations, and work within them for policies and legislation that support midwives and the mothers they attend. It would be easy to conclude that only professional midwives, with their greater access to high technologies and international networking systems, can achieve the *informed relativism* I am highlighting as the primary characteristic of the postmodern midwife. But traditional midwives in many countries are undergoing radical changes, to which they often respond with an emergent, critically engaged postmodern consciousness.

CHARACTERISTICS OF THE POSTMODERN MIDWIFE

- An informed relativism that encompasses science, traditional midwifery knowledge, professional midwifery knowledge, and complementary or alternative (holistic) practice systems
- A desire to keep learning, growing, and incorporating new techniques
- Cultural competence and sensitivity
- Willingness to collaborate with other types of midwives and practitioners
- A sense of mission around preserving midwifery in the best interests of women and babies
- A sense of autonomy as practitioners
- Dedication to the midwifery model of care and to midwifery and women's health care as social movements
- Local, global, and historical awareness of the past and present context of midwifery
- A vision for the future of midwifery both locally and globally
- Political engagement, including work with governmental authorities and participation in local, regional, national, and international organizations to try to achieve that vision

A Short Story: How I Came to Identify and Understand "The Postmodern Midwife"

I am grateful to two midwives—one traditional and one professional—for helping me to more deeply understand the meaning of the word "postmodern" and to conceive the notion of "the postmodern midwife." In 1991, midwife and anthropologist Janneli Miller and I were both participants in a MANA conference held in El Paso, Texas. It was the first MANA conference in which Mexican midwives were well-represented; Alison Bastien, a professional direct-entry midwife from San Miguel, Guanajuato, Mexico, had found scholarship money to bring a group of traditional Mexican midwives to this conference, where they presented their own workshops and talks.

Wanting to honor these "wise elders," the American midwives prepared a form of Blessingway ceremony, placing four chairs with their backs to each other, with each chair facing one of the four cardinal directions. The four eldest Mexican midwives were seated in the chairs; the mostly much younger American midwives made a circle around them, one-by-one kneeling in front of them, and offering them small gifts, murmuring words of appreciation, and bathing their feet with corn meal.

As the ceremony progressed, I was reflecting on the anthropological irony of young, mostly white, American midwives who, though certainly not wealthy, had far more money, far bigger and nicer homes and far more possessions than the Mexican midwives they were, effectively, worshipping, and who probably had no idea of how those midwives lived—some of them in dirt-floored huts serving women who could barely pay them, if at all. And I was wondering what those Mexican midwives were thinking about during the ceremony. Meanwhile, Janneli turned to me and exclaimed softly, "How postmodern!" And suddenly I understood, in a visceral, emotional way, what "postmodern"—a word bandied about in anthropology in hundreds of complex contexts—really means.

That understanding was deepened at the end of the ceremony, when my unasked question about what the Mexican midwives were thinking was answered by Doña Enriqueta Contreras, an accomplished traditional midwife and well-known speaker, who stood up and said (in Spanish with translation) in her clear and carrying voice, "We did not know what we signified to you.

Doña Enriqueta Contreras, who has recorded her extensive healing knowledge of plants and other techniques in her beautiful book *Medicina Tradicional: Doña Queta y El Legado de Los Habitantes de las Nubes* (2009), which contains color photos of every plant she describes. Photo taken in Robbie's home in Austin, where Queta had been invited to teach a workshop for Mexican American women to help them "get back to their roots," and another for a group of psychologists who felt the need for more connectedness and spirituality in their lives. She told me that "healers are often the ones most in need of healing."

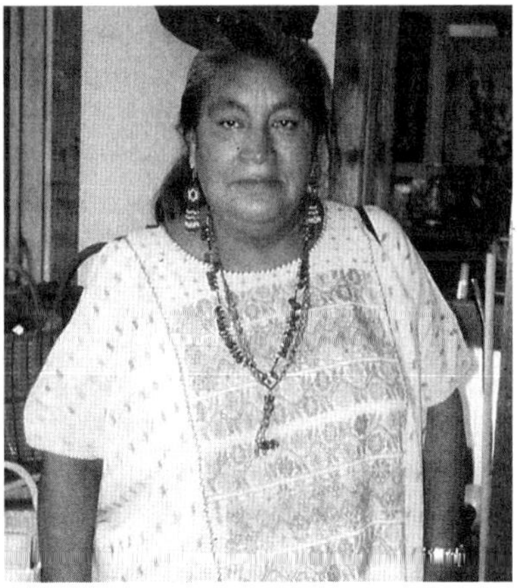

Now we understand that for you, we represent connection to Mother Earth, and to community, and to tradition, and to the ancestors who came before us. We are honored to represent those essential elements of life to you, and by your gracious honoring of us. Thank you, from our hearts!" (my translation, from memory). With those words, Doña Queta, as she is fondly known, made it clear that she understood, in an entirely postmodern way, what the American midwives had intended to accomplish in that ceremony, and that she in no way blamed or judged them for their much higher socioeconomic status nor for the fact that some form of ongoing financial support would have been far more helpful to those traditional midwives than tiny gifts and cornmeal. It was the spirit and the intention that counted, and Doña Queta made it clear that she "got it," with a graciousness that remains unmatched in my experience.

Postmodern Traditional Midwives

Previous studies of traditional midwives have painted them as unself-conscious participants in their local folk systems, as structurally subordinate practitioners relative to modern biomedical practitioners, and/or as essentially obsolete—that is, as phased out altogether by the advent of biomedicine. These descriptions seemed inadequate to capture the self-awareness, relativistic perspective, political savvy, and drive toward autonomy I was encountering in my research on American and Mexican midwives (Davis-Floyd 1998b, 2000b, 2001a, b, 2003a, 2006, 2010). I formulated the notion of "the postmodern midwife" to encompass the informed relativism of not only the various internationally-oriented professional midwives but also of the increasing numbers of traditional midwives who are trying to renegotiate their identities and to articulate new ways of practice and new rationales for maintaining themselves as viable practitioners.

Anthropological research on birthing has shown the heterogeneity in the roles of folk specialists who provide birth assistance worldwide. Some are respected healers who offer both maternity and general health care. Others are low-status birth attendants who simply perform the "polluting" tasks associated with birth, while decisions about how to manage labor rest with the family, as in some parts of South Asia. Some perpetuate physiologically harmful traditions like using cow dung to seal the umbilical stump or laying the baby on a pile of dirty rags until the placenta is born (perceived as the moment of greatest danger in many indigenous societies due to the possibility of hemorrhage); others (or sometimes those same practitioners) perpetuate physiologically beneficial traditions like birth in upright positions. Some folk or traditional midwives operate from within relatively closed knowledge systems (see Davis-Floyd 2004b), while others expand their traditional systems to encompass a wide range of concepts and practices from other systems.

While some traditional midwives are compassionate and woman-centered, others crossly order women to comply with their commands. For example, Jordan (1993) reported how midwives in the Yucatan sometimes stuffed a birthing woman's braid down her throat to make her gag so her pushing would be more effective, and Graham (1999) documented the occasional slap a traditional Ugandan midwife might administer to snap a woman out of self-pity during labor. Traditional midwives do not all share in "the midwifery model" of woman-centered care, and the only real unity that can be found among them is their international classification as "traditional birth attendants" (TBAs).

By contrast, the traditional midwives I am identifying as *postmodern* hold and adhere to "the midwifery model of care"—indeed, I developed the concept of the postmodern midwife as a way of bridging the definitional gap between TBAs and professional midwives who share the same essential characteristics, including humanism, a sense of autonomy, a high level of political engagement, and most especially, informed relativism.

Postmodern Traditional Midwives in Mexico: Negotiating Knowledge Systems

Imagine my surprise when I rounded a corner in a birth center owned by Doña Facunda, a *partera tradicional* in Morelos, Mexico, and encountered a flat marble delivery table, complete with metal stirrups. Laughing as I expressed my amazement, Doña Facunda, with a mischievous glint in her eye, pointed out that the fathers, mothers-in-law, and grandmothers who accompany her clients believe in the efficacy of the hospital and its procedures, including giving birth in the lithotomy position. "If they want me to act like a little doctor (*mini-médico*)," she said, holding up her blue hat and booties, "I

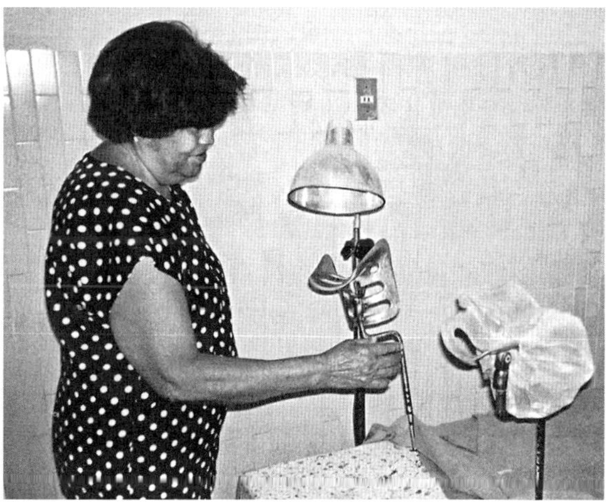

Doña Facunda and her marble medical delivery table.

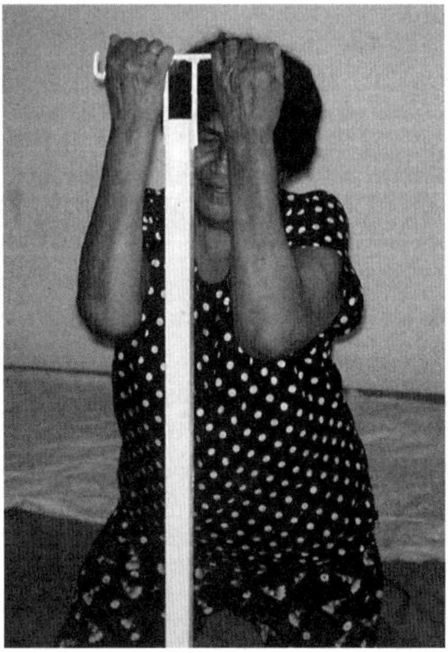

Doña Facunda demonstrating using her IV pole for the "hanging squat" birthing position.

can do that! But when the mother-in-law says, 'Shouldn't she get up on the table now?' I say, 'No, it's not time yet,' and I encourage her to keep walking around or to rest comfortably in my big double bed. Most of my mothers give birth sitting, kneeling, or squatting. Very few want the table. It's here if they do, but its main use is just for show!" She added, "If having an IV makes them feel safer, for an extra 100 pesos I'm happy to insert it. . . . But I encourage them to wait before they get up on the table, until they are really pushing well, and then they find they like being upright." In what I have since come to think of as the perfect postmodern midwifery moment, Doña Facunda added, "So this is what we mostly use the IV pole for!" as she grabbed the metal handles from which the IV bag would be suspended and used them to support herself in the upright birth position known as the "hanging squat."

Irony compounds irony in the postmodern midwifery world! Doña Facunda was fully aware that the hanging squat (which usually involves the woman squatting in front of a support person, who sustains her under the arms and sometimes by the knees) is not per se a traditional birthing position—most of which involve the woman squatting or kneeling alone or on a birthing stool or chair, often pulling on a pole or rope. Rather, the hanging squat had been named and displayed around the world by French physician and author Michel Odent. Facunda had attended one of his lectures in Mexico City a few years before. Her self-conscious transformation of the biomedical IV pole into a support mechanism for the hanging squat perfectly exemplifies what I mean by "postmodern midwifery": a traditional midwife appropriates a biomedical artifact (1) to implicitly critique its normative use in modernist medicine; (2) to reinforce her traditional birthing system (which has long utilized upright positions for birth); and (3) to expand it to include a birthing technique currently in vogue in the international birth activist and midwifery communities.

Such examples (I could cite many!) confound the overdetermined association of "midwife" with "tradition." They confront us with novel combinations, ironies, and unexpected juxtapositions. They highlight the fact that exchanges of knowledge and technology across locales increasingly muddle our attempts to find "authentic" cultural practices and value systems. Most of all, they underscore the inadequacy of the modernist tale of linear "progress" that has for so long been used to narrate the relationship of midwifery to the biomedical management of birth.

TBA training courses and other forms of exposure to biomedicine have resulted in fundamental alterations in practice for many traditional midwives in Mexico. Across the country, it is now common for traditional midwives to give pitocin injections to hurry labor, insert IVs for hydration, and wear blue biomedical garb when attending births—practices that they themselves think of as "modern." Combining such practices with the traditional *sobada* (massage), herbal treatments, and religious beliefs, Mexico's contemporary traditional midwives practice at the intersection of various cultural domains. These trends have particularly influenced midwives who practice in urban areas, as my extensive interviews with Doña Facunda and her colleagues who

Michel Odent using the hanging squat to support a birthing woman, with the midwife patiently waiting to receive the newborn. According to Michel (personal correspondence 2017), "This picture was taken unexpectedly in 1982 by a Japanese visitor (Lyu Anabusa) who had half opened a door by mistake. It was published in *Birth Reborn* (Pantheon, NY, 1984). (An important visible fact: the electric radiator has been switched on at the very time when the baby's head was visible as a way to facilitate the release of a vital peak of oxytocin within 2 or 3 minutes after birth to help ensure safe delivery of the placenta.) Although I was reluctant, the editor of Pantheon had convinced me about the importance of photos at that phase of the history of human births. Since that time, in a dozen books (including *The Functions of the Orgasm*), I have never presented photos and I have written about cameras as the most dangerous tools one can introduce in a birthing place. The issue is neocortical inhibition, a key to understanding human nature in general and human birth in particular. Have you tried to make love in front of cameras?" [Robbie's note: I don't agree with his position—I don't think taking pictures of a birth interferes with it—from personal experience, I can say that during labor, you are so focused on the task at hand that the camera is completely irrelevant. But I thought his words deserved to be heard.]

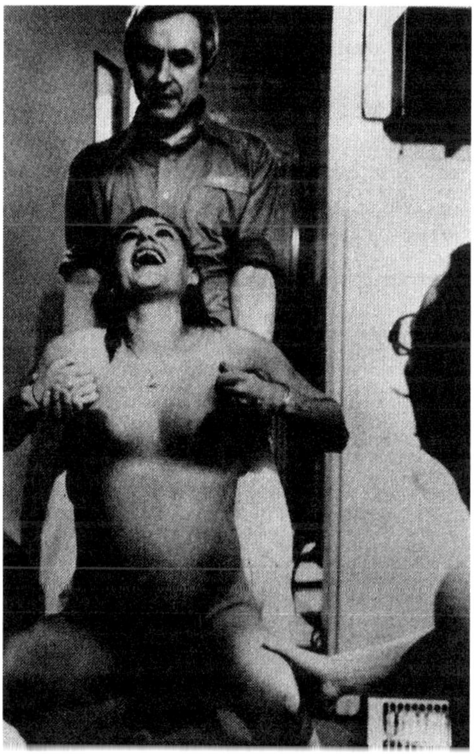

live and practice in the city of Cuernavaca (in central Mexico) reveal. Most of these traditional midwives are in their 50s, 60s, and even 70s, attended only elementary school, and many became fully literate in their 30s. For around three decades, they have been incorporated into the state health care system in Morelos through bimonthly seminars on family planning and other topics.

All of them went through a period of using allopathic interventions like oxytocin injections and experiencing complications as a result, so they returned to the use of traditional herbs—in other words, they went through a process of modernization and came out, as they themselves say, "on the other side." Marina Rodriguez, who is both a nurse and a traditional midwife, explained the difference between the biomedical and traditional systems as follows: "Allopathy is powerful, but it does too much. Its interventions are too extreme. Our traditional herbs take longer to work, but their effects are much more subtle and more precise." (It is worth noting that when these midwives use herbs to stimulate, or slow, labor or to stop a hemorrhage, they often give the mother not just a cup, but usually a thermos-full or more. Thus the beverage serves also as hydration and to aid in electrolyte balance.)

Today traditional Mexican midwives like Marina routinely send women out for ultrasounds when they diagnose a breech or transverse (side-lying) presentation and offer their clients an eclectic potpourri of traditional and biomedical techniques. Into this mix they add multiple "New Age" or "alternative" modalities that they have studied (reflexology, homeopathy, iridology, Reiki, etc.). Many have birth centers attached to their houses, complete with autoclaves, sterile equipment, and two double beds, one for the birthing woman plus an extra one for family members. Some of them own Dopplers, and use them with delight to exhibit their technological expertise and to let the pregnant woman and family members hear the baby's heartbeat. Their walls are covered with laminated diagrams of fetal positions and the female reproductive cycle, and with certificates from the dozens of continuing education courses they have taken at local universities on topics from anatomy to aromatherapy. Their shelves are filled with homeopathic remedies and herbal oils and salves they have learned to make in such courses. Most of them by now have computers, email addresses, and smartphones.

Dancing fluidly at the interface of biomedicine, holistic alternatives, and traditional birthways, these midwives are strategically negotiating the boundaries between knowledge systems and creatively producing a hybrid and increasingly well-articulated knowledge system of their own. These postmodern midwives of Cuernavaca elide and confound the usual distinctions between professional and traditional midwives: trained through traditional apprenticeships, they are presently engaged in a visible process of self-professionalization. Their efforts constitute a very conscious attempt to preserve homebirth in the face of biomedical hegemony: practicing as they do in a city whose hospitals have cesarean rates of over 70%, they are very aware that they often constitute the *only* alternative to a cesarean.

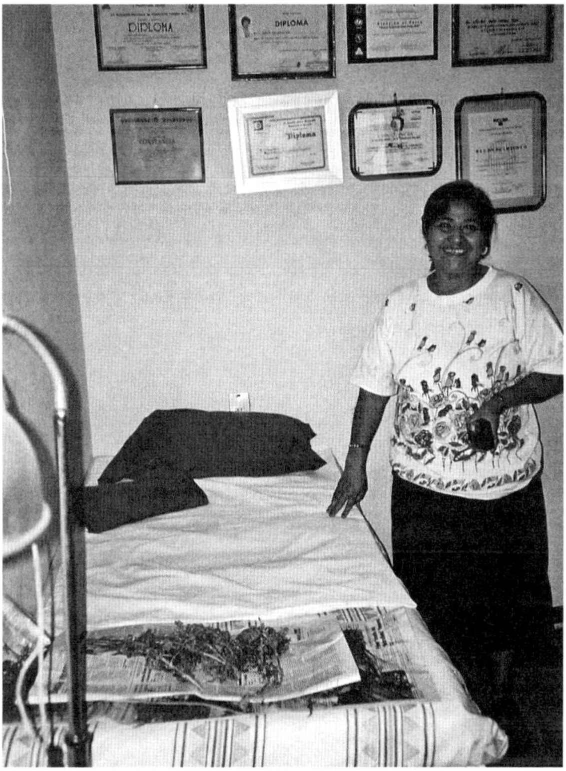

Marina Rodriguez in her prenatal exam room, which is part of her house. Note the traditional herbs drying on the professional exam table and the continuing education certificates displayed on her wall—there are dozens more in drawers. They demonstrate her commitment to learning and growing, even though there was no national certification that she could achieve.

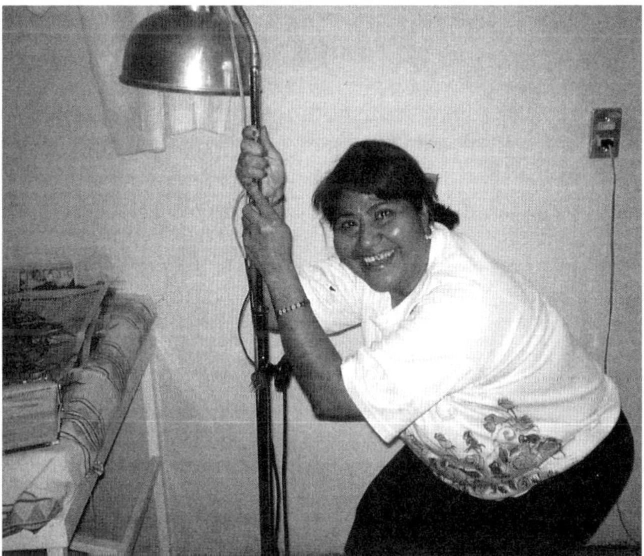

Marina demonstrating using her lamppost as an artifact to assist a squatting position for birth.

Many traditional midwives still practice autonomously, except when they need to transport a client to the hospital (see Chapter 10). Thus their major desire is not for autonomy, which they have, but for some form of governmental or professional recognition above and beyond the status of "TBA." Aware that professional midwives have such recognition, and of the many benefits it confers, postmodern traditional midwives like Doña Facunda and Doña Irene of Morelos, and Doña Queta and Doña Nieves of Oaxaca, long for national certification and state licensure as the professionals they feel themselves to be, in spite of their lack of governmentally accepted training. But their status as TBAs has kept them in limbo, blocking them from recognition as professionals.

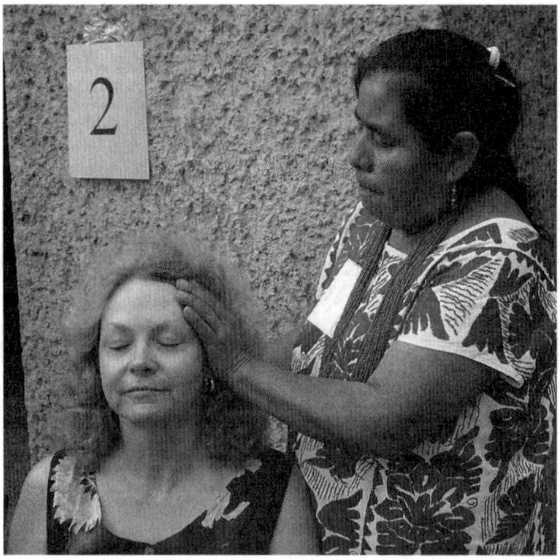

Doña Nieves giving me an herbal head massage to restore my energy at a Midwifery Today conference in Oaxaca City. She kindly offered because she noticed that I was exhausted—I had just given two long workshops back-to-back and was about to translate for another one. Before the massage, I simply felt too drained to go on; after it I was completely reinvigorated! Photo by Jan Tritten

I have personally met and spoken with traditional midwives from Costa Rica, Nicaragua, Honduras, El Salvador, Guatemala, Brazil, and Russia who also exemplify my profile of the postmodern midwife, so I know that the postmodernity of these Mexican midwives is not unique in the world. I suspect that their efforts to renegotiate their identities and restructure their practices to meet the demands of a changing world are mirrored by other postmodern traditional midwives in many countries, and therefore I suggest that much more ethnographic research on such postmodern traditional midwives should be conducted. To that end, I provide the following brief portrait of a postmodern traditional midwife from Morelos, Mexico, with whom I worked and interviewed over the course of years and whom I came to value as a treasured colleague and friend.

Portrait of a Postmodern Traditional Mexican Midwife: Doña Irene Sotelo

For decades, Doña Irene Sotelo was the most highly respected traditional midwife and healer in the state of Morelos. She was born and raised in the state of Guerrero in El Puente Rio San Juan in the *municipio* of Cocula and completed primary school. She began assisting the aging village midwife at the age of 16 and then served as community midwife for 11 years. She attended births for over 40 years. In 1977, when the sugarcane factory in which her husband worked closed, she and her family moved to the big city of Cuernavaca. She lived in the *barrio* of Tejalpa, in the municipio of Juitepec, just east of the city, for over 30 years in an attractive house built by her construction worker husband, Don Bolivar. Attached to the house on one side was a spacious birth center with two twin beds, a few tables and chairs, and a closet where she kept her midwifery equipment. Unlike most of the other traditional midwives in this urbanized region, Doña Irene did not wear blue medical garb to attend births; she wore street clothes over which she tied the plastic apron given to her by UNICEF upon completion of the requisite two-week TBA training course.

By the time she took this course (1991) to obtain her official government registration, she had attended over 3,000 births. During the week of in-hospital training that was part of the course, she was called in to quiet a woman in labor who had been scheduled for a cesarean because of a transverse presentation. Recognizing Irene as a traditional midwife, the mother pleaded with her, "Don't let them cut me!" So Irene closed the door and performed an external version, turning the baby to a head presentation. When the baby crowned, Irene ran to call the physician (she was not allowed to catch babies in the hospital), who arrived just in time. About this experience, she said that she was very glad she had been able to save a mother from an unnecessary cesarean but regretted deeply that the doctor, who wanted her to learn about medical procedures for birth, had no respect for her traditional knowledge. She said that physicians believe versions (the manual turning of the baby in the uterus) are dangerous, but that in her experience the safety of versions depends on the context.

Her method for external versions first involved both the mother and the midwife sharing a beer (remember Maggie's story in Chapter 7?) to ensure that both were relaxed. Then she would give the mother a full-body massage so that Irene's hands would know the mother's body and the mother would be as relaxed as possible. Then she would have the mother turn onto her hands and knees and wrap a *rebozo* (traditional shawl) around her bottom while Irene held both ends in her hands; she would then stand at the mother's head and perform a *manteada* (shaking), pulling the rebozo back and forth to loosen the baby from the pelvis so that it would be as free-floating as possible. Then Irene would have the mother lie on her back, and Irene would begin moving her hands on the mother's belly, gently pressing to turn the baby, and talking to the baby all the while, asking it to turn. If she felt any resistance, she would stop, because that might mean that the cord was too tight for the baby to turn or could cause the placenta to detach.

Once while attempting a version some years ago, she was having great difficulty getting the baby to move and suddenly a song came into her head. Irene sang the song twice and the baby turned, and so since then she has sung it to babies she is seeking to turn, many times with great success. Once she

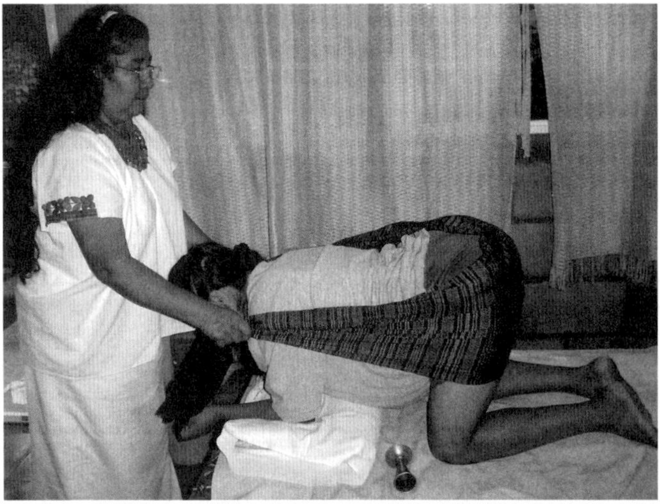

Doña Irene performing the manteada prior to attempting a successful external version.

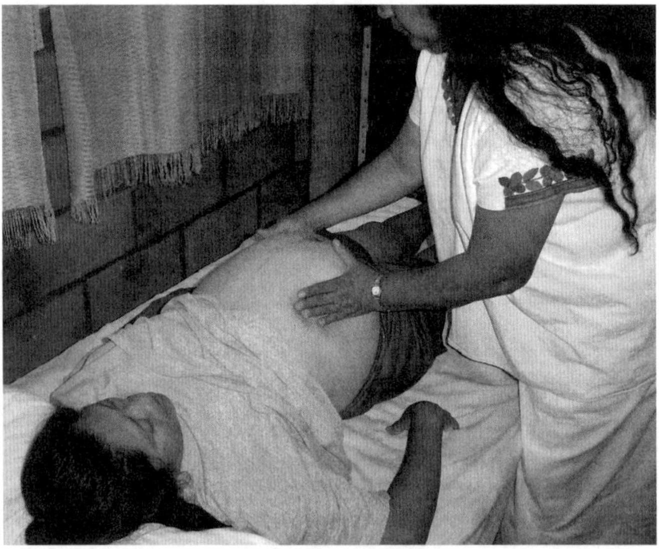

Irene performing an external version after the beer, the full-body massage, and the manteada.

sang it at a conference onstage—I had put the words on PowerPoint for her so everyone could sing along—and of course, all of us in the audience cried. I perform this song in my talks whenever relevant, in an effort to keep it alive and spread it around the world as widely as I can. And here it is for you:

Bebé, acomódate bebé (Baby, accommodate yourself baby)
No es hora de nacer (It's not time to be born)
No lastimes a Mama (Don't hurt Mommy)

Bebé, acomódate bebé (Baby, accommodate yourself baby)
Te esperamos con amor (We are waiting for you with love)
Pedazito de mi ser (Little piece of my being)

Below is the musical score for the song, created for me by musician Brian Hudson:

Acomódate Bebé

Doña Irene Sotelo

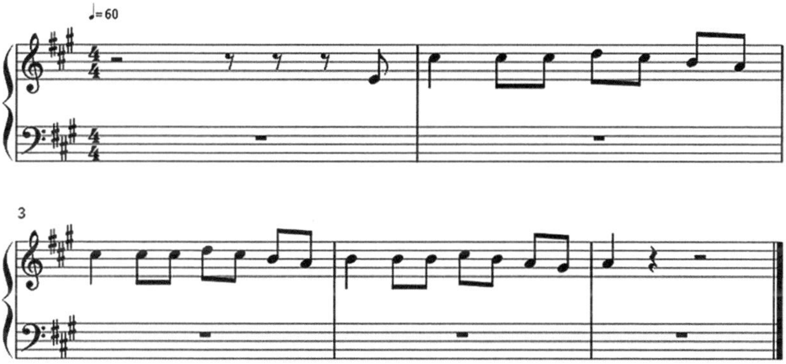

My translation above is literal but does not match the melody. Here is my non-literal translation, which does match the melody—should you wish to, please feel free to use as is or make up your own version in your own language:

Baby, please turn around now Baby
It's not time yet to be born
You don't want to hurt your mom

Baby, please turn around now Baby
We wait for you with love
Little piece of my own soul [or, if you want it to rhyme, you can change this line to:
Little gift from God above]

Irene's working day might begin in the middle of the night with the arrival of a woman in labor (on average she attended around five births per month), but usually began around 7:00 AM with the ringing of the front bell. Soon a line of clients would be waiting in her small garden, sitting and chatting in the plastic chairs she provided. She greeted them individually at a wooden desk in her exam room; the light and airy room contained two high exam tables topped with soft foam mattresses and pillows. She carefully recorded each client's history, then invited him or her onto a table for a check over. She treated a wide variety of ailments, from kidney infections and ingrown toenails to broken arms, which she set and coated with a special clay that hardens quickly, and then put in a sling. The one time I got to watch her do it was for a little boy who had broken his arm playing soccer. She told him she could either fix it on the spot but it would hurt, or he could go to the hospital and get a shot for the pain. He chose to endure and was fixed up in no time. She was widely regarded as an expert in massage for conditions from headaches to sore backs to pregnancy; she said she learned most of her massage techniques from her own instincts, from experience, and from God. She charged on a sliding scale; her average fee per visit was 100 pesos (approximately $10 USD). Chronically ill patients often came to stay for various periods of time in her guest rooms on the second floor; she developed individualized treatment programs for such patients, including tailored diets of organic foods.

During prenatal exams, in addition to the traditional *sobada*, Irene checked urine and vital signs and used a Doppler to amplify the fetal heart rate so that the family could also hear it; she was also quite expert with the Pinard—an ancient cone-shaped device used around the world that can be made of wood or metal; you put the small end into your ear and the large end on the woman's lower abdomen and concentrate hard. Beginners like me

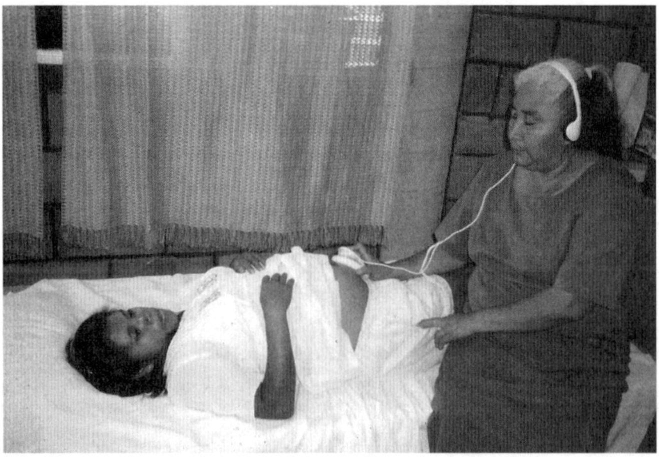

Doña Irene using her Doppler.

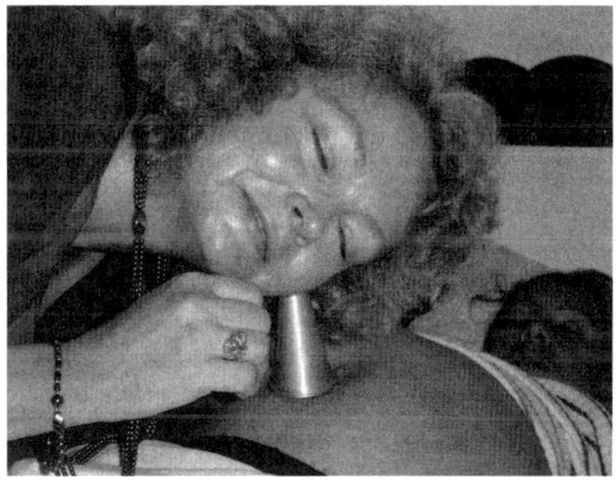

Robbie learning to use the Pinard in the birth center of Angelina Martinez Miranda, an internationally renowned traditional midwife and a close friend of Doña Irene; we met Lina at the beginning of this chapter. Photo by Debra Pascali-Bonaro

have to really work to shut out all external sounds to hear the sound of the heartbeat—it took me about 20 minutes of trying to finally learn to focus deeply enough.

Irene sometimes sent women for ultrasounds to confirm her manual diagnosis of a problematic presentation. During labor, she prepared nutritious foods for the mother; encouraged her to eat, drink, and move around at will; and to labor in upright positions. She performed cervical checks when she felt it necessary, always using sterile gloves. She was committed to what she called "a clean birth" and often trained other midwives in sterile technique. If labor stalled, she prepared labor-stimulating herbal teas; she rejected the use of pitocin to speed labor because of the dangers of a ruptured uterus. After the birth, she waited for the cord to stop pulsating (to ensure maximum oxygen and nutrient flow to the baby), tied it with sterile string and cut it with sterile scissors, immediately handed the baby to the mother and carefully checked its Apgar score, weighed the baby in a soft cloth sling, and then went to the kitchen to prepare a cleansing tea for the mother and hot chocolate for the whole family in celebration.

Well trained in medical protocols, she referred women to the hospital if she considered them too high-risk—unless she was sure that she was better prepared to handle a particular complication than medical personnel. She had a good working relationship with several physicians who knew and respected her. When asked, "Why do women in this city pay you for births instead of going to the hospital where it is free?" Doña Irene replied, "Because we attend them much better than the hospital! We attend one woman so beautifully that she tells a friend, and we attend that friend beautifully, and that is how the chain keeps growing. Here in my community I've attended almost everyone's births, although there are plenty of doctors—but the women don't stay with the doctors, they come to me." Irene also provided ongoing postpartum services, which are not provided by the Mexican health care system. The people of her community called her *la doctora corazón.*

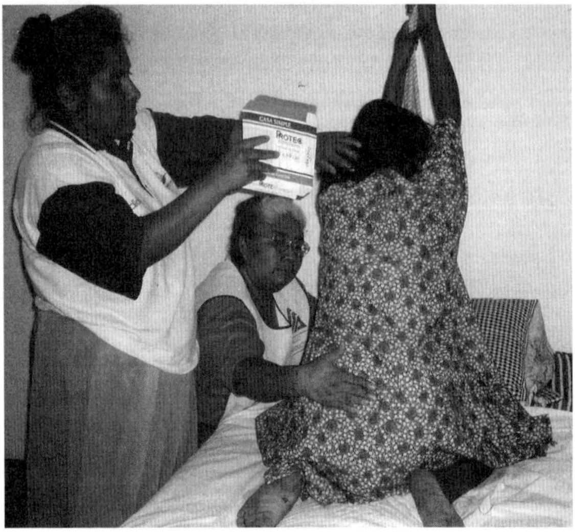

Doña Irene attending an upright labor in her birth center while she herself is kneeling, applying back pressure to help the mother with the pain. I was staying with her and had gone out to dinner with friends; as I drove in she came running out to call me to the birth. As with the other photos taken by me in this anthology, the mother gave me permission to take them.

Doña Irene installed the rope you see in the picture above after attending a presentation I had given at a local conference on traditional positions for birth. After my talk, she exclaimed to me that almost all the women in her prior mountain community had given birth squatting and pulling down on a rebozo that they had thrown over the center beam in their round huts. "*Ya me urbanize*" (I got urbanized), she noted ruefully, saying that she had forgotten about those traditional upright positions for birth, as most of the city women she attended expected to give birth on their backs. She went straight to a store and purchased a strong metal pipe and a rope. She had her husband, Don Bolivar, install the pipe catty-corner across the right-hand back corner of her birth center, solidly grounded in the plastered brick walls, and hung the rope, doubled, from the bar so that it would have two handles that the laboring women could hold onto. She would push the twin bed on that side of the room under the rope so the women could kneel or squat on the bed while holding onto the rope, or move the bed aside if the mother preferred the floor. She was thrilled to "rediscover" this traditional technique, while I was delighted at the highly postmodern irony of an anthropologist helping a traditional midwife to reclaim one of her own traditions.

In 1998 when Hurricane Mitch caused tremendous damage in Nicaragua, Doña Irene went by bus with a group of 40 medical students and nurses and five traditional healers from Morelos and stayed there for a month attending over 350 people with various ailments, including diarrhea from contaminated water, and teaching them to prepare their own remedies with local plants.

Because of her reputation as a skilled midwife and healer, Doña Irene was frequently invited to give talks and seminars at midwifery conferences in Mexico and the US. She attended the first MANA conference in Mexico in

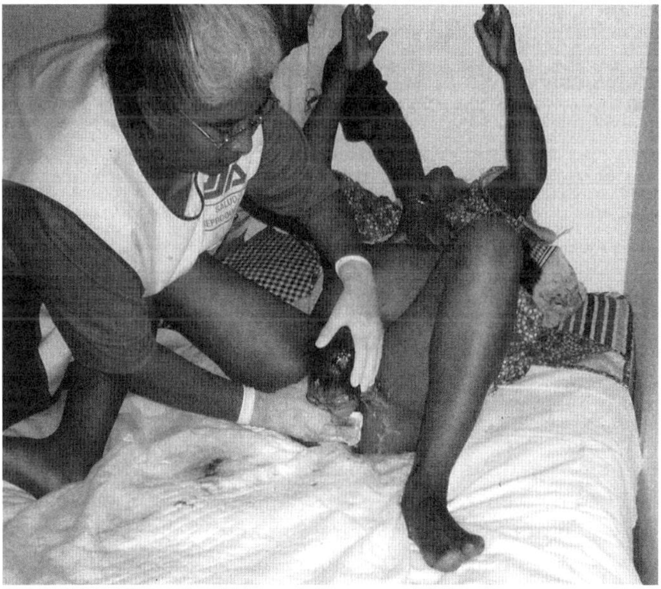

Irene receiving the baby's head—note that the woman has turned over and is giving birth in the lithotomy position. Later on, when I asked Irene why, she explained that she had been on the floor for hours doing back pressure and massage, and her knees were killing her! Two issues are salient here: (1) sometimes midwives need to take care of themselves; and (2) if you have been mostly upright and moving around a lot during labor, the exact position you are in when you give birth is not that important.

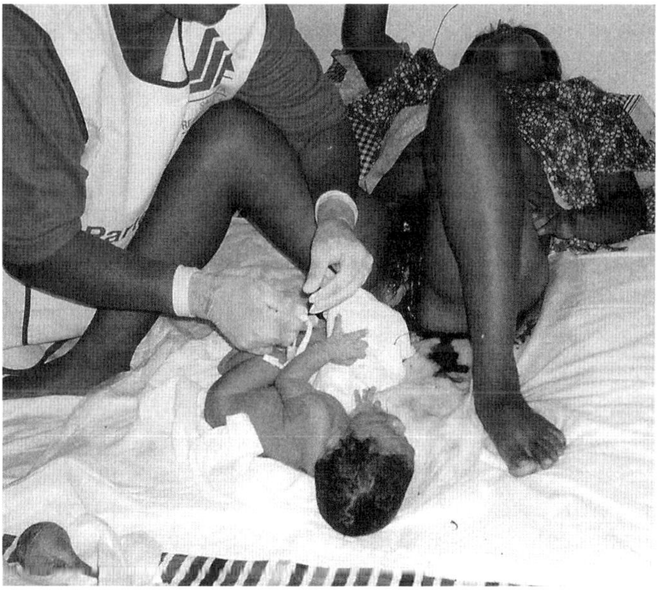

The baby is born and Irene is untangling the cord before she passes the baby to the mother.

Xalapa in 1995 and taught at many others over the years. Her workshop on *sobada* and *manteada* at the MANA conference in Puebla in 1997, for example, was attended by almost all of the 90 or so traditional midwives at the conference, who were eager to expand their knowledge base and reported that she knew far more massage techniques than they. She also taught at midwifery conferences in the US, Canada, Trinidad, and Tobago. Thoroughly postmodern in her eclectic manipulation of multiple knowledge systems, she had taken various university continuing education courses in indigenous and alternative medicine, and received a Diploma in Herbal Medicine from the Universidad Autónoma del Estado de Morelos. She often prepared homeopathic remedies and herbal soaps, salves, and massage oils for her clients. She purchased a computer some years ago, on which she recorded her herbal and medicinal recipes and remedies.

Postscript. Doña Irene and her husband Don Bolivar were robbed in their home some years ago, perhaps in 2011—I am not sure of the date. Two people knocked on their gate in the wee hours of the morning asking for help for an illness, and of course she came running to oblige. But after gaining admittance into the home, the two pulled out weapons and tied Doña Irene and her husband to chairs in their living room while the robbers ransacked the house, carrying out all the electronic and kitchen equipment. After they left, Irene and Bolivar remained tied to their chairs for some hours until someone came in and freed them. I was told that Doña Irene was greatly saddened and discouraged after that and subsequently retired from practice for a while and moved to a small house in the countryside, saying that she was done and all she wanted to do at that point was care for "*mi viejo*"—her husband Don Bolivar. She was greatly missed by the community she attended so faithfully for so long. Since Don Bolivar's death, she has returned to a more minimal practice, helping only those she knows.

Postmodern Professional Midwives

Although the most recent trend at WHO and UNICEF is toward diminished support for traditional midwives coupled with increased support for professional midwives, recent anthropological ethnographies call into question the appropriateness of this approach. A distressing cross-cultural trend is showing up in the growing body of anthropological literature about midwifery and birth in the developing world. From Croatia to Tanzania to Papua New Guinea, anthropologists who observe professional midwives giving prenatal care and attending births increasingly note that, far from the midwifery ideal, professional midwives often treat women very badly during birth, ignoring their needs and requests, talking to them disrespectfully ("Why are you complaining now? You should have thought about this when you were having fun making this baby!"), ordering them around, and sometimes even yelling at them and slapping them. At the same time, and in direct correlation, the professional midwives are themselves often treated badly by the health-care systems in which they work. They are almost always underpaid, are frequently mistreated by physicians, who rank above them in the medical hierarchy, and generally work long hours under stressful conditions that often include inadequate facilities and equipment and too many women with too few midwives to care for them well. In short, many professional midwives are trapped in the biomedical health care system, a system that is failing to meet the needs of birthing women in developing countries.

Although unlike traditional midwives, professional midwives have the structural benefits conferred by government certification, access to certain technologies, and the status-conferring white coat, they still must struggle with the pressures imposed on them by the modernist and colonialist biomedical model, which defines biomedicine as structurally superior to traditional medicine, doctors as superior to midwives, and professional midwives as superior to traditional midwives. Where doctors are few and midwives predominate, professional midwives have opportunities to establish themselves as relatively autonomous practitioners and can make culturally and individually reasonable choices about how to interact with the local traditional midwives. Where doctors are many and professional midwives are clearly subordinate to them in medical hierarchies, they often find that their only route to biomedical status and respect involves rejection of, and often downright rudeness too, traditional midwives and their clients.

Studies show that in some places, professional midwives trained in government-approved two-year courses and sent to rural villages work hard to get to know the village women, to give them nurturant care, and to cooperate with the local village midwives (Chen 1977; Kroeger 1996; Kwast 1992). But in others, professional midwives adopt an attitude of arrogance and superiority, and treat the village women disrespectfully (Allen 2002; Byford 1999; Iskandar et al. 1996), in effect discouraging further referrals to the hospital. It is a paradox of contemporary midwifery that while some professional midwives are working hard to help traditional midwives creatively adapt biomedicine to their native systems (Daviss 1997; Graham 1999; Davis-Floyd 2000b, 2001a, b; Barclay 2009; see also Chapter 9), other professional midwives and most physicians have long been working equally hard to further marginalize or fully eliminate their traditional predecessors (Whittaker 1999; Dietiker n.d.; Sieglin n.d.; Geurts 2001; Jenkins 2001).

Postmodern professional midwives as I am defining them very consciously strive *not* to engage in such behaviors. When they interface with TBAs, they apply the same relativistic perspective to the knowledge system of the traditional midwife as they do to the knowledge system of biomedicine. In other words, they seek to identify and support efficacious aspects of the traditional birthing system and, respectfully and sensitively, to change harmful practices. I could cite hundreds of examples of professional postmodern midwives. But for the sake of space and simplicity, I will confine myself to describing midwives in Mexico, Japan, and the United States who fully exemplify my profile of the postmodern *professional* midwife.

Postmodern Professional Midwives in Mexico

My ethnographic research in Mexico (Davis-Floyd 2001a, b, 2003a) documented the emergence of an entirely new kind of midwife, the thoroughly postmodern *partera professional.* These women of diverse sociocultural backgrounds initially sought training from American direct-entry midwives in the independent out-of-hospital midwifery model; since then they have been reformulating that model for Mexico. Through their own practices, intensive liaison work with traditional midwives, and organizing national midwifery conferences and meetings, they are creating midwifery as both an emerging profession and social movement in Mexico. Some of them operate outside the medical system while others are carving a niche within it. In my article "*La Partera Profesional*: Articulating Identity and Cultural Space for a New Kind of Midwife in Mexico" (Davis-Floyd 2001a), I described the first 20 of these new professional midwives—all the ones I was able to identify at the time. By 2005, there were 50 or so professional midwives whom I could identify; today there are many more. These women face a long struggle to define their identities, legalize their practices, and generate a sustainable space within the emergent Mexican technocracy. To their intense dismay, this struggle must take place within the context of the disappearance of Mexico's traditional midwives, who have long been vanishing at a rapid rate (in the 1970s, traditional midwives attended over 40% of Mexican births; today that figure is around 3%, and the majority are over 65 or 70 years of age). Mexico's new professional midwives live in constant tension between their desire to preserve traditional midwifery and the need to create a sustainable form of professional midwifery because, in effect, traditional midwifery cannot sustainably be preserved in most regions of the country—so many traditional midwives are retiring or dying out without passing on their knowledge and skills that there are now none left in some states. Mexico's newer professional midwives cope with this tension by adding to their professional knowledge base many traditional birthing techniques (such as the use of herbs and of the *rebozo* to shift the baby's position or to ease labor pain). And they help traditional midwives as best they can through foundations, joint conferences, skills-sharing workshops, and government advocacy.

This effort to respectfully combine professional and traditional knowledge systems is particularly visible at the CASA School for Professional Midwives in San Miguel de Allende, where students undergo a professional three-year training program that combines didactic classroom work, clinical work in the CASA hospital and in some of the public hospitals in San Miguel (which they find extremely traumatic because women are treated so badly there), and five three-week apprenticeships with traditional midwives in small and remote rural villages (Davis-Floyd 2001a, b; Mills and Davis-Floyd 2009; Goodman forthcoming). These apprenticeships not only allow the professional students to incorporate traditional techniques into their practices, but also prevent them from developing the attitude of arrogance and superiority that many professional midwives around the world exhibit toward traditional midwives. Living in the homes of the traditional midwives, helping with their daily routines, and observing their forms of care instill an attitude of deep respect and admiration for these elder midwives in the younger professional midwifery students, and a strong desire to follow in their footsteps while making the path they traced viable in the postmodern technocracy.

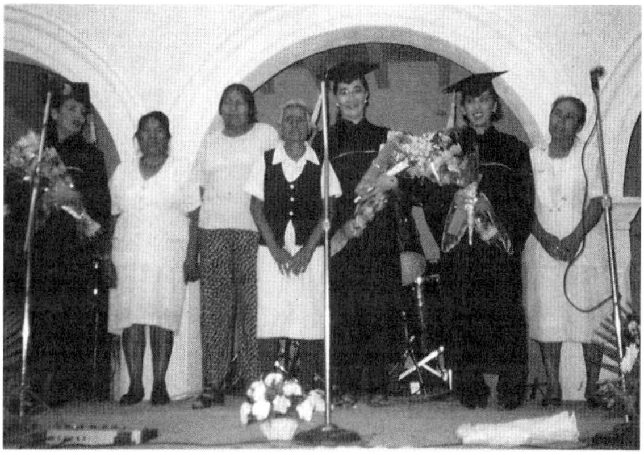

The graduation of the first class from CASA. The graduates were handed their diplomas by four of the traditional midwives with whom they had apprenticed. These midwives are now deceased, as are all of the traditional midwives who used to practice in the state of Guanajuato.

Postmodern Professional Midwives in Japan

Japanese anthropologist Etsuko Matsuoka (2001; Matsuoka and Hinokuma 2009) demonstrated how the shift in Japan from agriculture to industrial production to the contemporary service and information economy (which I call “the technocracy”) has been mirrored by a shift from birth at home, attended by traditional midwives, to hospital births, attended primarily by professional midwives, to the emergence of new midwives who are beginning to offer Japanese female consumers a plethora of options for childbirth. In premodern Japan from the 1880s on, well-trained, licensed, independent midwives attended the majority of births, usually in maternity homes (a form of birth center where the midwife and her family also lived). Japan’s modernization period took place after WWII from the 1950s to the 1970s as the country experienced rapid economic growth. In those days professional nurse-midwives went into hospitals to produce babies just as workers went into factories to produce goods. But since the 1980s, with the advent of the natural childbirth movement, a new type of postmodern Japanese midwife has emerged.

The midwives who have been playing a prominent role in this natural childbirth movement are different from either of the two previous types of midwives: they practice independently but cooperate with and learn from each other. Many of them have worked in hospitals for years but have passed in their thinking about birth beyond the limitations of the medical model and have "come out on the other side." They pursue their own midwifery model of care and are developing new identities. Some have their own maternity homes or "birth houses," and others work in hospitals trying to introduce a better way within a medical setting. They are mediators, crossing the boundaries between obstetric care and alternative care, home and hospital, modern and traditional, local and international, and thereby increasing options for women. Ironically, these options include the reincorporation of elements associated with "traditional" birth, such as out-of-hospital birth and the use of upright positions.

The primary reason these Japanese midwives give for leaving hospital practice is the damage to mother and baby they observe to be caused by the application of routine technological interventions to the process of parturition. Their personal evolutions through hospital practice to attending births in birth centers and homes contradict modernist evolutionary notions that defined the movement of birth from home to hospital as "medical progress." As described by Matsuoka and Hinokuma (2009), these independent postmodern Japanese midwives' primary value during labor is *patience*. They see the labor process as "metamorphic"—each contraction works not only to bring the baby but also to transform the young woman into a mother (a process that researcher Denis Walsh [2006] has named "matrescence"). Therefore the pain itself has value and is to be honored for its transformative qualities, at the same time as the laboring woman is to be held, caressed, and nurtured through this metamorphic process.

Tomoko: A Postmodern Japanese Midwife by Japanese anthropologist Etsuko Matsuoka

> Tomoko's maternity home is an ordinary three-story residential house located in the center of Osaka with a small signboard placed outside the door. On entering I was ushered, after passing a corridor decorated by pictures of couples and babies on the wall, into a small room where futon mattresses were folded up at one corner. Tomoko says this is the room where she talks to women and gives antenatal checkups as well as delivers babies. When a woman comes into this room for delivery, it is made dim by light from a lantern, which sometimes progresses labor immensely, as the woman feels more relaxed in this dark but cozy small tatami space.
>
> Tomoko set her mind to become a midwife after delivering her third child at a maternity home where she met a midwife over 70 years of age,

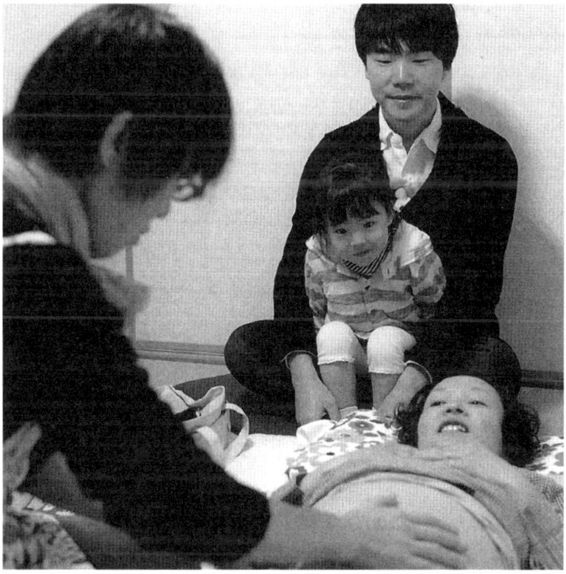

Antenatal checkup at maternity home. Midwife Tomoko talks to the baby, the pregnant mother, a sister, and the father while she performs the exam. Photo by Azusa Nakao

who was working passionately, being respected and thanked by women in the community over generations. Her fascination with midwifery as a woman's job led her into a university again in 1993 at the age of 35. As she already had her own experiences of birth in hospital, clinic, and maternity home, the midwifery education based on a medical model at school seemed very much apart from her "real" experiences of birth. So while studying to get a license, she explored alternative ways of practicing as a midwife, visiting a Japanese midwife in Africa and building close connections with independent midwives in Japan, thereby extending her options for practicing midwifery in different ways from what was taught at school.

Before becoming independent in 2004 at the age of 46, she worked in two general hospitals for five years and a maternity home for one year. In hospitals she gained as much knowledge as possible in preparation for future independence; not only in the obstetrics section but also in NICU, internal medicine, orthopedics, ophthalmology, and even terminal care; she also gained experiences in premature baby care, intravenous drips, the use of different drugs, and so forth. But after those five years of biomedical experiences, she realized that the births she encountered in the maternity home were full of fresh discoveries and some even seemed like miracles. Tomoko states that hospital care and maternity home care are two completely different things, saying, "I am amazed by the perineum of a postnatal woman when she leaves a maternity home. Did she really deliver a baby? It is intact and beautiful, so different from that in hospital. I was also surprised by the natural growth of the newborn baby who had not been fed any formula milk in the maternity home before discharge. Mother's breast milk is enough. That was a sheer discovery."

Since 2009 she has lived and worked in her maternity home with two beds on the third floor of her house. Luckily when she was in the process of setting up this institution, one retiring independent midwife offered Tomoko expensive medical equipment such as an ultrasound machine, fetal monitor, saturation monitor, and others. Tomoko admits that those technological gadgets are protecting her by providing important information, especially in transferring a woman to a hospital. Currently in Japan an independent midwife with maternity beds is obliged by law to have both a backup obstetrician and a linkage hospital, a law that hampers many midwives from establishing or maintaining a maternity home, because obstetricians are usually reluctant to engage in this kind of linkage. Thus she thinks that technological information from a midwife facilitates communication between the two professionals and helps to build trust between them.

Another thing that pushes Tomoko forward is her relationships with senior independent midwives from whom she learned her skills. Whenever she feels unsure whether she can keep monitoring a pregnant woman whose risk factors place her in a gray area (not low-risk but not clearly high-risk either) or if she should transfer her, she phones a senior midwife who is available to her 24 hours a day. The senior midwife, after hearing her detailed accounting, usually says, "Wait some more and it will work out." This kind of advice empowers her with confidence. If a similar situation took place in hospital, a doctor would say, "Rotation problem. Impossible," words that work as an ultimatum to take birth away from the midwife's hands. Because of her ability to depend on senior independent midwives, Tomoko feels that her midwifery care is part of a large reservoir of skills and experiences that have been accumulated by many experienced midwives over many years.

Tomoko consistently demonstrates the key characteristic of a postmodern midwife as defined by Robbie Davis-Floyd: informed relativism. Tomoko utilizes information based on technology to facilitate communication in biomedical language with obstetricians, while her energy and confidence are nurtured by a large reservoir of midwifery tradition. She combines both worlds within her thinking and praxis, thereby making her midwifery practice viable in a world dominated by technocratic thinking. She was also a mother first, before starting her career as a midwife; she feels that her experience as a mother puts her on a par with her clients whose worries and problems she can understand, so she makes a skill of listening to women, rather than focusing on giving them professional advice.

Her first prenatal session with a new client lasts at least two hours, during which she listens intently and works on freeing women from their fear of birth. She calmly answers queries about emergency transports, deploying her extensive knowledge of the scientific evidence to alleviate their concerns. She says that those maternity homes whose midwives cannot explain with words will not survive, because her clients themselves anticipate the possible need for a combination of two worlds—the world of one-to-one midwifery care and the biomedical world they may have to face in case of an emergency. I learned from Tomoko that not only postmodern midwives themselves have an attitude of informed relativism but also *pregnant women demand this attitude.* They want to know that their midwife can move fluidly between these worlds, these separate but overlapping knowledge domains. In this sense postmodern midwifery is a product of three elements: (1) a vast and ancient premodern midwifery art and craft in which professionalization has taken place only recently; (2) the development of modern obstetrics and its hegemonic domination over birth; and (3) women's desires to have their midwife embody the best of both of those worlds in a fully comprehensive and postmodern way.

Postmodern Professional Midwives in the United States

In Chapter 6, I provided a full overview of American midwifery. Here I simply remind my readers that cumulatively American midwives attend around 11% (CNMs attend 10% [Declerq 2015], while CPMs attend 1%) of all births, and that small percentage has been reached only after many decades of often fighting, and sometimes working with obstetricians who, starting in the early 1900s, tried very hard to keep midwives, any midwives, from any kind of practice in the US. Thus, midwives' mere existence in the United States constitutes a radical postmodern critique of technomedicine, not to mention the midwifery model of care that most of them work hard to practice (described in Chapter 11). This section contains a profile of an American postmodern midwife, Melissa Cheyney, a short story about the process of creating the CPM—the certification Missy holds—and a consideration of the highly postmodern preservation of age-old apprenticeship-training in the requirements for receiving that certification.

A Daya*'s Omen: Chronicling Melissa Cheyney as a Scholar, Postmodern Midwife, and Activist*
by Holly Horan, Bonnie Ruder, and Courtney L. Everson

In her nascent years before applied anthropology, midwifery, and maternal and infant health advocacy, Melissa (Missy) Cheyney was an undergraduate student at Calvin College earning a bachelor's degree in premedicine and ancient history. To complete the requirements for her ancient history degree, she enrolled in an archaeological field school in *Umm el-Jimal*, a village in northern Jordan. During this field school, an ancient burial site was discovered beneath the village after a horse had fallen into a hole. Missy, with extensive coursework in anatomy and physiology as a result of her premedicine background, was asked if she

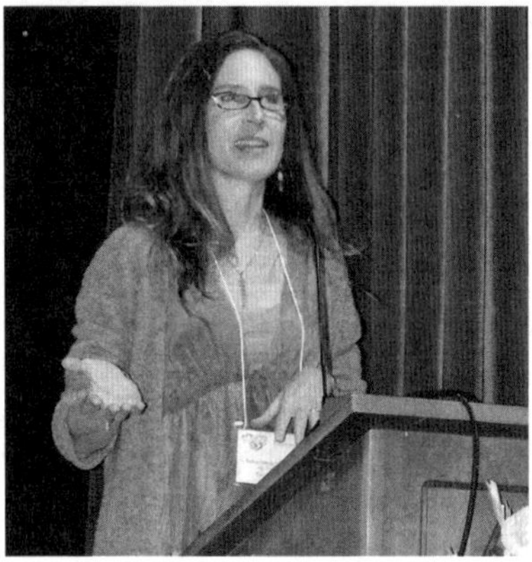

Missy Cheyney, giving a talk at a MANA conference. Photo by Colleen Donovan-Batson

was interested in excavating this site. Thus, Cheyney's undergraduate honors college thesis project was born and her career in anthropology began.

Ultimately, she decided to pursue a master's degree in bioarchaeology and forensic anthropology at Western Michigan University (WMU). In this program, she continued to work at Umm el-Jimal, leading four different field seasons, excavating cemeteries and collecting data for her master's thesis. In addition to her work on past populations, Missy's frequent visits and extended stays in this village made her a community member of the Bedouin, the people who live in and around the ruins of Umm el-Jimal. Living in such close proximity, the Bedouin were integrated into the excavation and continuously welcomed Missy and her returning recruits of students and colleagues to work at the site.

After several trips to Jordan, Cheyney had grown close with a *daya*, the local Arabic word for "midwife" in this village. She learned that dayas were revered and special members of the community, as biomedical birthing options were only offered in the closest city, *Mafraq,* 17 kilometers west of Umm el-Jimal. Bus transportation to Mafraq was only available once a day and the journey was slow—inadequate conditions for a laboring woman. During one of Missy's field seasons, the daya observed the love and admiration Cheyney received from the local Bedouin children and told Missy, "You're going to become a midwife." The budding bioarchaeologist was unfamiliar with the concept of midwifery, but the seed had been planted and her interest in working with extant populations began to grow.

Cheyney's passion for studying medical anthropology in living populations was solidified by the economic imbalance she witnessed between high- and low-resource nations. During one field season, the daya asked Missy how much money was spent each year on their excavations. As she tallied up the numbers, she realized that an enormous amount was spent on the field school, including money for bringing students from the United States to Jordan, the tuition costs for each student in the field school, and the costs incurred during the six-week program. Cheyney reflects on the daya's support for her work while also vocalizing the needs of the local community: "She always welcomed me and the students, saying 'Our home is your home, our artifacts are your artifacts. But, if you really want to know what we want, we need a more reliable source of clean water, food through the hunger season and access to medical care and education.'" It was in this existential moment that Missy realized that she was called to work with living populations.

By the end of this field season, Cheyney had graduated with a Master of Arts in bioarchaeology, and had just finished the first year of her doctoral program in bioarchaeology and dental anthropology at the University of Oregon (UO). Coincidentally, she was enrolled in a medical anthropology course the following term. Given her premed background and the blessing of the daya in Jordan, Cheyney seriously considered a career change to midwifery as a life-calling and aimed to integrate her dissertation research with midwifery education. Cheyney's advisor was supportive of this shift and advocated that her midwifery education and training be considered for the skills requirements in her doctoral program. Over the next six years, Missy simultaneously completed her doctoral degree in anthropology and became a Certified Professional Midwife (CPM), conducting her thesis research while apprenticing and attending births for her midwifery certification. Later, she obtained her Oregon state licensure in midwifery. Yet after finishing both her doctoral degree and her midwifery educational requirements, Cheyney could not see a way forward to remaining both a practicing midwife and scholar, and planned to pursue a tenure-track job as a medical anthropologist with a focus on maternal and infant health.

Early in her professional career, however, Cheyney became a tenure-track faculty member in Oregon State University's (OSU) anthropology program, an opportunity that almost miraculously enabled her passion for anthropology and midwifery to coalesce. Upon hiring Missy, OSU's anthropology program chair asked how Cheyney would manage being a midwife while also fulfilling the requirements of a tenure-track career. She responded that she did not believe that maintaining the two professions was possible. The department chair disagreed and offered full support for Cheyney to pursue both careers, recognizing that her unique positionality as a midwife would provide an emic (on-the-ground, local) perspective into her midwifery research and an avenue to understand, conduct, and apply her research more effectively. The department chair also felt that being a practicing midwife would make her a more eclectic and engaging professor, one who could share with her students in class a description of the birth she had just attended, for one example.

Since the beginning of her academic career, OSU has supported Cheyney by providing her with lab space and graduate students. This robust support network has allowed Cheyney to feel comfortable stepping out of her academic career when being called for a birth—a sense of support that was strongly reinforced during her first year at OSU. She was scheduled to give a presentation but was called to a birth just hours before. With the support of the department and a graduate student,

Cheyney was able to attend the birth while her student, who was working with her on the research project, gave the presentation. Missy reflects on the anxiety she had as a new professor, saying, "I thought, 'OK, this is where the support ends,' having to miss a presentation last minute." The following week, Cheyney was surprised as colleagues asked her about the birth without providing any backlash about the missed presentation that was successfully covered by her graduate student. This response confirmed for Missy that she indeed had an essential support network at OSU that would allow her to maintain both of her professions and to continue her research.

When Cheyney was up for tenure, OSU again demonstrated unwavering support. Academically, Missy was well published; her long list of articles in peer-reviewed journals includes "Reinscribing the Birthing Body: Home Birth as Ritual Performance," published in *Medical Anthropology Quarterly* (2009), and two coauthored articles on home to hospital transports, published in *Qualitative Health Research* and the *Journal of Midwifery and Women's Health.* Works such as these enhanced her status in the national midwifery community, as did her appointment by MANA to become the director of MANA's Division of Research—she is trained in both qualitative and quantitative research methods. Increasingly, she is becoming one of the "public faces" of homebirth midwifery.

Probably for this reason, during the tenure process she began to be targeted by a retired obstetrician who is an outspoken opponent of CPMs and their attendance at homebirths. This obstetrician has a small group of rabid anti-homebirth followers (many of whom had bad homebirth experiences) who consistently persecuted Missy on the Internet in the form of negative blog posts and hate mail, and via letters these women wrote to her university leaders urging them not to give her tenure because she "killed babies." They also accused her of ethical violations in her research, resulting in an Institutional Review Board (IRB) investigation that found no violations. Cheyney and her daughter's safety were also threatened by members of this "anti-Missy Cheyney" group, some of whom followed her both around campus and around town carrying posters of her photo with the caption "BABY-KILLER"—simply because she attends homebirths herself and advocates for keeping the homebirth option alive by supporting certified midwives who attend homebirths. (Missy herself has never lost a baby during her years of practice.)

Despite the potential for negative publicity for OSU, the university continued to support Cheyney's work, providing her with public representation staff, public safety assistance, and any other legal professionals she needed to continue to safely and successfully continue her research. She did successfully obtain tenure during this intense period in her professional career, a further testament to the institutional support she has received for her work.

For a time, the prosecution died down. However, in 2014, Cheyney was the lead author on the largest study to date on outcomes of care for midwife-led planned homebirths in the United States. This article, which was published in the highly reputable *Journal of Midwifery and Women's Health* (Cheyney et al. 2014a), reinvigorated the obstetrician's "witch hunt," and the hate mail again began pouring into Missy's in-box. In the midst of these personal attacks, OSU granted Cheyney the "Scholarship Impact Award," one of the most prestigious awards a faculty member can receive. Much to her credit, Missy also transformed the negative energy she received from the persecution into actual research: she conducted a thematic analysis of commonly reoccurring themes in the hate mail and blogs. She presented this work at the American Anthropological Association (AAA) meetings in 2012, where Robbie Davis-Floyd, the discussant for this AAA panel, expressed strong support for Cheyney and her work, and also invited Missy to become the coauthor for the complete revision and update of Davis-Floyd's first book, *Birth as an American Rite of Passage* (2003 [1992]), because she believes there is no one better qualified to undertake this task. Moving beyond Robbie's original focus on white, middle-class women (because they seemed to have the greatest degree of choice), Robbie, Missy, and her graduate students are currently at work on conducting 100 new interviews with a much more diverse array of women who have given birth since 2000. They hope to complete this revision in 2018.

Cheyney is grateful that due to her robust support network, she has successfully maintained two professions: midwife and anthropology professor and researcher. She believes these two professions are for her inextricably linked and essential for continuing her career path, which focuses on improving maternal and infant health in the United States, where the majority of medical resources are used. She stated: "We spend $110 billion on maternity care only to have some of the worst outcomes and the lowest rates of access to care among high-resource countries; that is very hard for me to accept. I am confident that we can find ways to spend less, increase access and improve outcomes."

Cheyney argues that as a result of the last decade of research and the increased accessibility of medical-testing procedures, it has become clear that maternal and infant health would benefit from the availability of systems-wide access to midwifery care for low-risk women. This shift in maternal and infant health care could massively reduce medical costs (see Anderson, Daviss, and Johnson forthcoming; see also Cheyney, Goodarzi, and Wiegers forthcoming) and provide a better model of care that could be emulated in other nations where the hegemonic, biomedical model of care and its associated inequities has spread.

Currently, Cheyney maintains a small-scale midwifery practice in Oregon in which she demonstrates her postmodern informed relativism, combining elements of the ancient skills she first witnessed with the Bedouin dayas who insisted that Missy should become a midwife with the contemporary knowledge and skills she learned during her education at a MEAC-accredited school and her additional year of apprenticeship training, while teaching full-time at OSU and continuing to serve as director of MANA'S Division of Research. Her current anthropological research focuses on knowledge sharing, with an emphasis on cultural humility and multiple ways of knowing among members of the maternal and infant health care provider community. She is also working to improve the evaluation of birth outcome data to provide midwives with feedback about their own statistics and mothers with more accurate information about models of care and birthing options.

The Postmodern Professionalization of American "Lay" Midwifery: A Short Story about Creating the CPM

In this section I provide one fascinating case study in the postmodernization of American midwifery by briefly describing a small part of the story of the creation of the professional certification Missy holds—the Certified Professional Midwife (CPM) credential. To briefly recap from Chapter 6, this certification was developed by the members of the North American Registry of Midwives (NARM), a daughter organization of MANA, assisted by the members of a Certification Task Force (CTF), in which any midwife who wished to could participate, as around 150 nurse- and direct-entry midwives did, in a series of meetings around the country (1993–1995). The parts of this story I will recount here focus on two primary issues: the highly postmodern preservation of apprenticeship as an educational model and the professional, modern, and biomedical question of whether or not to require the ability to insert IVs as an entry-level skill of all CPM candidates. In the heated debate over whether to require the ability to administer an IV as an entry-level skill, the depth of these midwives' commitment to preserving midwifery as it was learned, understood, and practiced by homebirth midwives—while at the same time professionalizing it through this new certification—was put to its greatest test.

It was January 1995. The members of the NARM board and the Certification Task Force (CTF), including myself (Robbie), were in a hotel on Captiva Island in Florida.[2] These midwives knew that this gathering was about creating a viable professional future for what had been known as "lay" midwifery, so a full 40 of them showed up at their own expense. The sun was shining and the beach was calling on that warm and breezy day. Nevertheless, we sat in a meeting all day long while everyone in turn spoke their mind on the important issue of which skills should be required for entry-level practice.

[2] At that time, the members of the NARM board, who held primary responsibility for developing CPM certification, included midwives Sondra Abdullah-Zaimah, Shannon Anton, Alice Sammon, Suzanne Suarez, Ruth Walsh, Pam Weaver, and Sharon Wells, and myself. Key committee heads included Ann Cairns, Susan Hodges, Abby Kinne, and Sandra MorningStar. I was invited to become a member of the NARM board in 1994, in the position of consumer representative. Before I accepted the invitation, I made it clear that if I accepted, I would want to be studying NARM's work even as I participated in it, a request that was approved by the board members, who have unfailingly supported me in my research efforts to this day.

Written on the board were "IV insertion," "catheter insertion," and "pitocin administration for hemorrhage" as the skills in immediate question. From a homebirth perspective, these were high-tech and highly medical skills. I listened with astonishment as midwife after midwife spoke in favor of requiring all of these skills for entry-level midwives.

Halfway into the process, I raised my hand and asked for a quick sense of the room—how many of the midwives present favored requiring all these skills? When 36 out of the 40 sets of hands went up, I was amazed to realize that I was bearing direct witness to the professionalization of lay midwifery. Even Ina May Gaskin, an irrepressible and eternal hippie and internationally known point person for "spiritual midwifery," argued for the IV requirement. Ina May noted that after many years of holistic midwifery practice, she realized she had been relying on EMTs (emergency medical technicians) on the Farm (the intentional community in which she lived at that time near Summertown, Tennessee) to insert IVs in those rare cases of severe postpartum hemorrhage, and had finally taken responsibility for learning the skill herself. She felt that it was now an invaluable part of her midwifery repertoire, and she stressed not only its lifesaving potential but also its positive value in terms of the public image of midwives, saying, "When we have a hemorrhage and we transport the woman with an IV already in place, we really look good to the hospital personnel who receive our clients. It helps them to trust us as practitioners."

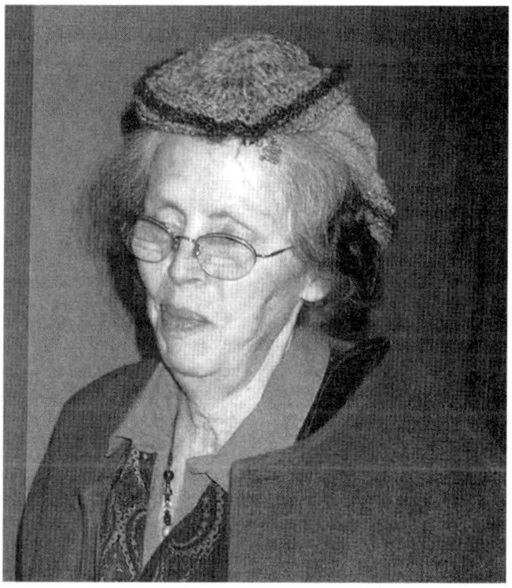

Ina May Gaskin, author of *Spiritual Midwifery, Ina May's Guide to Childbirth*, and *Birth Matters*, is arguably the most famous midwife in the world, as her work has been published in many languages and she has long been an international speaker traveling the globe to teach her innovative midwifery knowledge and skills. These include the famed "Gaskin Maneuver," which she learned from traditional midwives in Guatemala; it consists of asking the mother to adopt a hands-and-knees position to widen the pelvic outlet for breech babies and shoulder dystocia (stuck shoulder), and is a very effective position for any type of normal birth.

Only four of the midwives there were in active opposition. Their primary spokesperson was Sandra MorningStar (now known as Sister MorningStar), a midwife from Missouri who had been sent to the meeting with a mandate from her state midwifery association *not* to allow IVs to be required as an entry-level skill for CPM certification. (In the consensus process used by members of MANA at that time, one person could block a proposal even if everyone else supported it.) As midwife after midwife tried to get her to change her mind, Sandi held fast, insisting that requiring IV insertion as an entry-level skill sent the wrong message to student midwives. She said that IV insertion was "an advanced, not an entry-level skill," because the proper first courses of action in case of a hemorrhage were, in this order, to speak to the mother, looking into her eyes and commanding her forcefully to "*stop bleeding now*!" (an intervention that midwife/anthropologist Janneli Miller [2000] has called "magical speech"), to administer the herb shepherd's purse, to utilize bimanual compression of the uterus, to give pitocin buccally (on a swab in the cheek pouch) or intramuscularly via an injection, and only after all that had been tried, to insert an IV and transport. Sandi herself had learned IV skills a decade ago, but she didn't want student midwives thinking that they should jump straight to the IV without learning all the other techniques that postmodern homebirth midwives have "rediscovered" for dealing with hemorrhage, because usually those less interventionist techniques are all that are needed. And the midwives in her state, who were practicing illegally, did not want to be required to carry IV equipment, as this would open them to the serious charge of practicing medicine without a license. So steadfast was Sandi in her insistence on blocking the IV requirement that, after four hours of trying to get her to change her mind, the others gave up, put the matter in the hands of the Steering Committee, of which Sandi was a member, and took a break before dinner.

At dinner I was curious to see how Sandi would be treated by those who had opposed her so vehemently only an hour before. (She had been in tears at one point, openly questioning whether she should even be a CPM.) When Ina May arrived at the dining room, she rushed over to Sandi, gave her a big hug, and thanked her for "speaking her truth" and "holding her space." Ina May said that when one midwife holds her space, it always works out better for everyone than if she had given in against her will and compromised her principles. And so the dinner went, with everyone hugging Sandi and expressing their appreciation. They still disagreed with her, but their trust in their consensus process was deep—experience had taught them that somehow it would work out.

By the time the Steering Committee met after dinner, everyone on it was exhausted, including me. We sprawled around the room and tentatively started the discussion. Sandi still wouldn't budge, until Becky Martin, a consumer representative from the Florida School of Traditional Midwifery, said, "Well, Sandi, if you knew that most of the midwives in the US wanted IVs to be required, would you still hold this position?" Sandi answered, "Of course not! I'm not here to tell the majority of midwives what they should do! It's just that I don't think the 40 women at this meeting [all of whom were midwifery leaders or directors of private midwifery schools] really represent the majority of practicing midwives—I'm trying to speak out for the ones who are not here, who don't think as you do." At that point, with dawning amazement, the group began to realize that we had just been handed a golden key. It occurred to all of us simultaneously that none of us could really say *what* the majority of practicing midwives thought about which skills should be required for entry-level practice, and so obviously we should *ask* them—and right away the Steering Committee began to actively and excitedly plan what soon turned out to be the largest survey of practicing midwives ever conducted in the US.

Some months later, after hundreds of volunteer hours of work, 3,000 surveys were mailed, and although they were so detailed they took over 12 hours to fill out, 800 or so of them were returned in usable form (Houghton and Windom 1996a, b).[3] As a result, the CPM certification process was based on midwifery as actually practiced by these 800 out-of-hospital midwives, not just by the 40 who had been present on Captiva Island that day. These grass-roots midwives themselves set the standards by which they were to be judged and thereby avoided two of (what they saw as) the primary potential downsides of certification—the many being co-opted by the rule-making few and the quality and individualized design of apprenticeship training being co-opted by mass standardization. Thus this process fully exemplified both the inclusive attitude and the informed relativism of the postmodern midwife.

The Postmodern Preservation of Apprenticeship in the Creation of the CPM

Licensure is not something that should be forced on recalcitrant midwives by a paternalistic government. It is something that should be created by midwives; it is the next step in self-actualization

— Ida Darragh, NARM board chair

By the consensus of the majority of midwives who participated in the survey, routes to the CPM include university education, private accredited schools, and what is known as "pure apprenticeship." The time-honored apprenticeship route, not considered legitimate by the ACNM, is highly valued by the members of MANA and the NARM board for the connective and embodied experiential learning it provides.[4] Apprenticeship training is a thoroughly individualized process, the shape and nature of which depends on the relationship that develops between apprentice and mentor. When it is suc-

[3] Regarding the IV question, a large majority of survey respondents indicated that IV insertion should not be required for entry-level practice, and so it was not and still is not, though CPMs must be able to identify when an IV is needed and either transport or get someone else to insert it if they cannot. (However, most of them do learn that skill, even though it is not a requirement for certification.) Another fascinating result of the original survey was in the category of "Well-Woman Care." Respondents indicated that they did not wish the category as a whole to be required; however, they did wish all the skills listed under it to be required. At first puzzled by this response, the NARM board eventually ascertained that its meaning was that practicing midwives wanted entry-level midwives *to be able to perform* all these skills, but not to be *required* to offer general well-woman (gynecological) care. See Davis-Floyd 2006 for a full description of the development of the CPM credential and certification process.

[4] See Jordan 1993, Ch. 7, for a detailed discussion of the differences between experiential and didactic learning.

cessful, the apprentice–mentor relationship provides a supportive and nurturant educational context within which the apprentice can learn about pregnancy and birth through the immediacy of touch and experience, and can supplement that embodied knowledge with reading and long discussions with her mentor and others. Apprentices accompany their mentors to homebirths, witnessing woman after woman give birth successfully on her own, and developing comprehension of the normal, untrammeled birth process. Where hospital training tends to focus on pathology and generate a fear-based approach to birth, homebirth apprentice training generates *trust.* Midwives who fundamentally trust birth are more likely to be able to create an atmosphere within which women can find their power and trust themselves to give birth. Thus, preserving apprenticeship—the route by which most traditional midwives around the world have always been trained—because of their postmodern awareness of its value in both the past and the present has been and remains essential to the ethos and ethics of MANA's and NARM's philosophy and practice (Davis-Floyd 1998b, 2010; Benoit et al. 2001). In 1997, speaking for all those who participated in the development of CPM certification, CPMs Pam Weaver, Elizabeth Davis, and Alice Sammon exclaimed, "We did it! We actually managed to develop a certification that encompasses everything we hold dear!"

Preserving apprenticeship has in fact generated many problems for contemporary CPMs, as those who graduate from formal accredited programs meet the international definition of a midwife, while those who learn via pure apprenticeship do not (see Chapter 6). For that reason, ACNM recognizes only about half of CPMs (those from formal programs) as "midwives" and codes the rest as "TBAs," refusing to recognize them or support legislation legalizing them. (They do this not out of malice but because they consider themselves bound by the ICM international definition.) And some states have followed suit, passing laws that legitimate CPM formal program graduates but not those who come from apprenticeship training (see Chapter 6). Nevertheless, for now the NARM board continues to keep the apprenticeship route open, continuing the legacy of its first chair, Ruth Walsh, who insisted during her retirement speech, "We must always protect and preserve this precious jewel called apprenticeship."

Professional vs. Traditional Midwives: The Ramifications of Definition

I have described the above aspects of the development of CPM certification in part because they make a great story, and in part because the issues of IV skills (which many traditional midwives such as Doña Irene, Doña Facunda, and others have easily mastered) and apprenticeship training bring up yet again the arbitrariness of the distinction between professional and traditional midwives. Any effort to make sense of the complexities of contemporary midwifery must deal not only with biomedical and governmental power structures but also with the definitions such structures impose upon midwives and the ramifications of these definitions within and across national and cultural borders. The international definition of a midwife requires graduation from a government-recognized educational program. Again, those who have not done so are not considered "midwives" (in English) but are labeled "TBAs." Since there are myriad local names for midwives in myriad languages (and many modes of birth assistance that occur but are not performed by named folk specialists), the impact of this naming at local levels can be hard to assess (Cosminsky 1977, 1983; Pigg 1997). But on the global scale, the ramifications of the distinction between midwives who meet the international definition and those who do not have been profound. Those who do are incorporated into the health care system (usually below doctors in the medical hierarchy and above nurses). Those who do not remain outside of it, and suffer multiple forms of discrimination as a result.

Many social scientists studying contemporary midwifery find the arbitrary distinction between TBAs and midwives to be highly problematic in terms of its cultural effects. From a social science perspective, a government-approved midwifery training does not necessarily produce a midwife—it may produce a "mini-doctor" instead. Thus social scientists tend to define midwives not only in terms of their attendance at births but also in terms of their social and community roles. In other words, for most social scientists, a "midwife" can be a practitioner who meets the international definition and/or one who is recognized as such by her community.

In general, social scientists do not assume that the roles and the practices of those considered "real" midwives according to the international definition are any more important to the welfare of women and children than the role of the practitioners officially classified as TBAs. Every social scientist who studies contemporary midwifery (including social scientists who are also midwives) is impressed by the ongoing contributions of "TBAs" and concerned by the colonialist and biomedical limitations of professional midwives, especially in low-resource countries where TBAs still attend a large percentage of births. (Social scientists who study midwives also support midwifery in general, as we know midwives to be the most-suited practitioners for the vast majority of births.) Traditional midwives have already vanished or are vanishing at a rapid rate in many parts of the world. Yet the many thousands who remain, from the *dais* of India to the Mexican *parteras tradicionales*, are providing vital services to the populations they serve, both rural and urban, and preserving knowledge systems that contain much that is of value and relevance in the postmodern world.

Defining traditional midwives as TBAs is a powerful statement that their knowledge does not count in the global system. And indeed in some cases their practices have been shown to be scientifically unsound, just as the practices of many medicalized professional midwives and physicians have also been shown to be. *The point is not to romanticize traditional midwives but to approach them with the same informed relativism that postmodern professional midwives apply to biomedicine.* A relativistic, postmodern perspective reveals that the same traditional midwife who uses cow dung to dry the umbilicus or tells a mother that her colostrum is bad for her baby (in fact it's the best possible nourishment a newborn can have) can often skillfully and successfully attend births that would confound professional midwives accustomed to obstetrical backup (see Chapter 9, pp. 271–272 for a prime example).

The same postmodern perspective reveals that professional midwives with years of government-approved training may withhold food and drink from laboring women and force them to deliver flat on their backs. Indeed, the surest marker that traditional midwives have had contact with medicalized professional midwives and government-sponsored trainings is that they suddenly begin to demand that their clients deliver in that most unscientific of positions. There is nothing postmodern about the willful eradication of traditional healing and birth systems, and everything postmodern about their preservation and their combination with science-based professional midwifery knowledge—precisely as the CPM credentialing process seeks to do. The CPM is the only midwifery credential in the world that recognizes and validates all types of midwifery education, insisting that it is *what midwives know* that counts, and not where they learned it, which can be in a university program, a private vocational program, or via apprenticeship. This uniqueness of the CPM surely makes it worthy of further academic study and research (for one example, see Cheyney et al. 2015); it stands as an example of postmodern possibilities. Creating this kind of combination, this synthesis of knowledge systems, is a challenge faced by all postmodern midwives, whether professional, or traditional, or an elision of both.

As I hope I have made clear, postmodern *professional* midwives in my definition are culturally sensitive and competent, work respectfully and cooperatively with traditional midwives and, like the CASA students, include traditional practices in their repertoire and either incorporate, or at least respect, the apprenticeship model of midwifery education, like the CPMs of the US, and also the CNMs, who often emphasize that their educational process includes a major preceptorship component very akin to traditional apprenticeship. Postmodern *traditional* midwives gain exposure to both biomedical *and* professional midwifery information and techniques and selectively incorporate these into their practice, learning as they go. Informed relativism characterizes both groups. Thus, as I have noted previously, the line between the professional and the traditional midwife is becoming increasingly

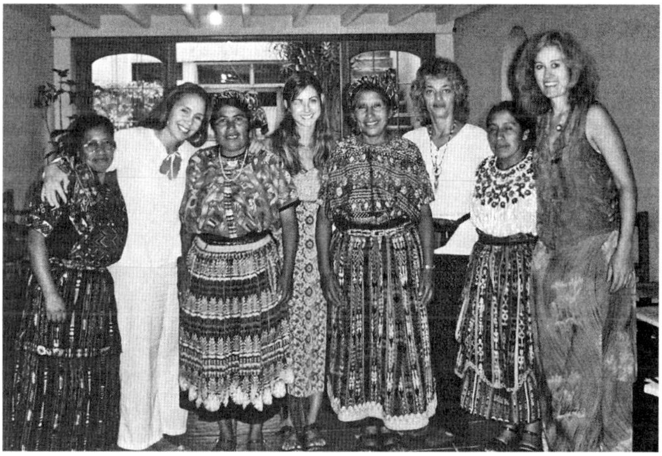

A rainbow of transnational interlinkages—Mexican and Guatemalan midwives with international birth workers and activists—coming together at a Midwifery Today conference in Oaxaca.

blurred. This fact affects the ongoing viability of the international definition of a midwife and the ultimate goal of all midwives—the welfare of mothers and babies.

The Postmodern Obstetrician: A Brief Note

The obstetrician should be the hero of the hospital!
— Marcos Leite MD

Of course, obstetricians can be postmodern too, when they are characterized by the informed relativism I have emphasized here as the primary characteristic of the postmodern midwife. I have little space here to address this issue (but see Chapter 5); I would just like to note that as my friend and colleague Marcos Leite (a very postmodern Brazilian ob/gyn who attends both home- and hospital births in private practice with his son Pablo in Florianopolis, Brazil) often says, "The obstetrician should be the hero of the hospital!" By this he means that midwives should be in charge of all normal births, while OBs should be ready to swoop in to save the day when their expertise in pathology is clearly needed. The postmodern obstetrician as I define him or her sees the proper ratio for birth attendance as something like midwives: 80%, and OBs: 20%. In the hospital in which Marcos worked for some years, this ratio was achieved. The nurse-midwives attended the majority of the births, referring to the OBs the high-risk cases that the midwives themselves identified. During his years in that public hospital, Marcos' personal CS rate was 75%; how, you ask, can an OB who considers himself humanistic have a CS rate that high? Because, of course, he attended only the high-risk cases referred to him by the midwives; thus he was quite proud that 25% of his deliveries were vaginal births, even though they were all high-risk.

This ratio has actually been achieved country-wide in New Zealand, where postmodern midwives proliferate. Ninety-two percent of New Zealand mothers choose midwives to be their primary pregnancy and birth attendants. The midwives refer the high-risk cases to the OBs, yet stay with the mother as well all during labor, even if she has a scheduled cesarean. All New Zealand mothers—100% of them—have a midwife present during their births even if an OB—for the high-risk cases—is in charge (see Hendry 2009; Guilliland 2017; Georges and Dallenbach forthcoming for descriptions of the New Zealand model). New Zealand obstetricians have come to understand that midwives are in fact better qualified than they to attend normal deliveries and that their role is best confined to true cases of risk; it is to be hoped that their excellent model will spread.

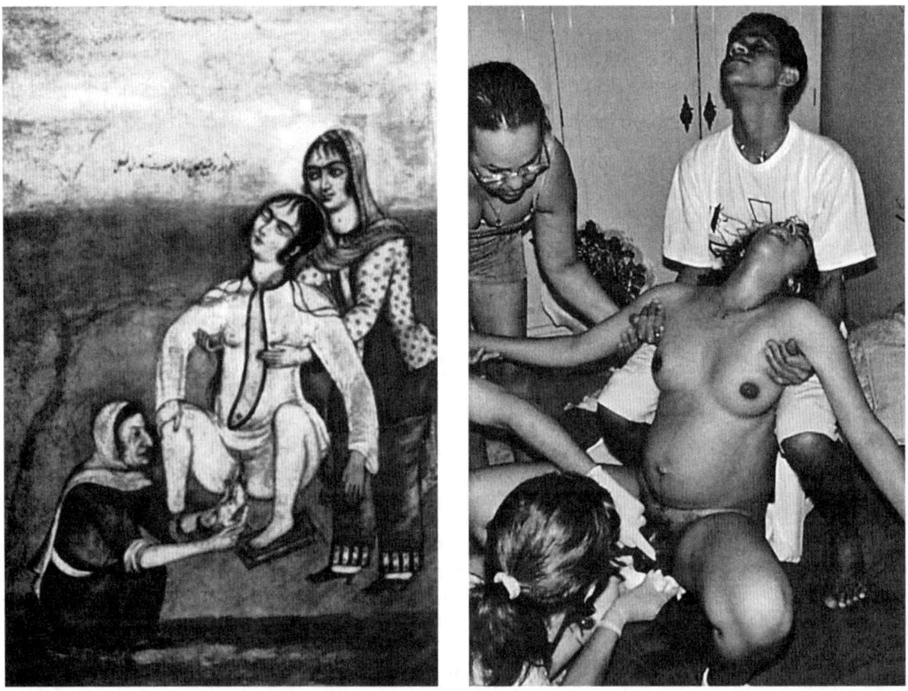

A painting of a traditional Indian birth and a photograph of a contemporary postmodern Brazilian birth, a juxtaposition that brings the best of the transnational past into the present. Note the precise similarities in birth position and the place of the midwife, and in the support provided to the birthing woman. Photo by holistic obstetrician Ricardo Jones (see Chapter 5). The attending nurse-midwife is his wife, Zeza, one of Brazil's most well-known midwives.

Conclusion: Daughters of the Past Redefining Themselves in the Present

Postmodern midwives, for all their value, often find themselves living in a constant state of stress, lobbying legislatures for the right to exist, struggling to balance conflicting ideologies and knowledge systems, and arguing with each other about appropriate standards for education and practice. In developed and developing countries alike, the tensions between biomedical, traditional, and alternative knowledge systems permeate professional midwifery training and praxis and generate conflicts between midwifery educators, between educators and students, and among practicing midwives and those who regulate them. The professional midwives of the industrialized North are accelerating their long struggle for autonomy even as traditional midwives in the less affluent countries of the South continue to lose the autonomy they formerly held. In short, today nothing is easy about being a midwife of any type. Yet motivated by a shared desire to offer viable long-term options to biomedical birth, these postmodern daughters of time and tradition continue their struggle, with varying degrees of success, but always

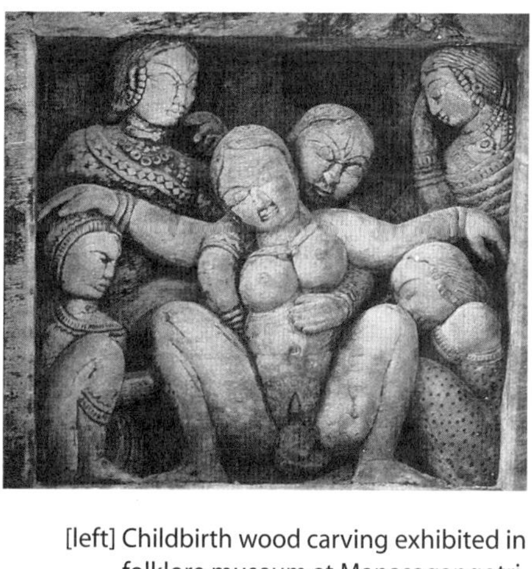

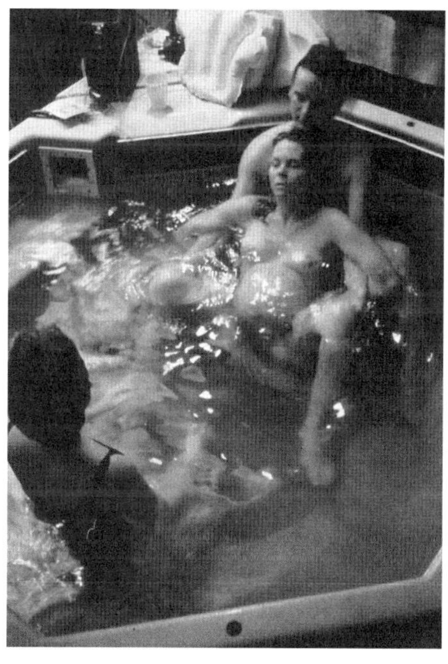

[left] Childbirth wood carving exhibited in folklore museum at Manasagangotri, Karnataka, India, showing a premodern, traditional midwife-attended birth. Photo by Dinodia Photos/Alamy Stock Photo. [right] Cathy, a postmodern American midwife supports me (Robbie) to labor in water. Note the similarities in position as I went "back to the past" to recapture ancient indigenous ways of knowing about birth in my own homebirth in 1984. Photo by Peter Gonzalez

with the necessary determination to make sure that midwives, with all their limitations *and* all their power, remain available to care for the mothers, babies, and families of the contemporary world.

Questions for Thought and Discussion

1. Explain, in Davis-Floyd's terms, the differences between the "premodern," "modern," and "postmodern" eras. Are these terms useful to you in understanding the unfolding of human history?
2. What does Davis-Floyd mean by "postmodern midwife"? What are the major defining characteristics of a postmodern midwife?
3. Can obstetricians, in Davis-Floyd's view, be postmodern too? What does that entail?

Recommended Films

Birth Story: Ina May Gaskin and the Farm Midwives: produced by Kate Roughan and Zachary Mortenson, 2012. See full description at the end of Chapter 6. Available at: http://birthstorymovie.com/the-film/

Guerilla Midwife: produced by Robin Lim and Deja Burnhardt, 2011. This film features midwife Robin Lim, who was voted CNN Hero of the Year for 2011, showing her work in Bali where she owns and operates a world-famous birth center called Bumi Sehat Bali, as well as her disaster-relief work and later construction of Bumi Sehat Aceh in Aceh, Indonesia, after the tsunami. Available at http://www.guerrillamidwife.com/

Acknowledgments

The members of the NARM board and the Certification Task Force were always tolerant of and helpful with my dual roles as participant and researcher, and I would like to express my appreciation to them for accepting me in both capacities. I again express my gratitude to Janneli Miller and Doña Queta for (unwittingly) helping me develop the useful notion of "the postmodern midwife." And many thanks to all my midwife interviewees, both in Mexico and in the US, for their time and their efforts to help me understand their ideologies and their practices.

9

Mutual Accommodation or Biomedical Hegemony?

A Brief Anthropological Overview of Global Issues in Midwifery

A Dysfunctional Maternity Care System

As I have previously noted in this volume, and need to re-address here, a distressing cross-cultural trend is showing up in the growing body of anthropological literature about midwifery and birth in low- and middle-resource countries. Around the world, and most especially in developing countries, anthropologists who observe professional midwives giving prenatal care and attending births in facilities such as city hospitals and rural medical clinics, increasingly note that, far from the midwifery ideal, professional midwives often treat women very badly during birth, ignoring their needs and requests, talking to them disrespectfully, ordering them around, and sometimes even yelling at them and slapping them (Miller et al. 2016). At the same time, and in direct correlation, the professional midwives are themselves often treated badly by the health care systems in which they work. They are almost always underpaid, are frequently mistreated by physicians

This chapter is adapted and expanded from my article, "Mutual Accommodation or Biomedical Hegemony? Anthropological Perspectives on Global Issues in Midwifery," originally published in *Midwifery Today*, March 2000, pp. 12–17, 68–89. Copyright Midwifery Today and Robbie Davis-Floyd.

who rank above them in the medical hierarchy, and generally work long hours under stressful conditions that often include inadequate facilities and equipment and too many women with too few midwives to care for them well. In short, professional midwives are often trapped in the biomedical health care system, a system that is failing to meet the needs of birthing women in developing countries.

To recap the ICM international definition: a midwife is one who graduates from a program duly recognized in its jurisdiction. In low- and middle-resource countries, this generally means a two- or three-year government training program. The women who attend these programs are usually young, often fresh out of high school, and have borne no children themselves. They are educated in an urban environment, then sent out to serve in a rural village, where they wear the white coat and expect respect from the townspeople for their professional, educated status. They usually work in the government-built clinic, but for an extra sum of money will sometimes attend a homebirth if they are called. These government clinics are usually underfunded and understaffed, and often the drugs with which they are supposed to be stocked are sold out the back door by clinic staff to compensate for the inadequate salaries they are paid. Anthropological ethnographies now spanning two decades describe indigenous women in India, Mexico, Tanzania, Papua New Guinea, and elsewhere, saying the same thing about the care they receive in these clinics: “They expose you, they shave you, they cut you, they leave you alone and don’t come when you call, and they won’t allow your relatives to be with you.” Here is a highly representative quote from an article by anthropologist Pauline Kolenda describing birth in a hospital near a small village in India:

> Before entering the hospital we have first to decide how much money we have to give. We are not admitted unless we first give them money. When the woman enters into the hospital, the doctor behaves rudely with her. Sometimes nurses beat her. They do not let close and affectionate relatives, who came from home with us, stand at our side. They themselves either do not stay near us. We wish that somebody hold us by the waist when pains come, but they do not do it. We have not even to moan, lest they talk sarcastically, make fun of us, which is very hurting, still we have to bear. If we moan too much, they may sometimes slap us. If we happen to say something, they retort by asking us whether they had invited us to come. “Why have you come then? You may go back home!” In hospital we have to lie down on the bed to get delivered. In the hospital they excise the vaginal wall with a blade for enlarging it. The body gets damaged unnecessarily. After delivery we feel terribly hungry, but we consider ourselves lucky if we get a cup of tea. (1998:6)

Not surprisingly, even though the governments of these countries have embarked on massive programs to bring birth into the clinics and hospitals, many rural women resist, choosing instead to birth at home with a community midwife. As described in Chapter 8, officially labeled "traditional birth attendants" (TBAs) by WHO and UNICEF because they do not meet the international definition of a midwife, these community midwives are usually older women who have given birth several times and who have become midwives by being asked to attend the births of friends and relatives, slowly gaining firsthand experience of birth. Some of them undertake long apprenticeships with experienced community midwives, while others learn simply by attending births. From the point of view of villagers and townsfolk all over the developing world, the biggest difference between community and professional midwives is that community midwives are recognized by their community as midwives, while the professionals are often seen as young and inexperienced women who have to prove their worth to the villagers before they can be trusted.

When the professional midwives make a sincere effort to learn about and honor local customs and traditions, when they approach local people with an attitude of respect and demonstrate willingness to work with community midwives, honoring them as colleagues, this partnership-oriented system

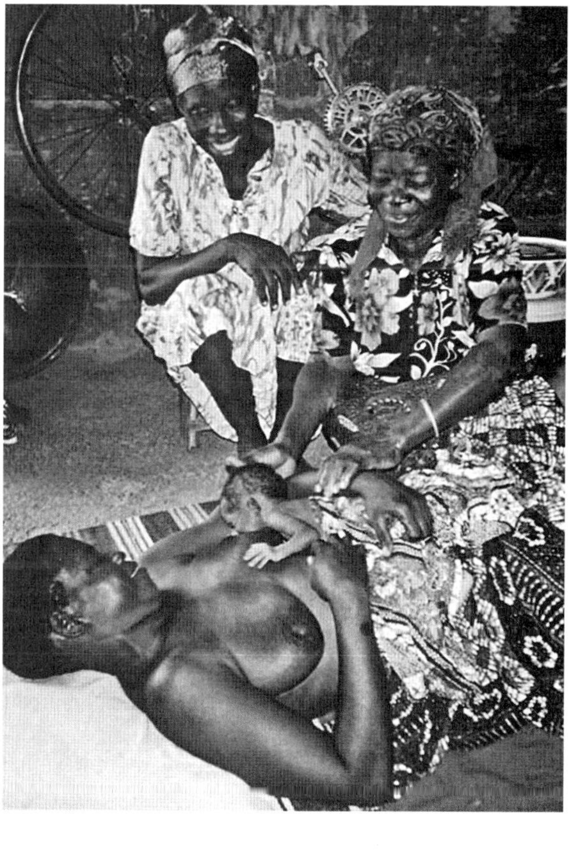

Breastfeeding after a homebirth in Ghana attended by a traditional midwife with an American CNM, Mary Kroeger, there as backup—an example of mutual accommodation. With hormones and pheromones flowing, the baby seeks the breast. If newborns are placed on the mother's stomach immediately after birth, they often will crawl upwards and bob their heads, searching by smell for the nipple that will give them colostrum they need. Photo by Mary Kroeger

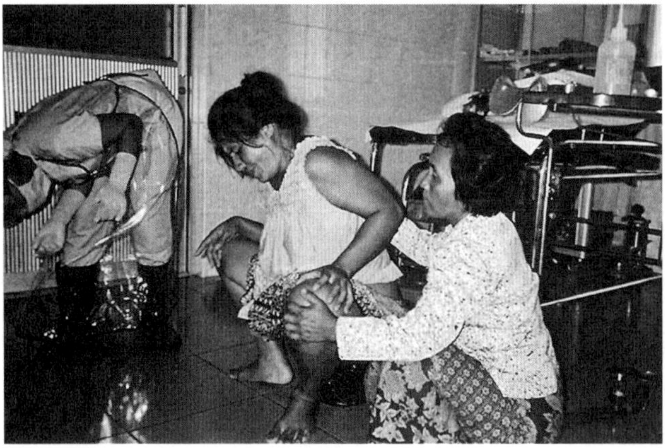

An example of mutual accommodation of birthing systems: A traditional midwife assists a woman giving birth on an inexpensive birthing stool inside a public hospital, while the doctor leans down to try to see if the baby is coming. Photo by Mary Kroeger

can function efficiently. In such cases, community midwives are generally very willing to advise women to go to the clinic or hospital in situations of risk and will often accompany them there if they are sure of being well received and of getting adequate care for their clients.

But when doctors and professional midwives approach the community with an attitude of arrogance, treat the TBA with disdain, and punish women who attempt homebirth by treating them badly when they do transport—an all-too-typical situation—a consensual agreement is made among mothers and their at-home attendants to avoid the clinic or hospital at all costs. Such a situation leaves the community midwife to cope with emergencies at home as best she can, often until it is too late to seek help. If disaster befalls, of course, it is she who takes the blame, when in fact the fault may lie in the dysfunctionality of the system.

Debora Barnes-Josiah and her colleagues (1998) showed that in Haiti, as in other countries, a lack of confidence in available medical options was a crucial factor in delayed or never made decisions to seek medical care. They suggested that improving the quality and scope of care available at existing medical facilities would prove crucial in reducing needless maternal deaths. Likewise, Soheir Morsy (1995) has shown that in the rural area of Egypt she studied, traditional midwives were getting blamed for the high rates of maternal mortality, when in fact most of the deaths occurred among women who had given birth in the hospital as a result of complications from cesarean sections. Here is a further and very clear description of the international situation from the recent *FIGO Guidelines for mother-baby friendly birthing facilities*:

> The majority of maternal mortality reduction programs encourage facility birth with skilled providers . . . including conditional cash transfers and other methods/strategies to improve facility-based delivery rates. However, many facilities, particularly in low- and middle-income countries are overcrowded, understaffed, and have few resources. Women

> often choose to avoid facilities because of abuse, coercion, or neglect. . . . Recently there has been increasing focus among international and national organizations on examining the quality of care, abuse/neglect of women in facilities during childbirth, and the lack of professional and social accountability among facility-based providers of care. . . . Evidence collected in a variety of settings has documented that the quality of care is related to the quality of maternal and newborn health outcomes, including mortality. . . Miller et al. [2003] noted that paradoxically high rates of maternal mortality persisted in the Dominican Republic, despite 98% facility delivery by skilled attendants. The results of the study demonstrated that *the lack of quality care and accountability was at the root of unnecessary maternal deaths*. A recent review series on quality of maternal and newborn care found that *improving access to facilities did not guarantee improved maternal outcomes*, and posited that poor quality of care was the most likely explanatory factor. (Bhutta et al. 2014:1; italics mine)

TBA Training: Another Dysfunctional Approach

UNICEF, WHO, and those once engaged in implementing the Safe Motherhood Initiative have for well over three decades centered their efforts to reduce maternal and perinatal mortality in the developing world around "TBA training"—short, usually two-week-long courses taught by medical personnel, usually doctors, nurses, or professional midwives to community midwives. The purpose of these courses has generally been to educate TBAs about the risks that require transport and to improve their prenatal and maternity care. Of course, these courses too have been plagued by the same systems failures as the situations I describe above. Almost always, these courses are designed by biomedical personnel trained in biomedical institutions to think about and manage birth in biomedical ways. Very seldom do the "trainers" enter a community and spend time there learning about the indigenous birthways before they try to intervene. Rather, they attempt to educate traditional midwives in medical ways of thinking that are often totally inappropriate to local circumstances and realities.

For example, perhaps the local custom is to cauterize the cord with a candle flame after cutting it, or instead of cutting it, to burn it apart—an extremely sanitary practice. Trying to replace that sustainable custom with Merthiolate (a topical antiseptic) in a place where supplies are scarce and Merthiolate is unavailable or expensive is an unsustainable and inappropriate intervention, but one nevertheless that typifies this training approach. Another example provided by Brigitte Jordan in *Birth in Four Cultures* (1993) is the Yucatecan practice of using a sliver of freshly cut bamboo to cut the cord—also a sanitary practice. But when the TBA trainers came to town, they tried to eliminate that practice by telling the midwives to use sterile scissors instead. But such sterility is impossible to achieve when you have to boil the water in the kitchen across the compound from the birthing room, then carry the scissors in the water in an unsterilized bowl—of course instances of neonatal tetanus started occurring where they never had before. Unfortunately, TBA trainers often think their job is done if they succeed in educating midwives about the multiple conditions that are biomedically deemed to require transport to a clinic or hospital (some of these conditions, such as "advanced maternal age" [over 35] appear absurd to the midwives). The training complete, the trainers leave, and the midwives get blamed if they do not transport for the risks they have just been educated about, even when transport is simply not available.

The Complexities of "TBA Training": Patricia's Story

I am not minimizing the difficulties of appropriate biomedical training for traditional midwives, and here is why, in a story told by Patricia Kay. Over 30 years ago after completing her training and becoming a well-respected licensed midwife (LM) in New Mexico, she moved to Mexico and became the first professionally trained US midwife to open a practice there. At CASA founder Nadine Goodman's request, she gave a three-year professional training course to four traditional midwives, including Antonia Cordova, who went on to become the clinical director at the CASA Hospital, a position Antonia held for decades. Out of Patricia's original pre-CASA class of four traditional midwives, she noted that Antonia had the least difficulty with didactics and attributed this to the fact that Antonia's earliest midwifery training did not involve hands-on apprenticeship but, rather, didactic training offered through the *Seguro Social*. Patricia concluded that this didactic training had predisposed Antonia to be comfortable with didactic learning and to be open to accepting new information.

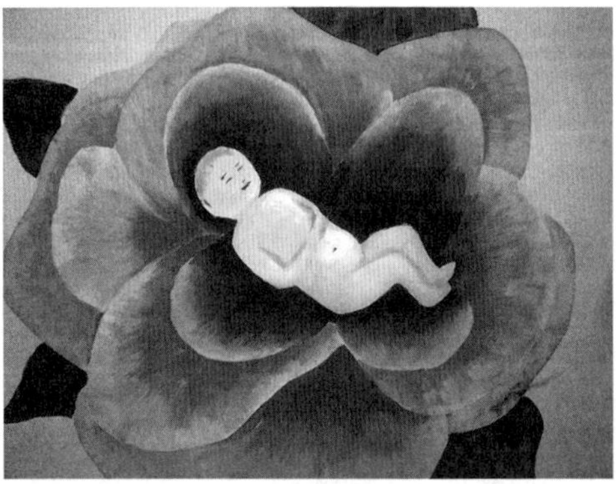

Antonia said that from Patricia she learned not only many lifesaving techniques but also the skill of visualization; she was renowned for "nearly hypnotizing" laboring women by having them imagine their uterus as a rose opening slowly, petal by petal, with each contraction. This photo depicts this image as it appears on the ceiling of Antonia's prenatal exam room, painted by a student as a gift to Antonia, so that women lying on the table could gaze up at the image and internalize it, making the visualizations more effective.

The three other traditional midwives who completed Patricia's three-year course in professional midwifery not only were older than Antonia but were empirically, not didactically, trained and also had been practicing for many years before they came to study with Patricia. She noted that they had grown accustomed to doing birth in particular ways and, thus, seemed to find it difficult to incorporate new information (much like obstetricians steeped in their own traditional ways). Their approach to birth was infused with beliefs and rituals grounded in their particular cultures, and it was upon these that they tended to rely in problematic cases. For example, Patricia described her experience with Esther, the most experienced of her group of four, as follows:

> Esther had already been working for 25 years as a midwife and a traditional herbalist, and her grandmother had been the one she learned from. Esther had worked way more than I had when I was training her. . . . I'm really convinced because of the traditional midwives that I've known here, it's almost as if the Creator puts these outstanding women in certain places on the earth where there is no one else, and they are given these amazing intuitive skills and they take women through the door and they do it. And they have amazingly good records, you know. They live out in the middle of nowhere, they have no medical backup, they work with very poor populations, and yet they have this power about them—a few of them, not all of them, I'm not romanticizing it either—that is steeped in wisdom, deep common sense and a deep connection with something else. And Esther's grandmother and Esther herself were two of these women.
>
> Esther probably had a third-grade education. So I developed all these ways of—we did hands-on teaching all the time, but, you know, Esther already had in her mind a way of approaching Mystery, so that the Western world doesn't really make sense to her, it never really made too much sense.
>
> But, just an example of the difficulty, I took her to a homebirth one time, and she had been a janitrice in the Seguro, which is where she learned to do IVs because she watched the nurses do them and she figured out how to put in IVs just by watching—I mean, that's how brilliant she is, you know. So I took her to this homebirth because I thought there would be a good match between her and this woman I was attending, who was a middle-class intellectual, but who had this kind of back-to-nature attitude and thought that herbs and midwives were a good idea.
>
> And it was a long birth, it was a difficult birth. And I thought that things were going along pretty well, and, after about seven hours of being there, Esther says she is really worried. "What's the matter, Esther? The birth is going slowly, but there is definite progress, and the baby is fine, the mom is fine." Esther said, "Yes, but it seems as if it's really slow." "So what would you do?" "What I would do is put aloe vera (*sávila)* on her—put it on her sacrum and it's going to make her sweat and she is going to dilate like that and you'll see, the baby will be here in an hour." I thought, "Fine, if you can make this baby come within the next hour"—because I was thinking at least another seven hours, you know—"I'm going to put a monument to you and to sávila," you know?

So she goes and finds a plant, and she gets the *comal* out, which is a Mexican round plate that we make tortillas on, and she is roasting the sávila and she is getting it nice and warm, and then she takes it and opens it and starts putting crosses all over this woman's body. The woman had agreed to the herb part of it, but she wasn't into magic and she wasn't into the religious part of it, you know? But Esther is invoking this saint and that saint and putting crosses all over her, and she finally puts the aloe vera on her sacrum and she kind of winks at me and she said, "You'll see, within an hour she is ready and she'll have this baby."

Great—an hour came and went and there was now sweat but there was no baby and we go on with this long labor. Esther is beside herself. So she goes out of the room and later, when she comes back, she says, "I just don't know what's happening. I have been praying to San Martín, and praying and praying and he's ignoring me."

So about seven hours later, when dilation is complete and this woman had chosen to squat. . . . And the pushing of course is long like the rest of the birth, so we are waiting and waiting, and Esther is like beside herself again. She said, "What she needs to do is to offer everyone something," so she runs into the kitchen and gets some cookies or something, wanting this woman in the middle of pushing to be offering cookies to everyone! I said, "Esther, relax, put the cookies away, sit down next to me, she is doing fine," you know? So the baby came out, it was a little depressed, and then the mother proceeds to have a massive hemorrhage.

So, since I had to revive the baby, I tell Esther to get an IV in the woman *now* [to administer pitocin to stop the hemorrhage]. And I'm working on the baby and I look over and I see that Esther is about to put a solution in her without draining the line, and I realized that she didn't have this part of it down, that she had never used a butterfly cath, and so I kind of—by then the baby was doing fine, so I go and put in the IV and you know—I thought, by the grace of God this woman has not killed someone, because she never understood the part about draining the line first (which of course I explained to her again, in detail, after the birth). So we got the hemorrhage under control and we wrapped the baby and everyone is fine and we go home. And Esther is just really upset that San Martín has failed her.

And I realized—I have thought a lot about this birth, because the cultural match that goes on, you know, of us who have a cultural background that has included school and doctors and nurses—you can't take that part of yourself out, it's there. So this woman, the intellectual woman who was giving birth, had that. But Esther didn't, and I don't doubt that if we had been in Dolores, where Esther is from—I visited her house and stayed in her birthing room, and there is a little statue with a little plug-in flashing light for San Martín—and you know, I have no doubt that within that whole milieu the sávila and the prayers would have worked.

[This quote is excerpted from Robbie's article "La Partera Profesional: Articulating Identity and Cultural Space for a New Kind of Midwife in Mexico" (Davis-Floyd 2001a.)]

This story resonates with the tensions between folk and professional systems of practice and belief, and between the culture of the *campesino* and the middle class. Patricia speaks to the difference site of care and cultural milieu can make in the experience of birth, acknowledging that, within Esther's accustomed cultural space, where she shared a mutual belief system with her clients, her approach would most likely have yielded results. It also highlights the absurdity of the two-week TBA trainings, which are purely didactic and thus often not intelligible to midwives used to hands-on learning. To fully teach a traditional midwife what she really needs to know would ideally require attending births with her to see what she has internalized from the lessons and where the gaps in her knowledge exist, or at least to conduct peer review with her, discussing some of her more difficult births. After completing Patricia's course, Ester returned to practice in her native town of Dolores, where she received an official commendation for detecting a placenta previa and transporting, thus saving the woman's life, which Patricia had taught her to do.

After completing Patricia's three-year course, Antonia herself became a teacher of a class of four traditional midwives, which was so successful that two of the members of her class, Belén and Manuela, were hired to work permanently at CASA, while the other two went back to continue to practice in their native villages. Traditional midwives are individuals with differing backgrounds and mind-sets; teaching them effectively means *first understanding what they already know and then identifying the gaps in their knowledge and filling them*. Many TBAs around Mexico and in other countries can successfully put in IV lines when necessary and do understand that you must empty the tube of air before inserting the IV.

When There Is No Transport: Stories from Doña Nieves and Doña Queta

In Mexico and other countries, UNICEF discontinued funding for TBA-training courses years ago when it was determined that maternal mortality rates had not dropped after 20–30 years of TBA training; the conclusion was that TBA training does not work. Of course it didn't work; as we have seen, the trainings given all over the world were almost always inadequate and dysfunctionally inappropriate to their cultural settings. This conclusion that training TBAs does not help was based on the assumption that mothers die because these "untrainable" TBAs give them bad care or fail to transport them in cases of need. But as we have seen, often it is the hospital that gives inadequate care. And often women in need are simply unable to reach the hospital. I remember well when Doña Nieves, a very short and very experienced traditional midwife from rural Oaxaca, Mexico, bravely stood up in the big auditorium in Mexico City in the middle of the Safe Motherhood Conference and said to all assembled:

> Do not blame us for failing to transport women. We know when we should transport. But none of us own cars, nor do our clients, the buses run very irregularly, there is no ambulance service and if there were our clients couldn't pay for it, and the only taxi driver in our town charges far more than our women can pay. How then do you expect us to get our clients to the hospital in the city an hour away? No, we can't, we just have to do the best we can with no help from anyone. If you want me to transport women who need to go to the hospital, give me a car!

She did get a huge round of applause, but no car.

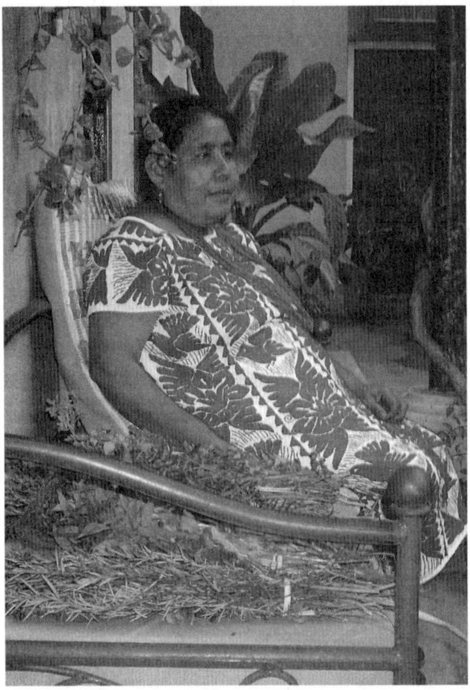

Doña Nieves with some of her traditional herbs, which she had with her to use in teaching a workshop at a Midwifery Today conference in Oaxaca.

Doña Queta, whom we have already met, described to me how a woman came to Queta's tiny village high in the Oaxacan mountains many years ago. The woman, nine months pregnant, had tripped over a log and fallen hard. As she got up, she felt the baby move once, and then no more. Afraid that the baby had died, the mother walked for two days over the mountains to get to Doña Queta's home. By the time she arrived, said Queta, the odor around her was foul and it was obvious that the baby was dead. What to do? The woman had arrived alone and penniless. Doña Queta went to fetch the one doctor within 100 miles, but he was away on a trip. So she spent the next three days pouring liters of antibiotic herbs into the woman and praying for her life. Finally the woman went into labor and gave birth to the dead fetus, and then almost died herself from massive infection. But Queta persevered with the antibiotic herbs and other nutrients, the rituals, and the prayers, and two weeks later the woman walked home alive and well. When the doctor arrived back from his trip and found out what had happened, he scolded Queta for taking on the care of this woman, but had to back off when he realized that he had left her with no other choice besides leaving the woman to die on the road. (See Contreras 2009 for descriptions of Doña Queta's herbal knowledge and healing techniques.)

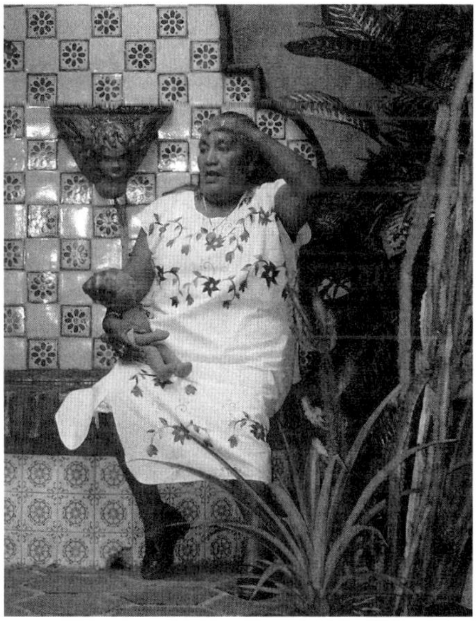

Doña Queta teaching birthing techniques using herbs, a plastic baby, and demonstrating hand maneuvers.

In an ideal world, and because *women want care in their communities*, the community midwife is the first line of care and is backed up by professional midwives, doctors, and the biomedical system. In the real world, often there is no backup or no way to get to it, and she must handle whatever comes as best she can. Clearly, the solution does not lie in giving her superficial training in biomedicine and expecting her to get women to the hospital when they need to go; rather, the solution must be found in a system-wide approach that requires as much flexibility of biomedicine as it does of the community midwife.

Achieving Functionality: Examples of Mutual Accommodation

Consider for example the case of a rural tribe of cattle herders in a remote corner of an African country. (This tribe must remain unnamed because of the current politics in that country surrounding "TBA" training—the program I am describing here might be shut down by the government if it becomes aware that it still exists, as low-resource countries everywhere work to phase out or eliminate "TBAs.") A British midwife whom I will call Susan went to this country some years ago to work in a public health clinic serving this tribe. Maternal mortality rates were high among this group, and Susan wanted to improve maternity care. She had been trained to think that the Western system was the best; nevertheless, it occurred to her that it might be a good idea to learn about the indigenous system before trying to change it. Slowly getting to know the local midwives, she eventually developed good enough rapport with them to suggest weekly meetings during which they could engage in mutual discussion of their different techniques. Susan discovered over time

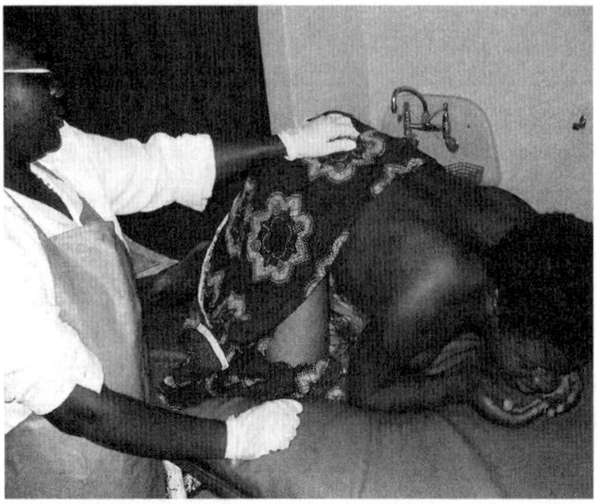

Functionality in mutual accommodation. A Malawi mother giving birth in the highly physiologic hands-and-knees position in a rural medical clinic attended by a compassionate nurse-midwife. Photo by Mary Kroeger

that these midwives had many skills; she came to realize just how many one day when a wizened elder midwife came running out to stop Susan's Land Rover, waving her hands excitedly. She told Susan she was very sorry that she would miss the meeting that day; she had to stay home as both her daughter and her daughter-in-law had given birth the night before to twins! One of the twins (the second to emerge) had been transverse, and she had had to do an internal version to get it out (the midwife has to reach into the uterus, grab the feet and pull them down, then sweep up the arms so they won't get twisted or stuck)—a situation that would have had most professional midwives, including Susan, in fits. Both mothers, and all four babies, were doing well.

It turned out, Susan found, that the indigenous system didn't really need changing; the problem lay, as it so often does, in the *interface between* the biomedical and the indigenous systems. Tribal midwives who transported were often rudely and dismissively treated, so they tended to hold on at home longer than was wise in order to avoid subjecting themselves and their clients to such disrespect. Susan's solution was to bring the clinic staff, two at a time, to the weekly meetings she held with the midwives. As the staff developed more respect for the community midwives, they invited them to the clinic for tours and get-acquainted sessions. Then when the midwives transported, their advice was respectfully solicited and listened to, and they were invited to remain with their clients and give labor support. This model of mutual accommodation, which Susan called the "partnership paradigm," was implemented over 17 years ago as a result of Susan's work and is still functioning well. (She wrote an outstanding article about it which, unfortunately, cannot be published because of the political issues I mentioned above.) Susan's partnership paradigm reminds me of the models American direct-entry midwives often develop with doctors and hospitals in their communities. After years of mistreatment by hospital personnel, over time they earn their respect and develop good working relationships that exemplify this partnership paradigm, as described in the following chapter on home to hospital transport.

All over the developing world, in spite of the massive dysfunctionality of most obstetric systems, it is possible to find models that work. The system that Dr. Galba de Araújo developed in northeastern Brazil is one prime example. Araújo was the head of obstetrics and gynecology at a tertiary care center in Fortaleza, Ceara, Brazil. Concerned about high mortality rates in the rural regions his hospital served, he went out to the rural communities and asked the midwives what was needed. Their answer was that women needed a clean and safe place to give birth; most of their houses had dirt floors, and cleanliness was almost impossible to maintain. So he created a system of maternity care clinics in numerous rural villages. These centers were equipped with donations from local villagers: anything was welcome, from a fork to a plate to a chair. Each center was equipped with the hammocks in which local women preferred to give birth, and with the drugs and equipment that Dr. Araújo felt the midwives should have. He also created an efficient radio and ambulance system, so that transport over long distances was as readily available as possible should the midwives call for it. Outcomes in these maternity centers were so good that Dr. Araújo began to study what the traditional midwives did and ended up incorporating hammocks, more patience, and upright positions for birth into the hospital. This system functioned efficiently until his death; it has since been dismantled due to lack of support and interest on the part of the younger obstetricians who replaced him. While it existed, this system was an excellent example of Susan's "partnership paradigm," or what Brigitte Jordan has called "mutual" or "fruitful" accommodation" between biomedical and indigenous systems.

Biomedical Hegemony: Examples of Its Consequences

In 1978 with the publication of the first edition of *Birth in Four Cultures*, Jordan issued a call for the replacement of top-down, culturally inappropriate, biomedically-oriented systems with models of mutual accommodation like the ones Galba Araújo and Susan created. But the worldwide hegemony of Western biomedicine has made this kind of mutual accommodation an elusive goal. Why bother to accommodate to a system you regard as inferior? Why not, as has so often been done, demand instead that the indigenous system change to accommodate biomedical ways of knowing and managing birth? The answer is quite clear of course: *biomedicine is an inappropriate model for birth in any culture. It is too costly, too interventive, too drug- and technology-oriented, and does too much harm to mothers and babies for it to be a viable model to which developing countries should aspire.* Nevertheless, because of the general global dominance of the West, the legacy of colonialism, and the dramatic successes of biomedicine in other arenas, all developing countries do aspire to meet the standards set by Western medicine, standards that are inappropriate for birth and indeed for many of the world's health needs.

Consider the following description of a clinic birth in rural Papua New Guinea (PNG) from the doctoral dissertation of Julia Byford, an Australian nurse-midwife who also became an anthropologist:

> Mispa, a young woman of twenty, was admitted to the hospital this morning [after walking for a whole day to get there]. She is seen by the Health Examination Officer, who does a vaginal exam and tells me that she is four to five centimetres dilated . . . and that she may commence a Syntocinon [pitocin] infusion. . . . The labor room is small and the air conditioning unit mounted high on the wall belches cold air at us. When it is on the room gets very cold; when it is off the room gets hot and stuffy. There is a sink but no plumbing to allow it to be operational. There is no water at the hospital today anyway. . . . Mispa asks to sit on the floor and is given permission to do this, but as her labour progresses the nurse says she must stay on the bed so the staff can do their observations. She acquiesces and does not ask for anything else. Most of the time she is left alone. She has not eaten all day and only drunk a small amount of water. Her lips are dry and swollen. The staff do numerous vaginal examinations but none of them are recorded [so when a shift changes, another exam is performed].
>
> During the second stage of labour, every time Mispa has a contraction, the Health Examination Officer inserts a few fingers into Mispa's vagina between the perineum and the baby's head in order to stretch the perineum. Mispa finds this excruciating and tightens her grip on my arm. . . . [After the birth] I am dismayed although not surprised to see that the baby is flat and pale and requires resuscitation. The HEO delivers the placenta by placing one hand on Mispa's abdomen and pulling on the umbilical cord with the other hand [a very dangerous practice]. . . . As soon as the placenta is out, Mispa has a large postpartum hemorrhage. The HEO asks me to increase the intravenous infusion rate and then inserts her hand high up into Mispa's vagina and manually removes some retained placental pieces. This is done without explanation or anesthetic.
>
> Perhaps the hardest thing for me to come to terms with is the lack of care offered to Mispa simply on a human level. She was never consulted, only told what to do and what not to do. . . . No one tended to her basic needs for food or fluids or inquired if she needed to go to the toilet. It was as if Mispa, the embodied person, did not exist. (Byford, 1999:186–190)

Unfortunately, this description is all too typical of clinic and hospital births in low-resource countries. Byford's dissertation describes the general poor health of rural Papuan women, who suffer from overwork, exhaustion, anemia, malnutrition, and a variety of diseases that result from their lack of access to clean water. She discusses research in public health, which shows that the single most important intervention that colonial health services could have brought to PNG would have been an adequate clean water supply. But biomedicine, here as elsewhere, prevailed, and instead of investing in clean water, PNG invested in doctors and hospitals in the cities, and rural clinics like the one Julia describes above are left with resource deficits, such as the lack of running water. This biomedical approach to health makes it appear that problems should be treated on an individual basis, patient by patient, hospital by hospital, obscuring the fact that the major causes of disease and death, among parturient women as among the general population, are *structural* and will benefit far more from large-scale systemic change than from diverting money into hospitals and clinics.

Given the difficulty of reaching the hospital and the poor treatment they receive once they get there, most rural Papuan women still choose to deliver at home—a trend paralleled around the developing world as rural women, disillusioned with clinics and hospitals, return to their community midwives and traditional birthways, leaving development planners to shake their heads over this unaccountable unwillingness to use modern facilities, attributing it to ignorance and close-mindedness. On the contrary, *birthing at home with a traditional midwife is often a considered decision that women make after weighing the risks and benefits of their options.* For example, Morsy (1995:168) noted:

> In villages of the Nile Delta, although modern medical facilities are available, women prefer to deliver at home with the assistance of a local midwife. This choice is not a result of reified "cultural attitudes" but a measured judgment about the inadequate health care extended to peasants and the urban poor in modern health care settings.

Anthropologist Denise Roth described this process of "measured judgment" in detail in *Bodily Risks, Spiritual Risks: Contrasting Discourses on Pregnancy in a Rural Tanzanian Community* (2000). Policy planners on high decided that each Tanzanian mother should have and be in charge of a card documenting the prenatal care she had received and her health and pregnancy condition. To make sure she carried the card, it was decided that she would have to show it in order to be admitted into the local clinic for labor and birth. In both the city and the small town Roth studied, this confronted each pregnant woman with a difficult decision: should she obtain prenatal care, which was costly, time-consuming, and often inadequate, in case she needed to go to the clinic during labor, or should she cast her lot with the traditional midwife, who was inexpensive and kind but would be unable to take her to the clinic without the card? Not surprisingly, after careful reflection, many women chose the latter option; if they then had problems during labor but could not go to the clinic, the traditional midwife would be blamed for the outcome.

Certainly, as Roger and Patricia Jeffery pointed out in 1993 and as previously stressed in this book, it is important not to romanticize indigenous midwifery and indigenous midwives; not all of them are skilled, not all of them give women good care, and some indigenous customs can be as harmful as many obstetric procedures. Those anthropologists most concerned about overromanticization of the traditional midwife, including the Jefferys, usually study birth in countries like India and Bangladesh, where women's status is low. In a cross-cultural study, Shen and Williamson (1999) point out that low status for women directly correlates with higher maternal mortality rates. Where women's status is low, their nutrition is poor, their overall health is poor, and community midwives are less able to develop effective knowledge systems, as Rosario (1998) and many others have shown. Where women's status is higher, community midwives are often able to develop long-standing and viable systems of indigenous knowledge about birth, as indicated in the growing body of ethnographic literature I cite in this chapter. This literature consistently indicates that community midwives (TBAs) usually give skilled and considerate care and remain, in many parts of the world, the only viable option for millions of women. As an anthropologist, again I question the wisdom of dividing professional midwives and TBAs in this hierarchical, biomedically-oriented way, which allows government agencies and development planners to support one group while trying to exterminate the other. Can't a "real midwife" either be recognized by her government *or* by her community as such?

"Midwifery Hegemony": What Happens When Professional Midwives Buy into the Biomedical Hierarchy?

In sum, the present policy of separating professional from traditional or community midwives has led to midwives' integration into a hierarchical, intensely colonialist system that has doctors at the top, professional midwives in the middle, and community midwives at the bottom, with no power and very little government support. In this system, doctors have most of the power. Professional midwives, who are usually biomedically trained, often buy into this hierarchy and work to impose biomedical models of birth on indigenous populations—a situation Australian midwifery professor and researcher Leslie Barclay (1998) calls "midwifery hegemony." The surest sign that such a system is in operation is when women who have birthed upright for countless generations are suddenly told by the midwife or doctor to lie down. Numerous studies now document the efficacy and superiority of upright positions for birth. Yet biomedicine in its arrogance insists that its way is best, and around the world is still working to eliminate the few remaining viable indigenous systems of birth, teaching even community midwives to make women lie down for birth and replacing home with hospital wherever possible.

In rural Thailand, for example, anthropologist Andrea Whittaker (1999) documented the escalating biomedicalization of birth. As more and more rural women spent large sums of money to have the more prestigious hospital births, the community midwife's role was reduced to postpartum care. Ironically, at the same time as indigenous birthways were rapidly vanishing in the rural areas, in Thai cities, where birth has long been biomedicalized, an incipient alternative birth movement finds some professional midwives now attending the births of middle-class women at home (Andrea Robertson, personal communication).

Conclusion: Midwives and the Possible Future

In the words of songwriter Joni Mitchell, "Don't it always seem to go, that you don't know what you've got till it's gone?" Must we lose the viable indigenous birthways that still exist before we rediscover how valuable many of them were? Must the professionalization of midwifery mean its colonization by biomedicine? In 2014, after a careful overview of the status of birth and mortality around the world, ICM and WHO issued a clarion call for 350,000 more skilled professional midwives, needed immediately. What kind of midwives will answer that call? Will they be biomedically-oriented modern professional midwives who buy into and foster the hierarchical agendas of technomedicine, or will they, in postmodern fashion, work to practice autonomously in collaboration with physicians, foster the globalization of the midwifery model of care in culturally sensitive ways, work in tandem and cooperation with traditional midwives, and become worldwide the agents of mutual accommodation and positive change?

Questions for Thought and Discussion

1. What does Davis-Floyd mean by the terms "biomedical hegemony," "midwifery hegemony," and "mutual accommodation"?
2. Why do many women, especially in low-resource countries, reject medical services in favor of utilizing the services of their local community midwives for birth?
3. What does the author see as a possible solution to the issues she raises in this chapter?

Recommended Films

Five Countries, Six Births, Seven Babies: Mother Nature's Design for Birth: produced by Love Delivers. Showcases homebirths in Guatemala, Costa Rica,

France, the USA, and Bermuda. The individual chapters in the film make it easy to use in classes, conferences, and lectures. Available at www.midwiferytoday.com

The Time Is Now/Birth and the Primal Period: The Path to Full Human Potential, Volume 1: producer/director Suzanne Arms, 2012. Features perspectives from Kenya, Brazil, the Peruvian Amazon, the Canary Islands, Spain, and the USA. 1 hr 45 min.

The Time Is Now/Birth and the Primal Period: The Path to Full Human Potential, Volume 2: producer/director Suzanne Arms, 2013. Features perspectives from Israel, Egypt, England, Sri Lanka, Mexico, Appalachia, and California.

The Time Is Now/Birth and the Primal Period: The Path to Full Human Potential, Volume 3: producer/director Suzanne Arms, 2014. Features perspectives from Mexico, Canada, Sudan, Venezuela, and the USA.

Birthing in Peace: producer British midwife Peggy Oolsthorn. This 32-minute film documents the successful fusion of traditional and biomedical obstetrical systems achieved by Brazilian obstetrician Dr. Galba Araujo, who organized the building of maternity clinics throughout northeastern Brazil, staffing them with local midwives who were given biomedical training but were strongly encouraged to continue with their traditional style of birth: the mother labors while walking or resting in hammocks and gives birth upright on a birthing stool with little or no insertion of hands into the vagina; after birth, the baby stays with the mother. Such practices, continued in the clinics, kept infection and mortality low, and were incorporated by Dr. Galba as far as possible into hospital practice in Fortaleza, Ceara, where he was Director of Obstetrics. http://www.worldcat.org/title/birthing-in-peace/oclc/36410096

10

Homebirth Emergencies in the US and Mexico

The Trouble with Transport

When we transport, we never know whether we are going to be welcomed or get a slap in the face! Hospital people don't freak out when they get a carwreck or a gunshot victim in the ER with no advance warning. Yet they get bent out of shape over homebirth transfers, even though we do alert them in advance. But they shouldn't. Taking care of people who really are in trouble—that's their job!

— Homebirth midwives from the US and Mexico, who both said almost exactly the same words

In Mexico, homebirth, while rapidly diminishing in frequency, still exists as a vital tradition and viable cultural option for many women; in the US, it was almost obliterated by the 1950s but in recent decades has formed the focus of a social movement of midwives, mothers, and childbirth activists dedicated to reclaiming homebirth and maintaining it as a viable option. As proponents of global maternal–child health initiatives have long stressed, in both the developing world where homebirth is often a necessity and the developed world where it is a choice, primary keys to safe homebirth include transport to the hospital in cases of need and effective care on arrival (Fullerton 2000). In this chapter, I examine what happens when transport occurs, how the outcomes of prior transports affect future decision making, and how

This chapter first appeared as an article in a special issue of *Social Science and Medicine*, called *Reproduction Gone Awry*, edited by Marcia Inhorn and Gwynne Jenkins 56(9):1913–1931, 2003. The version that appears here has been significantly revised and expanded.

the lessons derived from the transport experiences of birthing women and midwives in the US and Mexico could be translated into improvements in maternity care. Once the need for transport becomes apparent and agreed upon, two aspects are critical to its viability: (1) Can the mother get there? In other words, is there a hospital within reach, can a vehicle be found, and are the roads passable? (2) What happens when she arrives? The first, availability of transport, is a major issue in rural Mexico and elsewhere in low-resource countries, and deserves separate and thorough attention. Here my focus is on homebirth in urban areas in Mexico and the US, where the trouble with transport is not its lack but rather what happens when transport places the mother, who had planned to give birth at home, and the midwife attending her, in interaction with biomedical personnel.

In both countries, biomedicine and homebirth midwifery exist in separate cultural domains and are based on overlapping but distinctively different knowledge systems. When a homebirth midwife arrives in the hospital with her client, she brings with her the general ways of knowing and style of practice that characterize her cultural domain and her specific prior knowledge about the woman's overall health, personality, desires, and labor process. This knowledge can be vital to the mother's successful treatment by the hospital system. But the culture of biomedicine in general tends not to understand or recognize as valid the knowledge of midwifery. Thus in the hospital, the midwife may have no authoritative status. Yet she must interface with medical personnel if she is to communicate information the hospital staff may need to provide appropriate and effective care for her client. Smooth articulation of the medical and midwifery knowledge systems facilitates the safest transition for the woman and her baby, but all too often, disjuncture and dis-articulation occur. The tensions and dysfunctions that result are displayed in midwives' transport stories, which I here identify as a narrative genre. In this chapter, I will seek to unpack these stories for the collision of worlds they encapsulate and the points of fracture and permeability in the crusts of those worlds that they reveal.

I will focus specifically on the transport stories told by two groups of midwives with whom I have conducted extensive interviews: American Certified Professional Midwives (CPMs) who attend homebirths and a small group of traditional Mexican midwives who practice in and around the large urban city of Cuernavaca in the state of Morelos, just south of Mexico City. After describing these two groups of midwives and the national contexts within which they learn and practice, I will narrate some of their stories, analyzing them as cultural terrains that reveal how reproduction can go unnecessarily awry when domains of knowledge conflict and existing power structures ensure that only one kind of knowledge counts. I will describe such encounters as (1) *dis-articulations* that occur when there is no correspondence of information or action between the midwife and the hospital staff; and (2) *fractured articulations* of biomedical and midwifery knowledge systems that result from partial and incomplete correspondences. I will contrast these two kinds of disjuncture with the (3) *smooth* or (4) *seamless articulation* of systems that results when "mutual accommodation" (Jordan 1993) characterizes the interactions between midwife and medical personnel. In the final section of the chapter, I will link these American and Mexican transport stories to their international context, describing how they index some of the cross-cultural markers for "the trouble with transport."

Articulation and Authoritative Knowledge: Biopower Meets the Homebirth Midwife

> ***ar·ti·cu·late*** *vt. (1) to put together by joints; (2) to arrange in connected sequence, fit together, correlate. vi. to be jointed or connected. n. a joint in a stem or between two separable parts, as a branch and leaf [or] a node or space between two nodes.*
> — *Webster's New World Dictionary*, 2000

My use of the term *articulation* at various points in this chapter comes from Gramsci through Lawrence Grossberg. In *We Gotta Get Outa This Place: Popular Conservatism and Postmodern Culture* (1992:54), Grossberg notes that the concept of articulation "provides a useful starting place for describing the process of forging connections between practices and effects." His starting place will be my ending place, as most of the stories I recount below illustrate connections that could potentially have been forged but instead were either never made or only partially constituted. These disjunctures in what could have been functional, smoothly bending joints stem from the dominance of biomedicine—a hierarchical system that has sought, in general, not to articulate with homebirth midwifery but rather to eliminate it through discounting its practices and knowledge base. In her chapter "Authoritative Knowledge and Its Construction," in *Childbirth and Authoritative Knowledge: Cross-Cultural Perspectives*, Brigitte Jordan (1997:56) noted that

> for any particular domain several knowledge systems exist, some of which, by consensus, come to carry more weight than others, either because they explain the state of the world better for the purposes at hand (efficacy) or because they are associated with a stronger power base (structural superiority), and usually both. In many situations, equally legitimate parallel knowledge systems exist and people move easily between them, using them sequentially or in parallel fashion for particular purposes. But frequently, one kind of knowledge gains ascendance and legitimacy. A consequence of the legitimation of one kind of knowing as authoritative is the devaluation, often the dismissal of all other kinds of knowing.

Jordan maps out what happens when one kind of knowing does gain ascendancy, thus opening up the possibility of asking, What happens when an ascendant knowledge system and a devalued one must interface? When I was trying to figure out the answer to that question, I phoned to ask Gitti (Brigitte Jordan), assuming she would already have that all figured out. Her response: "I have no idea—you're going to have to figure that out for yourself!" So, in working on formulating an answer, and after listening to a lot of transport stories, I came also to ask, why do adherents of a dominant knowledge system sometimes dismiss what adherents of a devalued system have to say, sometimes give them partial credence, and other times honor them, act promptly on their recommendations, and include them in the process? The stories I analyze below illustrate all of these possible scenarios, and answer my questions above.

In the process of describing how Western biomedicine gained its cultural ascendancy, Michel Foucault identified the cultural authority it carries as a form of "biopower," which he defined as "disciplines of the body," used as "numerous and diverse techniques for achieving the subjugation of bodies and the control of populations" (1978:140). This subjugation and control include the biomedicalization of bodily processes like childbirth and the development of institutions within which such processes are supposed to take place, along with formalized structures for managing them. Jordan (1997:57) augments Foucault's notion of biopower with her focus on the status of particular knowledge systems:

> It is important to realize that to identify a body of knowledge as authoritative speaks, for us as analysts, in no way to the correctness of that knowledge. Rather, the label "authoritative" is intended to draw attention to its status within a particular social group and to the work it does in maintaining the group's definition of morality and rationality. *The power of authoritative knowledge is not that it is correct but that it counts.*

Although the midwives in the US and Mexico whom I have studied treat their own knowledge system as authoritative in the home context, they are acutely conscious of the larger and higher authority carried by biomedicine not only inside the hospital but also in the culture at large. As we have seen in previous chapters, much of the time these midwives do not accept biomedical knowledge as truth or fact; many of their practices and much of their midwifery knowledge system constitute a radical critique of obstetrics, challenging its claims to the authority of fact and truth. But these midwives also understand that in the hospital as in the wider culture, including in courts of law, their radical critique goes largely unheard and *their ways of knowing do not count.* Faced with this formalized system of biopower that discounts their individualized approach to maternity care, during transport midwives nevertheless must seek to communicate what they know, in the interests of securing the care for which they brought the woman to the hospital, which they deem to be necessary for their client's safety and well-being. So as they enter the hospital, they extend into that system what I term *fingers of articulation* in an effort to generate a productive interface. The following detailed examination of midwives' transport stories intends to illuminate what happens along a spectrum of possibilities from dis- to seamless articulation, from the dismissal of these outreaching fingers to their clasping by a biomedical hand. Through examining this *spectrum of articulations* between knowledge systems, I hope to augment Jordan's (1997) explanations of what happens when one system of knowledge discounts another with a more nuanced consideration of how, in specific situations, the dominant system can come to take the subaltern system into a partial or fully accommodative account.

Methodology: Why and How I Chose to Study Midwives' Transport Stories

Articulation is a continuous struggle to reposition practices within a shifting field of forces.

— Lawrence Grossberg

This chapter is based on my years of research on American midwives (1991–2009) and on traditional and professional midwives in Mexico (1997–2009). The focus of this research was primarily on midwifery politics, practice, and the complex interrelationships among the various types of midwives in each country (Davis-Floyd, 2001a, b, 2002, 2003a, 2010; Davis-Floyd and Johnson 2006; Chapters 6–9 and 11, this volume).[1] This research did not specifically focus on transport stories as a genre or on transport as a salient issue. But during its course (which involved hours of formal interviewing and even more hours of "hanging out" with midwives, during which I became fully immersed in their subculture), I heard many transport stories told, only some of which ended up on tape by luck or circumstance. Thus this chapter in no way pretends to constitute a comprehensive exploration of transport stories, a task I suggest to future ethnographers. Further research should include thorough quantitative and qualitative studies on the treatment of transported women and their midwives and its specific outcomes. For even though they had not constituted a specific research focus, over time these transport stories

[1] During the course of this research, most of which was funded by the Wenner-Gren Foundation for Anthropological Research (Grants #6015 and #6427), I interviewed approximately 50 American nurse-midwives, 45 nurse-midwifery students, 50 direct-entry midwives, 30 direct-entry midwifery students, 20 Mexican professional midwives, and 7 traditional midwives in Morelos who are professionalizing. I have also spoken informally or conducted short interviews with over 100 traditional Mexican midwives from all over the country.

began to emerge for me as a narrative genre that richly encapsulates clashes of power and ideology between the biomedical and midwifery systems and their potentially devastating consequences for mother and baby.

The particular stories I present here, told by American direct-entry midwives and Mexican traditional midwives, were chosen both for their representative nature and for the transnational similarities they index. These similarities include exclusively out-of-hospital practice and concomitant marginalization vis-à-vis the biomedical system, and thus they embody the collision of worlds I seek to analyze.[2] In both countries, there are a few primarily hospital-based professional midwives who attend both home and hospital births; their transport experiences are somewhat different, especially when they practice and carry authoritative status in both domains. I suggest them as potential subjects of a future study.[3] The following sections will describe the two groups of midwives on whom I focus here and the larger national and transnational contexts within which they work.

Background and Context: Obstetrics and Midwifery in the US and Mexico

The effects of any practice are always the product of its position within a context.
— Lawrence Grossberg

To recap from previous chapters (I ask my readers to remember that I intend each chapter in this book to make sense if read separately from all the others; achieving this goal requires a certain amount of repetition), in the US, obstetricians, together with some family practice physicians, attend approximately 90% of all births. Their discourse around childbirth centers on "managing risk"—from an obstetric point of view, every birth is a potential disaster and must be managed authoritatively and preventively to ensure the best possible outcome. (Hamilton et al. 2015). As I and others have previ-

[2] Other factors involved in the marginalized status these midwives hold in relation to physicians include differences in formal education, credentialing, and social class with wealth as proxy; in Mexico especially, gender is also an important factor.

[3] Ideally, nurse-midwives' transport experiences should be seamless but often are not. While there are excellent data on the statistical *outcomes* of nurse-midwife-attended births in the US, including home-hospital transports (MacDorman and Singh 1998), I know of no research on American nurse-midwives' transport *experiences,* except for Cheyney, Everson, and Burch 2014c. In Mexico, nurse-midwives do not really exist as a class of practitioners. Rather, nurses who choose to specialize in obstetrics undergo an additional year of university training. Officially titled *Licenciadas en Enfermeria y Obstetricia* (colloquially known as *las LEOs*), these women mostly work as high-tech labor and delivery nurses, in addition to performing administrative work and teaching. But they do attend births and function like American nurse-midwives in a few private hospitals and clinics in central Mexico.

ously described (Martin 1987; Miller and Shriver 2012; Rothman 1982, 1989; van Teijlingen et al. 2009; Part 1 of this book), the performance of birth in American hospitals tells a cultural story about the female body as a defective machine in need of assistance by technical experts and other more perfect machines. It also enacts and displays the technocracy's supervaluation of speed, efficiency, control, high technology, and the flow of information through cybernetic systems.

Technobirths are typical and normative in American hospitals through a consensual, biopowerful process jointly driven by physicians, who tend to be trained exclusively in that approach, and women, who tend also to supervalue technology, control, and most especially the elimination of labor pain (see Chapter 3). Generally speaking, the interventive American approach exists by mutual agreement between women and physicians steeped in the core values and overall approach to life characteristic of technocratic culture.[4] Both groups believe this approach offers comfort and safety in the face of an unpredictable natural process that proceeds more safely when carefully controlled, in the same way that a river subject to flooding seems improved when a series of dams and floodgates are installed.

To hospital practitioners steeped in this approach, the choice for homebirth appears to be a choice for pain and random chaos in contrast to order and control. Most hospital-based practitioners have never seen a homebirth and know little about the knowledge base of homebirth midwives, in part because of a near-total lack of contact. The many safe and woman-centered births that take place at home are invisible to the medical gaze; biomedical discourse tends to center around "botched homebirths." I have often heard this phrase bandied about by medical practitioners who tend to assume that any homebirth that ends up in the hospital must be "botched," even if it is the result of an appropriate transport.[5] Of course, the midwifery response is usually a sarcastic comment about enormous numbers of "botched hospital births"; women who have had "botched" hospital experiences and later choose homebirth are an important source of such accounts. This trading of insults is an in-group phenomenon: hospital practitioners complain to other

[4] In "Media Representations of Pregnancy and Childbirth: An Analysis of Reality Television Programs in the United States," researchers Morris and McInerney (2010) described the results of their content analysis of 85 reality-based television shows depicting 123 births, aired in the US on *Discovery Health* and *The Learning Channel* in November 2007, concluding that "women's bodies were typically displayed as incapable of birthing a baby without medical intervention."

[5] Medical practitioners who only see problematic homebirths that are transported to the hospital tend to think that all homebirths are "botched." The rate of problems derives as a function of a numerator (number of cases with problems) and a denominator (total number of cases—the majority—that have good outcomes). If one only sees the numerator, it is impossible to realize that the rate of transports is actually very low compared to the number of successful homebirths: again, only around 10 out of 100 planned homebirths end up requiring transport, and only 3 out of every 10 transports are emergencies.

hospital practitioners about homebirth and midwives; midwives complain to other midwives about hospital practitioners. Dialogue between these groups is rare; mostly, their members inhabit separate worlds that only intersect when a homebirth goes awry and a transport is the necessary result.

Throughout most of the 20th century, the movement of birth was from home to hospital, as technomedicine became increasingly dominant and cultural notions of safety became increasingly tied to the technomedical management of birth (see Declerq et al. 2001). Reacting to what they experienced as "overmedicalization," in the 1970s thousands of American women began to move their births away from the hospital and back to the home; a new class of practitioners emerged to serve them in what came to be known as the "lay midwifery renaissance." By the 1990s, many of these lay midwives had been practicing for over 20 years and had ample opportunity to create a distinctive knowledge base for out-of-hospital midwifery (e.g., Frye, 1995; Davis 1997; Gaskin 1990 [1977]; Rooks 1997). As part of their process of professionalization, they dropped the appellation "lay" in favor of the European term "direct-entry," which indicates that they entered directly into midwifery education without passing through nursing first (see Davis-Floyd 2010 and Chapter 6, this volume).

The exact number of direct-entry midwives practicing currently in the US is not precisely known; educated guesses place it at around 3,000. Most of these 3000 homebirth midwives have obtained certification as a CPM (Certified Professional Midwife) (see Chapter 6). Almost all of them work exclusively out-of-hospital, attending 1% of births.[6] Approximately 7,500 nurse-midwives practice mostly in hospitals, attending around 10% of all births (Declerq 2015).[7] CPM certification honors multiple kinds of midwifery education, including apprenticeship, which seems to many homebirth midwives to most effectively teach the experiential, intuitive, noninterventive, and trust-based approach they value as deeply as their technomedical knowledge and skills. CPMs and other independent direct-entry midwives

[6] In 2001, the American Public Health Association called for increased access to home- and birth-center births attended by legally regulated and nationally certified midwives (APHA 2002). At that time, less than 1% of all births in the United States were occurring out-of-hospital. However, over the last decade, out-of-hospital births have increased by 56% (MacDorman, Declerq, and Matthews 2013; MacDorman, Matthews, and Declerq 2014), reaching 1.36% of all US births in 2012. Of these, 66% (n=35,184 in 2012) were homebirths primarily attended by direct-entry midwives, including CPMs.

[7] Most of the 7,500 or so practicing nurse-midwives in the US attend births in hospitals; approximately 500 of them attend births at home. The ACNM officially supports homebirths, and many of its members would like to be able to attend them. But ACNM-certified midwives must have physician backup and insurance, and many are unable to attain these for out-of-hospital births. For hospital births their services are covered by private insurance companies in all states, as well as by Medicaid and managed care. In 1998, 96% of the births CNMs attended took place in hospitals (Rooks 1997; Paine, Dower, and O'Neil 1999; Curtin 1999); that percentage remains about the same today.

practice legally in 30 states, and a-legally or illegally in the rest.[8] In most a-legal and illegal states, they are fighting uphill battles for legalization (Davis-Floyd and Johnson 2006). In some states where they are licensed, their services are covered by private insurance companies and by Medicaid (and sometimes managed care). But in most states, homebirth attended by direct-entry midwives is still an out-of-pocket expense—a factor that exercises a significant limitation on its growth. (In states like Washington and Florida where homebirth is reimbursed, the percentage of homebirths is on the rise.) While their practices are not uniform, most CPMs practice according to specific protocols (sometimes individually arrived at, sometimes mandated by state regulation, and sometimes consensually established by local or regional midwifery associations) that include lists of specific conditions and circumstances that warrant hospital transport. The National Association of Certified Professional Midwives (NACPM) has created more uniform national standards for the increasing numbers of midwives achieving CPM certification.

In Mexico, biomedicine has not only taken over childbirth but is redefining its very nature. While high technologies like electronic fetal monitors are not as readily available as in US hospitals, in vaginal deliveries extreme interventions like fundal pressure (*Kristeller*) and manual extraction of the placenta are common, and Mexico's cesarean section rate is extremely high, standing in 2010 at 43.9% (according to OECD health data; see Niino 2011:140).[9] A common argument against midwifery made by government officials and MDs is that there are plenty of doctors and nurses in Mexico, that the poor are entitled to the same care as the middle class, and that therefore progress in maternal health care should entail giving everyone access to hospitals and doctors. This argument is representative of what has been called the "mega-rhetoric of developmental modernization" (Appadurai 1996:10), which identifies a single point in a given area toward which development should be progressing (Appiah 1997): in health care, that single point is Western biomedicine.

As Marcia Good (2000) has shown, Mexico's high cesarean rates stem in large part from physicians' deeply held belief that birth is a dangerous process that can cause harm to mothers and babies and that technological interventions like cesarean sections are the best way to ensure the safety and well-being of mother and child. Such physicians see midwives as a hangover from the undeveloped past, a temporary evil that must be replaced as quickly as possible with the vanguard of the future—modern health care. In the US and

[8] For updates on these numbers, see www.mana.org/narm.

[9] In public hospitals in Mexico, the cesarean rate increased from 13% in 1990 to 25% in 1997—and from 25% to 37% in Mexico City, in private hospitals the national average in 1997 was 52% (Comité Promotor por una Maternidad sin Riesgos 1997). Research indicates the doctor-driven nature of this excess of cesareans, which social scientists are now calling an "iatrogenic epidemic" (Castro, Heimberger, and Langer 2001). In 2016 the overall CS rate in Mexico was around 42%.

other developed countries, a postmodern discourse (one that stems from multiple points of reference, that does not assume the superiority of any one method; see Chapter 8) around the benefits of professional midwifery care and certain indigenous approaches—such as walking during labor, upright labor and birthing positions, and herbal remedies—occasionally punctuates the national dialogue about birth. This discourse is barely heard in today's Mexico, outside of some branches of the public health sector. In the US, nurse- and direct-entry midwives, backed by supportive consumers and often by public health officials, due to their record of good outcomes and cost-effectiveness (Rooks 1997; Cheyney et al. 2014b), are engaged in active campaigns to increase government and public awareness of the multiple benefits of midwifery care. In Mexico, a new breed of professional midwife has made great legal strides (Davis-Floyd 2001a, b; Goodman forthcoming; Mills and Davis-Floyd 2009; Chapter 8, this volume), while Mexico's traditional midwives are rapidly being phased out of practice.

Nevertheless, many working-class women resist government initiatives to bring birth into clinics and hospitals, choosing instead to birth at home attended by a midwife.[10] Officially labeled "traditional birth attendants" (TBAs) by WHO and UNICEF, these midwives refer to themselves as *parteras tradicionales* ("traditional midwives": see Chapters 8 and 9 for more detail). They are usually mothers who have given birth several times and who have become midwives by being asked to attend the births of friends and relatives, slowly gaining firsthand experience of birth. Some of them undertake long apprenticeships, while others learn simply by attending births. Between 1995 and 1996, traditional midwives attended less than 17% of births in Mexico (INEGI 1999). In 1994, the majority were over 65 years of age (SSA 1994); many are now dying without training replacements. Young people in Mexico today prefer to seek formal education into a profession; they also see the hospital as the progressive place to go for birth.

TBA training courses and other forms of exposure to biomedicine have resulted in fundamental alterations in practice for many traditional midwives in Mexico. Across the country, it is now common for them to give pitocin injections to hurry labor, to insert IVs for hydration, and to wear blue biomedical garb when attending births. Combining such practices with the traditional *sobada* (massage), herbal treatments, and religious beliefs, Mexico's contemporary *parteras tradicionales* practice at the intersection of various cultural domains.

These forces and trends have particularly influenced midwives who practice in urban areas, as my extensive interviews with seven traditional midwives who live and practice in various *colónias* in or around the city of

[10] Homebirth is almost completely nonexistent as an option for Mexican middle-class women, most of whom would not think of using the services of a traditional midwife; see Davis-Floyd 2001a; Dixon et al. forthcoming; Goodman forthcoming; and Mills and Davis-Floyd 2009 for exceptions describing the small number of middle-class Mexican professional midwives.

Cuernavaca reveal. These urban *parteras tradicionales* (unlike many of their rural counterparts) have long been incorporated into the state health care system in Morelos through bimonthly seminars on family planning and other topics; the government uses them as agents of family planning and birth control, a service desired by women, which both the government and the midwives are happy to provide. All seven went through a period of using allopathic interventions like oxytocin injections to induce stronger contractions; experiencing complications as a result, all returned to the use of their traditional herbs. Today they routinely send women out for ultrasounds when they diagnose a breech or transverse presentation to confirm their diagnosis, and offer their clients an eclectic potpourri of traditional techniques like external version (turning the baby manually) and biomedical options like sending a woman to a doctor they know and trust for a cesarean section. Dancing fluidly at the interface of biomedicine and their traditional systems, these midwives are strategically negotiating the boundaries between knowledge systems and creatively producing a postmodern, hybrid and increasingly well-articulated knowledge system of their own.

In this endeavor, they are assisted by a new group of equally postmodern *parteras profesionales* (professional midwives) some of whom are CPMs; I have described them elsewhere (Davis-Floyd 2001a; Mills and Davis-Floyd 2009; Chapter 9). Mexico's midwives, both professional and traditional, who used to work closely with the US-based organization MANA (see Chapter 6) have recently created their own professional organization—*Asociación Mexicana de Partería*; see www.asociacionmexicanadeparteria.org/.

Significant differences in lifeworld, knowledge base, and practice styles distinguish American and the few Mexican CPMs from the urbanized traditional midwives of Cuernavaca, along with equally salient differences in social class and access to wealth, education, and other resources of the technocracy. But their similarities are also relevant here. The transport stories they relate below can most effectively be interpreted in light of the understanding that the members of both groups do not practice in conceptual or geographic isolation, as some midwives do, but rather exhibit all the characteristics of what I have called the "postmodern midwife"—one who balances and evaluates knowledge systems in a relativistic way, and who participates in transnational networks of community-building and information exchange (Davis-Floyd, Cosminsky, and Pigg 2001; Chapter 8, this volume). Like American homebirth midwives, the traditional-yet-professionalizing midwives of Morelos are busy balancing knowledge systems and constructing hybrid identities in urban areas in which they must constantly engage in strategic negotiations with physicians. Their former membership in MANA gave them access to international midwifery networks; participation in these networks helped them to form a state association to support traditional midwifery in Morelos, and later, in tandem with Mexico's professional midwives, to form their own new national organization.

From an anthropological point of view, both the Cuernavaca *parteras tradicionales* and the American CPMs in my study elide and confound the usual distinctions between professional and traditional midwives: some of the American CPMs were trained through apprenticeship or self-study; the Cuernavaca midwives were trained the same way but were considered lay practitioners by their government, yet were engaged in an unnamed but nevertheless visible process of professionalization (see Davis-Floyd 2001b). Their ethnic, economic, and class differences are salient; yet despite these differences, and because of their mutual dedication to the welfare of women and belief in the safety and efficacy of homebirth, it is fair to say that the members of both groups are inspired by the transnational ideology of homebirth and "sisterhood" in midwifery that MANA sought to foster. Both groups critique the failures and limitations of biomedicine and have a strong sense of mission about preserving homebirth in the face of biomedical hegemony. They believe in women's ability to give birth with little intervention most of the time, in the superiority of homes and birth centers as the sites of birth, and in the efficacy of their own knowledge systems and skills.[11] They do not undertake transport lightly, and when they do transport, their intent is to do all in their power to make the medical system respond in ways they consider appropriate. Thus their transports usually involve at least two people from outside the biomedical realm: the mother who needs help and the midwife who will not abandon her even when she is no longer in charge of her care.[12]

All midwives who practice out-of-hospital must occasionally transport. I could find no national statistical data on midwives' transport rates for Mexico, but in the US, homebirth midwives have a transport rate of about 10% (Cheyney et al. 2014b; Johnson & Daviss 2001, 2005). In other words, 90 out of 100 of their clients give birth safely at home, while 10 are transported to the hospital during or after labor for various reasons: 6 out of these 10 are transported for precautionary reasons like failure to progress in labor, meconium staining in the amniotic fluid (possibly but not necessarily a sign of fetal distress), or a retained placenta after the birth. Only approximately 3 of these 10 are transported for potentially life-threatening emergencies. (My Cuernavaca interviewees anecdotally reported similar rates.) The transport

[11] My Cuernavaca interviewees keep notebooks recording their outcomes, and turn statistical forms into the Department of Health. It would be an excellent research project to compile their statistical data, including the outcomes of their transports.

[12] A caveat: To my knowledge, most American homebirth midwives who transport enter the hospital and stay with their clients for as long as they are allowed. But I have heard critiques from some hospital practitioners of homebirth midwives who "dump their clients at the door and take off." Such midwives live in states where their practice is illegal or in places where local hospital personnel are known to be particularly negative and unreceptive. Leaving their clients at the door can be viewed as an extreme form of dis-articulation stemming from midwives' fear that any interaction with the hospital system at best will result in serious harassment and at worst will send them to jail—a powerful argument for the legalization of midwifery, which certainly facilitates the development of systems of smooth or seamless articulation.

stories I have culled from my interview data and selected to recount below cluster inside that 3%; I urge my readers to keep in mind that the circumstances recounted here are *quite rare* and not representative of the vast majority of births. These experiences are most likely to be encoded in narrative because they are so unusual and also because of their heavy emotional charge. Stories give meaning and coherence to experience; midwives who transport under frightening circumstances often need to find that coherence and to evaluate through narrative, with the benefit of hindsight, their own actions and those of the mother and the biomedical personnel.

In transport situations, there are various ways in which "awryness" can occur: (1) The fact that transport is indicated means that the natural process of birth has in some way gone awry, or seems likely to; (2) the midwife may wait too long to summon transport, either because of prior bad experiences with transport, as we will see below, or because of the midwife's lack of knowledge of indications for transport;[13] (3) the hospital staff taking the call may not understand the urgency of the mother's problems; (4) EMTs may fail to respond appropriately, or there may be disjunctive communication between the midwives and the EMTs; (5) arrival at the hospital can go awry for the mother and the midwife if either is ignored or mistreated; (6) even well-intended biomedical interventions can at times do more damage than they fix; (7) not all natural disasters are fixable by biomedical means, so even with the very best of care, the death of mother or baby can occur.

Only some of these possible levels of awryness are articulated in the stories I tell below. I selected these particular six stories because they are typical: they represent the range of possible outcomes of transport and are emblematic of many other situations and possibilities I do not have room to treat here. Since I have no way of ascertaining the truth or untruth of these stories, for the purposes of this chapter I take them at face value and unpack them for what they reveal about midwives' perceptions of and the meanings midwives attribute to events as they unfold.

Midwives' Transport Stories

Analyzing an event involves (re)constructing it or, in Foucault's terms, fabricating the network of relationships into which it is articulated, as well as the possibilities for different articulations.

— Lawrence Grossberg

[13] Some midwives do fail to transport because of lack of familiarity with medical indications for transport. I cannot speak to such situations because all of my interlocutors for this chapter—American direct-entry midwives and the professionalizing traditional midwives of Cuernavaca—are thoroughly schooled in indications for transport.

In this section, the stories as the midwives recounted them to me are not direct quotes but my retellings, unless otherwise indicated. (The stories themselves are indented; my analyses of them are not.)

Dis-Articulations

Carrie's First Story: Unnecessary Delay

Carrie Smiley (a pseudonym) is a Certified Professional Midwife (CPM) who had, at the time of this study, practiced in Atlanta, Georgia, for over 18 years, attending during that time over 850 births. Her practice is "unlawful" (meaning that it is punishable as a misdemeanor). Most of the homebirths she attends are for white middle-class couples. She does prenatal care out of her own home, a two-story house at the edge of a small lake in an attractive Atlanta suburb. She began her birth career in the late 1960s working as a volunteer in labor and delivery, and then took training as a biomedical assistant, working in labor and delivery and for a pediatrician for several years. Starting in 1977 she began attending the homebirths of friends; in the early 1980s she undertook a year-and-a-half apprenticeship with another homebirth midwife who later became her partner. The following episode took place in 1984, during the early years of Carrie's homebirth midwifery practice. But it should not be regarded as dated, as it typifies many transports that presently occur, especially in "illegal" states.

> Carrie and her partner are attending a mother pregnant with her first child, laboring at home and planning a homebirth. After about eight hours of labor, the mother has reached ten centimeters dilation and is starting to feel the urge to push. Monitoring the baby's heart tones, the midwives detect decelerations, a sign of fetal distress. Hoping to get the baby out quickly, the midwives ask the mother to push a few times to see if the baby will come down. When they realize that the mother is not going to be able to get the baby out with sufficient expediency, they get her into a knee-chest position, put her on oxygen, and call the EMTs. When ten minutes pass and the EMTs have not yet arrived, the midwives help the mother into their car, planning on driving her to the hospital themselves. Just as they are ready to go, the ambulance pulls up and blocks the driveway. Announcing, "We're here now, we'll take it from here," the paramedics pull the mother out of the midwife's car and help her into the ambulance. But they refuse to heed the midwives, who are urging that they must rush the mother to the hospital, insisting that first they have to get a history. Asking questions like "have you had any nausea during this pregnancy?" the EMTs are wasting precious time. Frantic at the delay, and knowing the baby might be suffering from oxygen deprivation, the midwives ask the paramedics to put the mother on oxygen. They refuse, wanting to continue with the history, so the midwives get their own oxygen tank out of the car, at which point the medics finally accede and hook the mother up to the ambulance oxygen tank. As

> the ambulance starts toward the hospital, the midwife riding with the mother asks her to get on her hands and knees to relieve any possible cord compression, but the paramedics get upset and turn the mother flat on her back. Knowing that this position will exacerbate cord compression and reduce blood and oxygen flow to the baby, the midwife compromises by turning the mother on her side, and continues to listen to the fetal heart tones.
>
> Arriving at the hospital, the midwives are told that there are several obstetricians present in the hospital, but only the one on-call is allowed to treat a "walk-in" and he is not in-house and will have to be called. Increasingly frantic, the midwives insist to the nurse in the ER that the baby is in distress. The nurse auscultates the heart tones, records them at 130, announcing this to the midwives and the mother, and tells the midwives that "Everything is fine; we will take over from here." She will not look at the records the midwives brought, which show the heart rate fluctuations, nor pay heed to their insistence that this is an emergency. The midwives are not allowed to remain with the mother in the ER or to accompany her to labor and delivery. Instead they are sent to the waiting room. Carrie says, "Every time we went outside the room, we noticed that everyone seemed to be looking at us and talking about us."
>
> Terrified that they will be arrested and sent to jail, the midwives finally head home. Later they learn that it took the doctor on-call one hour and 45 minutes to show up. In the meantime, the nurses caught the baby, who was stillborn. (The "fetal heart rate" of 130 heard earlier had likely been the maternal pulse elevated by the anxiety of transfer.) The cause of death was listed on the hospital record as "prolonged fetal distress." The EMT records said that the mother had been antagonistic and refused oxygen, which the midwives insist is untrue. The nurses said the mother refused the electronic fetal monitor (she did). The hospital pushes the mother to file criminal charges against the midwives, but the mother tells the hospital personnel that this death is clearly the hospital's fault, that the midwives acted appropriately and bear no blame, and that if the hospital should try to harass the midwives in any way, she will sue the hospital, not the midwives.

In Carrie's view, she and her partner did their best. Trained to detect fetal heart rate decelerations and to recognize which ones are dangerous, they responded appropriately to the signs of fetal distress. But in retrospect, Carrie wishes that they had taken the woman to the hospital themselves. When I asked her why they called 911 in the first place, Carrie responded, "We were really dumb—we thought that was the appropriate thing to do."

From Carrie's point of view, blocking the driveway and announcing "We'll take it from here" demonstrated the EMTs' authoritative, even arrogant attitude, which at first glance seemed to leave no further role for the midwives to play. She feels she and her partner demonstrated strength in their refusal to accept this dismissal. Rather, they flexibly and creatively tried to work with the EMTs to help the mother get what they felt she needed. Frustrated by their inability to convince the EMTs of the need for haste, they experienced their success in getting the mother back on oxygen as a small victory. They had good reason to believe the baby was oxygen-deprived, so when the EMTs refused to act, the midwives resorted to the nonverbal yet eloquent strategy of getting their oxygen tank out of the car, figuring the EMTs would rather use their own oxygen than accept it from the midwives.

One possible reason for the baby's lack of oxygen might have been that the cord was compressed. Cord compression, or other forms of reduced blood flow to the fetus, is often exacerbated when a woman lies flat on her back, so the midwives wanted to put the mother in the knees and chest position in the ambulance, as this is the position most likely to take the most pressure off the cord. (In addition, the flat-on-the-back position can cause supine hypotension [low blood pressure] in women because it occludes the vena cava, resulting in inadequate circulation of blood [which carries oxygen] to the placenta and baby.) But a woman on her hands and knees in an ambulance is a strange and unsettling sight and most likely did not match the medics' internal maps of proper patient position or behavior, or of safety while driving. So the midwives had to give up on the most physiologic position; here again they creatively compromised, finding a position that minimizes both cord and vena cava compression while not challenging the medics' views of how a patient should be positioned. For Carrie and her partner, these stand as examples of midwives' ability to think around situations to get the system to meet the woman's needs. Such creativity has been demonstrated to be typical of subaltern groups, who must be as aware of the features of the dominant group as of their own in order to successfully navigate inside the dominant system (Schaef 1992).

Several obstetricians present in a hospital, but only the one on-call is allowed to treat "walk-ins," and that one is not in the hospital: here Carrie's voice dripped with sarcasm. For her this situation evidences hospitals' tendencies to be highly structured, category-oriented, and rule-bound. Her outside gaze notes that people who have a place inside the biomedical system, having contracted with a private obstetrician, are more likely to get an immediate response than the anomalous, unplaced "walk-in." The fact that the nurses would not look at the midwives' records seems analogous to the medics' refusal to heed the midwives' insistence on haste. Instead, the EMTs wanted to take a history, which of course the midwives already had. But the information the midwives had obtained *did not count* for these biomedical personnel, who valued only the knowledge they themselves obtained. It seems to Carrie that reality as defined by biomedical categories (taking a history, allowing only one OB to attend a walk-in, counting only information obtained by biomedical personnel) was more salient here than reality as the midwives, the mother, and the stillborn baby experienced it.

Tragically, the mother's refusal to be put on the electronic monitor denied the biomedical system an indicator on which it might have acted. This refusal likely stemmed from the distrust of the biomedical system and its technology that led the mother to plan a homebirth in the first place. When the ER nurse announced that the heart tones were at 130, the mother took this news to mean that the problem had resolved itself and "everything was fine." Carrie later learned that in the labor and delivery unit the fetal heart rate decelerations were noted and recorded by the nurses who were auscultating; however for some reason they never told the mother that they could hear the decelerations, so she continued in the belief that the heart tones were still OK. Emphatically, Carrie stated that if the midwives had been allowed to remain with the mother, they would have convinced her to allow the monitor; she said, "We would have done everything from cutting a huge episiotomy to jumping on her tummy to get that baby out. But we were sent away."

Carrie's sarcasm extends to the "lie" the EMTs told on their official records, a lie she is sure they told to cover themselves in case of a lawsuit. It is likely that the paramedics assumed that as biomedically trained practitioners, their word carried more authority and cultural weight than the words of the midwives and the mother, so their notes were more likely to be seen as valid. *Practicing inside a hegemonic cultural space can facilitate one's claim to truth.* Practicing outside that space not only calls one's veracity automatically into question but also puts one at risk of legal action: Carrie and her partner feared being sent to jail since their practice is unlawful in Georgia. They have dealt with this threat through their excellent outcomes, on which they keep careful statistics; through obtaining CPM certification, which is not recognized in Georgia but at least shows that they have been tested and have demonstrated the requisite competence; and through publicity: every few years, a local paper publishes a several-page spread on Carrie and her practice, showing pictures of her and of the happy couples she has attended. She feels this high level of visibility affords her far more protection in the form of community support than would hiding underground.

Reality is as one perceives it, and the effects of any given event depend not on the actual circumstances of that event but on how they are narrated. On both sides of this particular biomedical/midwifery//biopower/counterpower fence, opinions were formed or reinforced by this experience. We can imagine that the story that circulated among hospital personnel about this birth was very different from the one the midwives tell: chances are it was a story about another botched homebirth attended by irresponsible midwives. On the midwifery side, it was one more story about the absurdity of biomedical bureaucracies and the arrogance and narrow-mindedness of biomedical personnel—nurses, physicians, and EMTs alike. And it was a story about the dedication and loyalty of the midwives' clients: when I asked Carrie why the mother did not sue the hospital, she responded, "Because she knew that if she did, the hospital would come after us."

Later Carrie added, "Before this experience, I always thought that if you *have* a problem, you call the paramedics. Now I know that if you *want* a problem, you call the paramedics." She notes that this experience made her much savvier about the limitations of the biomedical system. Specifically, it taught her and her partner to always make sure they transported only to hospitals with on-call physicians in-house, and not to involve paramedics if there was any way the midwives could transport the client on their own. And, as we will see below, it led Carrie over time to work to develop a network of relationships with individuals in the hospitals to which she now transports, in order to enhance her ability to prevent this kind of dis-articulation of systems, and to facilitate the kind of smooth articulation that can save lives.

Paz's Story: A Transnational Parallel with a Different Ending

Maria de la Paz Puebla Alvear ("Paz" for short) is a traditional midwife with over 30 years' experience who attends homebirths in the impoverished *barrio* of Santa Maria, just north of the city of Cuernavaca. (All other names in this chapter are pseudonyms except for Paz, Marina, and Irene, who asked me to use their real names.) Paz and her family live in a crowded one-room shack made of wood and corrugated tin, with a dirt floor. They are building a much bigger house of brick and cement next door; they have been working on it for 25 years and it is finally near completion. Years ago, the family chose to pour the resources they could have put into the house into the construction of a birth center behind their one-room shack. The shack is hot, small, and unadorned; the cement-floored, brick-and-plaster walled birth center is spacious, cool, and breezy.

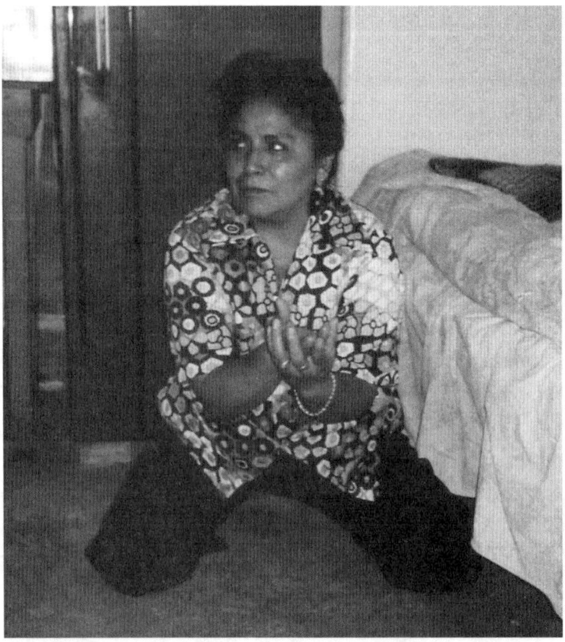

Paz in her birth center, demonstrating the position she is usually in when she receives the baby.

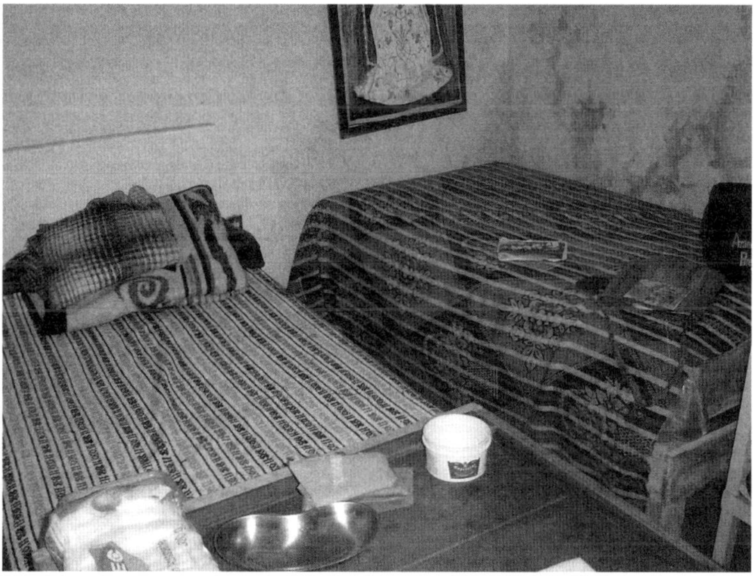

Paz's birth center behind her home. The climate is extremely humid so, although she repaints every few months, there is usually some mildew on the walls.

The two beds shown above allow family members to keep women company during labor; Paz's autoclave and midwifery equipment rest on the table at the foot of one of the beds. The women of her barrio like this birth center and prefer it to their own houses. There Paz attended four to five births per month. In the summer of 1999, Paz told me the following story:

> A woman who had not come to Paz for prenatal care showed up on her doorstep one day in labor. Paz does not like to attend women she has not seen before, but nevertheless took her in. Listening to the baby's heart tones through her fetoscope, Paz heard the heartbeat drop from 135 to 100, then rise back to 135, then drop again. She called a taxi. (Cuernavacan midwives almost never call 911 for an ambulance because of long delays in arrival. Taxi drivers' fees are low, and they arrive quickly because they are familiar with local neighborhoods.) Paz transported the mother to the hospital, where she carefully explained to the nurse on duty that this was an emergency. In spite of her entreaties, she and the laboring woman were ignored. Paz insisted to the nurse that the baby was suffering, and the nurse said "How do you know that?" "Because I am a midwife with 30 years' experience," Paz replied, "and I checked this patient and I know she needs to be in the hospital because the baby's heart tones show distress. And she has just come to me for the first time with no prenatal care, and you tell us to refer in such cases, and so for

these two reasons I am referring." "Sit down for half an hour," responded the nurse. "The doctors will be with you when they can." "No, call the doctor now!" insisted Paz. "The baby is in danger, it is very big and is not coming down, she needs a cesarean." Paz continued:

> We were there one hour and a half waiting. I could hear the doctors laughing and laughing down the hall—they were drinking their coffees. When I knocked on the door, they were putting away the cups. And still they made us wait. And I got really angry and I said to her husband, "Do you have money?" And he said, "Well, I've been working so I have some." And I said "OK, well go and get it, because you're going to need it—I am taking her away from here." And so I called the doctor who is a friend of mine at a *sanatorio* (private clinic), and he said "OK, you can bring her in and I will do the cesarean." And we took that woman to his clinic and he did the cesarean. It cost a lot, but we got out of that problem, didn't we? They tell us to "refer at the first points of alarm," so that the baby or the mother won't die because of my ineptitude. Ha! *El plan de trabajo mio es lograr a que viva la gente, no a que se muera.* (My plan of work is to succeed at people living, not dying.)

Like Carrie's story, Paz's story is about a midwife responding appropriately to dropping heart tones yet being ignored by biomedical personnel. In both stories, the midwives express their efforts to get attention and their enormous frustration at being ignored. Paz went so far as to appropriate the lexicon of TBA trainings when she listed to the nurse not one but two reasons for referral. "You tell us to refer in such cases": the plural "you" indexes the biomedical trainers who told her that she should send patients to whom she has not provided prenatal care to the hospital if they show up in labor, and that consistent fetal heart decelerations are an indication for transport. Taking the biomedical system at its collective word, Paz used those same words to try to get the system to respond. Yet like Carrie and her partner, in spite of the "30 years of experience" Paz invoked in an attempt to garner authority, she was ignored—an act that constituted a de facto dismissal of Paz from having *any* kind of authority, and which she resented deeply.

Not willing to sit passively and wait, Paz went so far as to knock on the door of the doctors' lounge, and was again dismissed. As in Carrie's case, this hospital was not going to respond smoothly or quickly to a "walk-in." But there was some benefit in trying, as this second dismissal convinced Paz that she was never going to get anywhere in that hospital, a realization that inspired her to search for an alternative. Exhibiting a creativity in hostile circumstances parallel to that of Carrie and her partner, but with better results, Paz conceived the idea to take the woman to a doctor she trusted and often worked with. His practice was private and would require financial payment, while the hospital, as part of the Mexican public health system, would have been free. So a prerequisite was to ask the woman's husband if he had money and could pay for the cesarean. His affirmative answer freed Paz to implement her plan that mother and child should "live and not die."

Like Carrie's story, Paz's experience highlights the frustration midwives often feel at the lack of obstetric recognition or valuation of their knowledge. Midwives see themselves as guardians of the normal. They are skilled at recognizing when a situation deviates from the normal and lands in the realm of obstetricians, who are experts in the abnormal. From a midwife's point of view, this professional demarcation system might work well if midwives' knowledge about normal and their ability to diagnose abnormal were regarded as authoritative by nurses and obstetricians. But as we have seen, in the face of biopower and biomedical knowledge, the midwife's knowledge and attempt to generate a response from the medical system often simply do not count; in this case, dis-articulation—no response from the hospital to the midwife—was the result.

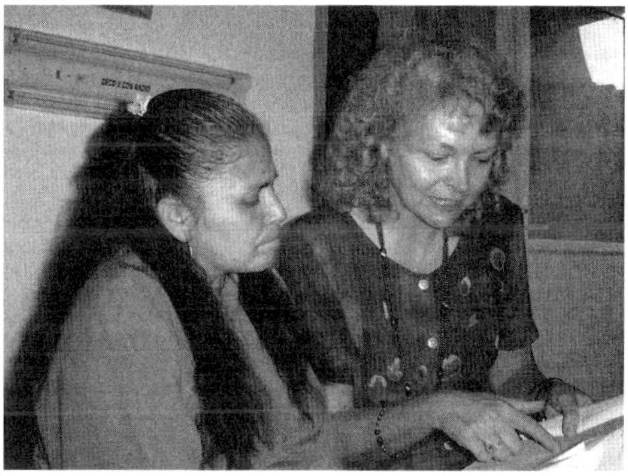

Robbie translating the part about Paz in her intuition article soon after it first came out, while Paz nods in agreement, noting that she would say the same things again! Photo by Debra Pascali-Bonaro

The fascinating difference between Paz's story and Carrie's lies in their endings. In Carrie's story, the dis-articulation of systems ended in the baby's death, and might have done so in Paz's story as well. But Paz found the opportunity to seek a smoother articulation. Over years of practice and referral, she had built a mutually respectful relationship with one private practice OB who did not question her diagnosis, but rather was immediately ready to respond. So she was able to create a radically different ending to this otherwise very similar story. Paz said, "What happens is that the politics are against us, so we have to be as creative as we can."

Fractured Articulations

Lana's Story: An Inaudible Voice

Lana Lane, an American direct-entry midwife, learned midwifery through a two-year apprenticeship in Fairbanks, during which, with her mentor, she attended over 100 births. Shortly after finishing her training in 1985, she moved to Wasilla, Alaska, where she went into partnership with Susan Eakin. By then the direct-entry midwives of Alaska had achieved their legislation and were practicing legally. This story, told to me by Lana's partner Susan, took place the following year.

> Arriving at the home of a woman in early labor who lived less than five minutes away from a tertiary care center in Anchorage, Lana performed a vaginal exam to check the degree of cervical effacement, dilation, and station (the position of the baby's head), and suddenly found the umbilical cord in her hand. Susan said, "The cord was just below the baby's head. Lana tried to slip it up away from the vaginal opening, hoping the head would block it, which can sometimes be done if too much cord doesn't wash down. But the cord just kept slipping, so all Lana could do was keep the cord from being pinched (which would cut off the baby's blood and oxygen supply) by splinting it between her fingers and pushing the head off it." While the mother assumed the knees and chest position and prayed, Lana used her fingers to push the head up and hold off the cord, telling her partners to administer oxygen to the mother and the father to call 911. He held the phone for Lana as she described the situation and begged them to have an operating room ready. At that point, the baby's heart tones were normal.
>
> The ambulance arrived in two minutes. The EMTs were cooperative and did not question the midwife's judgment. Lana straddled the stretcher below the mother, applying counter-pressure to the baby's head with one hand and with the other using the Doppler to monitor heart tones that were steadily dropping. They were inside the hospital within minutes. But upon arrival, they found that nothing had been done to prepare for the cesarean. For 30 minutes, Lana knelt on the stretcher holding the head in place and listening to the heart tones drop—50, 40, 30. She lost her voice from screaming for the hospital staff to hurry. But by the time the cesarean was finally performed, the baby had died.

A prolapsed cord is life-threatening to the baby—when the cord is in front of the baby's head, it is compressed, thereby cutting off blood and oxygen circulation. Unless the baby can be birthed immediately or a cesarean quickly performed, the baby is likely to die. In this situation, wherever it occurs, the mother must get into the knee-chest position, which takes the pressure off the cord, while the practitioner kneels behind her and applies counter-pressure to the baby's head so that the cord is not compressed between the head and the woman's pelvis. Keeping her hand inside the mother's vagina, the practitioner must hold up the baby's head until the baby is delivered by cesarean—a dramatic scenario to say the least, the success of which depends on how quickly the cesarean is performed.

This story resonates with pain; indeed Lana's partner Susan, who first recounted it to me, was crying as she spoke. She did not know exactly why Lana's pleas for speed were ignored, but she felt sure that it had something to do with the hospital staff's disapproval of homebirth. The worst-case scenario would interpret hospital personnel as deliberately ignoring this "walk-in" from outside to prioritize the women inside and/or to punish her for trying to give birth at home. Prior and subsequent experiences have ensured that Susan holds this worst-case view. She said:

> In my opinion, the reason no one came to the rescue is because it was a planned homebirth gone bad. I don't think they "believed" Lana knew a thing. More than once we've been forced to wait on circumstances they would normally be scampering to fix. I could tell you several stories in which the medical staff tried to hang us, instead of acknowledging that we transported appropriately.

In contrast, the scenario that attributes the best intentions to the hospital practitioners has to do with the logistics of hospital procedures. When a cord prolapse occurs in hospital, the practitioner who identifies it issues a crash call, the obstetric team flies into action, and when all goes well the baby is rapidly delivered by cesarean. But getting everything in place for a cesarean usually takes about 30 minutes "from decision to incision" (often about the same amount of time required to get to the hospital) and is expensive in terms of the personnel and equipment needed. And many hospitals have experienced doctors, paramedics, nurses, and/or midwives telling them to prepare for a cesarean when one really isn't needed. Setting up unnecessarily ties up rooms, obstetricians, and anesthesiologists and may keep them from being available if needed elsewhere. Thus it is logical that a hospital would want to assess the situation before taking action, especially on the word of a person unknown to them (which might include a private physician) (Judith Rooks, personal communication; see also Rooks 1997).

This transport took place in 1986 but cannot be dismissed as anachronistic—similar scenarios still play out around the country, especially in states where midwives practice illegally, but also in states where they are legal but not well accepted by or well-known to biomedical practitioners. It illustrates the dysfunctions generated by partial, fractured articulations between the biomedical and homebirth midwifery systems. The biomedical system's first response was appropriate—the EMTs supported the midwife to continue her work and did not challenge the validity of her knowledge or approach. And on the phone the hospital promised a response. But somewhere between the promise and the mother and midwife kneeling on the stretcher in the hall, a fracture occurred in what had promised to be a system of smooth articulation, and it was the baby who fell through the crack. Both the worst-case scenario (that the hospital deliberately delayed action to punish the midwives and the mother for attempting a homebirth) and the best-case scenario (that, given the expense and difficulty of preparing the OR, hospital practitioners didn't feel they could risk taking these unknown midwives at their word) point up the importance of prior dialogue and relationship between the hospital and the midwives in order to establish mutual trust and systems of smooth articulation well in advance of this kind of emergency.

Marina's Story: A Public Humiliation

Marina Rodriguez defines her primary identity as that of a traditional midwife; she also is a registered nurse. Her friend and colleague Paz lives to the far north of Cuernavaca, while Marina's residence is in a barrio called Tejalpa to the east of the city on the road to Tepoztlán and Cuautla, not far from the former home of her mentor and friend Doña Irene, whom we met in Chapter 8. Marina became a traditional midwife because she resented the subordination of the nursing role and found allopathic biomedicine entirely too interventionist for her taste. She attends four to five births a month, mostly in women's homes but also in the bedroom she uses as a birth center; she has a separate room for prenatal exams. Every time I visited, wild herbs lay drying on her prenatal exam table, a visual elision of boundaries and juxtaposition of worlds that is characteristic of the hybrid nature of these midwives' practices (see photo on p. 233).

> One night Marina received a phone call from the family of a distant cousin of her husband, from a small rural town. The cousin was six months pregnant and the family was worried about her and wanted to know if they could bring her to Marina for a check-up. Thinking they mean at some future date, Marina agreed. At about six the next morning the woman arrived on her doorstep. Marina was already in her nursing uniform, about to head out on a campaign to offer Pap screens to rural women. She didn't like the way the woman looked and immediately took her blood pressure; the diastolic pressure was 170, suggestive of pre-eclampsia. Marina immediately called a taxi and accompanied the woman to the hospital. By the time they arrived, the woman was convulsing. The hospital staff put her into intensive care, while Marina waited outside in the waiting room:
>
>> And every so often the doctor came out and told me that I am this thing and that thing, saying, "Useless midwives, why do you take these cases when they are serious and high-risk?" yelling at me in front of all the people in the waiting room. And the second time he came out he said more things to me and threatened me and in truth made me feel very bad. "Don't leave," he said. "Because if she dies right now we're going *to see about you.*" And I got scared. I didn't do anything besides take her blood pressure and bring her straight to the hospital. And after a while her family arrived and I told them that she started convulsing all of a sudden. I told them that I hadn't done anything, that I had been headed somewhere else and took a detour to accompany her.
>>
>> And finally the family spoke with the doctor and explained everything to him, and I spoke with another doctor there who knows me and has always helped us midwives. That first doctor was a real despot. And yes he finally apologized to me, because the doctor who is kind to me and respects me is the head of obstet-

> rics at that hospital, and made him apologize. But he apologized to me in private in a little back room, and he insulted me in public in front of everyone. The whole thing made me feel sick. But in the end they did save her life and the baby's life. In the ultimate case, I wasn't the one who was important, right? She was, and the baby was. But yes, my morale did go way down. What did I do wrong? Why would I keep her here and have her die on me? That despot wouldn't even let me tell him what I had found.

As a nurse, Marina has often served as first assistant at cesareans; she has good relationships with several physicians who respect her, and so the doctor's belittling remarks took her by surprise. Even worse than the insults, from her point of view, was the doctor's complete unwillingness to listen to the facts of the case; he blamed and judged her without even knowing what had happened. As with Carrie, Paz, and Lana, the midwife's knowledge and prior experience did not count—in Marina's case, indeed, they did not exist inside the system. The other midwives at least verbalized what they knew, even if they were not heeded, while Marina's voice had no chance to be heard. So even in this case, where the hospital recognized the gravity of the situation and immediately took over the care of the woman in appropriate ways with a good outcome for mother and child, the midwife was punished. As she narrated these events, which took place six months before our interview in summer 2000, Marina's face turned red and tears came to her eyes. She was grateful that the doctor and hospital staff saved the life of mother and child, but kept returning to the personal damage done to her. The doctor's apology seemed to her too little and too late—the humiliation was public, the apology forced and made in private.

From the biomedical point of view, it is important to understand that the doctor's specific question, "Useless midwives, why do you take cases that are serious and high-risk?" reflects his understanding that traditional midwives are taught a series of risk factors in training courses and told that they should always refer such cases. Earlier we saw Paz mention two of these risk factors as reasons for transport: fetal heart rate decelerations and unknown prior history. Preeclampsia is another such risk factor. Although in this particular case, the doctor's insult was unfounded, he had other reasons to make it. The traditional midwives I have interviewed in Cuernavaca often *do* take high-risk cases, choosing to ignore the protocols they have been taught, because of the circumstances under which they practice. Doña Irene explains:

> In a given moment the woman comes knocking on my door with eight or nine centimeters of dilation, and I can't turn her away even if it is a case of high-risk—I have to attend her. And we have moved forward with plants, with massage, we give all that is within our reach to give health to the parturient woman so that everything turns out well. . . . When the case is high risk because the baby comes breech, in the moment of the

> birth we have to be doing *maniobras* [hand maneuvers] to turn it, and if it can't be done, we have to receive it as it comes, even if the person never went to a prenatal consult. . . . A low-lying placenta is a high-risk case, right? What we do is push the placenta to one side and the baby can come through and be born. Only when really the placenta comes first, and then the baby—placenta previa—then we have to take her to the hospital, because that truly is a case of high risk.

Marina, too, acknowledges that she has often attended women that would be labeled high risk by the biomedical system. For example, it is not uncommon for poor Mexican women to avoid prenatal care—they resent the long waits at the hospital and the impersonal treatment they receive, so many of them just don't go. Perhaps such a mother would prefer receiving prenatal care from a midwife, but she may not feel she can afford it or may think it unnecessary, especially if she has had other children already. So then she comes to the midwife in labor, having avoided paying for prenatal care but preferring to pay for a midwife-attended birth over having a hospital birth for free. Or perhaps the midwife lives close by, and labor comes on precipitously, and there is no time to reach the hospital. So then, as Doña Irene says, what is the midwife to do? These midwives share an ethic of care that involves service to women; most traditional Mexican midwives (and some American midwives—see Chapter 12) will not violate that ethic by turning away a laboring woman they have not attended prenatally before they even check her. And if they check her and encounter a problem they feel they can handle, especially later in labor, they are very likely not to transport in order to save the woman from the otherwise inevitable cesarean.

Although many Mexican traditional midwives accept the notion of biomedical superiority and devalue their own skills in relation to biomedicine, Marina and her postmodern colleagues in Morelos do not. Like American professional midwives, they see their own knowledge system as more appropriate than technomedicine for all normal and some high-risk births, and they engage in a radical critique of technomedical limitations, pointing out that most doctors in Mexico have no idea how to turn a baby in utero or deliver breeches vaginally; they simply perform a cesarean. Women who come to traditional midwives in urban areas are usually there because they do not want to have a cesarean birth, which has become almost normative in urban Mexican hospitals. Urban women who go to a traditional midwife could have gotten biomedical care for free; they want her care badly enough to pay for it. The postmodern midwives of Morelos charge around $15 USD for a birth—a far cry from the $3,000–$6,000 or so that American direct-entry midwives often charge (for a full course of ante- through postpartum care). But for the urban and rural poor who seek the traditional midwives out, their fees, even though usually offered on a sliding scale, can still be a challenge to pay.

Home- or birth-center birth with a traditional midwife in an urban area like Cuernavaca, where hospital birth has long been the norm, is thus a deeply desired alternative choice in the same way that it is in the United States. It was the existence of this alternative, which many doctors would like to eliminate in the cities at least, combined with the even more provocative willingness of midwives to ignore the protocols they are taught in their training courses, that had the doctor already so angry at traditional midwives in general that he blew up at Marina without even bothering to learn the facts of this particular case. His knowledge system insists that cesareans are the solution in almost all high-risk situations and that the midwives' *maniobras* (hand maneuvers) are both ineffective and dangerous. This physician's successful management of the mother's eclamptic seizure, which the midwife could not manage, is of course one of the lifesaving skills that allows him to maintain his belief that only his knowledge counts.

It is worth noting that in each of the earlier stories, the biomedical staff would have had to trust the midwife's knowledge to take quicker action, as in the complications resulting from fetal heart rate anomalies detected by the midwives, but not by biomedical staff, and a cord prolapse that only the midwife had confirmed by touch. We can speculate that the reason why Marina's cousin got such quick attention when the other women we have heard about did not was the visible, unmistakable, and dramatic nature of her condition, which required no reliance at all on the midwife's knowledge to diagnose.

As in Carrie's story, the threat of legal action against the midwife hovers in the air in Marina's story. Unlike Carrie, Marina practices legally with her identification card from the health department, issued to her upon completion of her two-week TBA training course. She also relies on her nursing registration for various aspects of her practice. There is no national certification as yet available that Mexican traditional midwives can obtain; Marina is highly supportive of midwives' current efforts to create one (see Davis-Floyd 2001a), as she has longed for years to be able to prove her worth to the physicians in town. In the meantime, like the other traditional midwives in Cuernavaca I have interviewed, she continually augments her education through workshops and seminars given by various organizations and continuing education courses at local universities. The walls of her prenatal exam room are covered with framed certificates from these courses (see photo on p. 233); she showed me a large drawer full of others she intended to frame. Such certificates are proudly displayed by all of my interviewees in Mexico as visible evidence of their commitment to education and their ongoing quest to improve themselves as practitioners.

Sadly, Marina noted that while these certificates do carry weight with her clients, she didn't suppose they would make a difference to the "despot doctor." She was truly terrified by his threat to "see about you" should the woman die; as I noted above, although Marina and her colleagues practice legally, when there is a death they are often arrested and put in jail until the investigation is complete. In Marina's story, as she is the first to point out, the *mother's* transition from midwife to hospital was smooth; the fracture occurred in the interaction, or lack of it, between the midwife and the doctor. This fracture made Marina realize that the certificates on her wall cannot protect her from biopowerful devaluation, and gave her a great deal of impetus to address this fracture by working to increase midwifery power through supporting the formation of a midwives' association and the legal fund its members hoped to generate.

Marina's story finds a transnational echo in one told to me by Dina Farraw, an American CPM from Arkansas, who transported a client after a homebirth for a retained placenta. The doctor did remove the placenta, but only after sternly telling the woman and her husband that it was "child abuse" to give birth at home with midwives. This insulting remark was most likely made out of sincere beliefs that midwives are ignorant and that homebirth is a highly risky enterprise. The statistics on the safety of homebirth in the US are not taught in medical school, and most obstetricians are simply unaware of the good outcomes homebirth midwives generally achieve (Rooks 1997; Johnson and Daviss 2005; Cheyney et al. 2014b). Ironically, the doctor's belief in the midwives' ignorance stems from his own.

The hegemony of obstetrics has forced midwives to educate themselves in its ideology and assumptions, protocols, and lexicon to enhance their chances of successfully interfacing with it and of being able to defend their actions in its terms. In contrast, the marginality of midwifery has allowed obstetricians to remain ignorant about it. Obstetricians tend to be unilingual in the language and technologies of biopraxis, while my midwife interviewees on both sides of the border tend to be multilingual. They manipulate the lexicons of both obstetrics and midwifery, as well as of various folk systems of practice and belief that inform the lifeworlds of the clients they attend. Midwives thus transgress and elide professional boundaries on a daily basis, while obstetricians tend to reinforce them. Fractures in attempts at articulation (like this doctor's insulting remarks) often result from this kind of obstetrical boundary reinforcement.

In both the US and Mexico, a few physicians are willing to elide and transgress professional boundaries in order to support homebirth midwives. Such support can be costly: In the US, some physicians have lost their hospital privileges, their insurance, and their ability to practice in their communities as punishment for working with homebirth midwives. Of course, the more physicians supportive of homebirth midwifery are marginalized within biomedicine, the less ability they have to create needed structures for smooth articulation.

Smooth Articulations: Good OB Backup and a Receptive Hospital

It is important to remember that for all the transports that go awry, many others go smoothly and most do not result in anyone's death, even when they are characterized by fractured articulations. Very few urban midwives in Mexico and the US ever lose a mother, but out of every 1,000 births, one or two babies will die no matter where they are born or who attends them. In the US, data indicate that planned home and birth center births for low risk mothers carry similarly low rates of mortality for babies whose births start outside of the hospital (Rooks 1997; MacDorman & Singh 1998; Johnson and Daviss 2005; Cheyney et al. 2014b). As this volume's reviewer Melissa Cheyney pointed out, there is yet to be a study that compares a matched sample of planned, low-risk home-, birth center, and hospital births in the US. The absence of this kind of study is yet another reflection of the technocratic paradigm in action: Why study the effects of birth location and provider type if you believe you already know the answer?

As I noted above, only 3 out of 10 transports are true emergencies; the same emergencies happen in hospitals (where it still takes 30 minutes to set up an OR). But clearly, transports that involve fracture or disarticulation between biomedicine and midwifery can amplify the problems already generated by the complication that motivated the transport; sometimes those disjunctures alone are enough to cause a death that would not otherwise have occurred. On the other hand, when a homebirth transport is treated as effectively as a problem that takes place within a hospital, the chances for survival of mother and baby are greatly enhanced. This more positive scenario requires smooth articulation between the biomedical and homebirth midwifery systems, which the following two stories will illustrate. They both come from my interview with Carrie Smiley, the afore-mentioned CPM from Atlanta, Georgia; I chose them because they are highly representative of those of other midwives.

> A mother pregnant with her second child, whose first birth had been very fast, started bleeding during mild early labor with contractions six to eight minutes apart. Carrie had sent her for an ultrasound at 34 weeks, which had been normal, so she knew she was not dealing with a placenta previa (the placenta does not move after 34 weeks). Carrie noted that "if the mother had not had an ultrasound, there is no way I could have checked her with that much bleeding at home." (In a case of true placenta previa, doing a cervical check can cause harm.) Carrie checked the baby's heart tones, which sounded good. Carrie was concerned by the dark red color of the blood, which indicated that it was not from a superficial cause. She called the hospital and talked to the nurse-midwife who works for Carrie's backup doctor, telling her it looked like some kind of placental abruption might be occurring. Carrie and her midwife partner drove the mother to the hospital, where the nurse welcomed them into the labor and delivery unit and put the mother on an electronic fetal monitor, hooked up an IV, and drew blood to type and screen in case she had to have a cesarean. The baby's heart tones remained steady and strong. The doctor came in about ten minutes after they arrived and said to Carrie and the nurse, "It looks like you have everything under control." Carrie expressed her concern about the color of the blood, but the doctor was not worried. He stayed for only about five minutes. After he left, the mother

> labored for another three hours. She spent time in the Jacuzzi, sat on the toilet and then the birth ball for a while; eventually, she got in bed to try to rest. Carrie and the nurse-midwife turned off all the lights in the room.
>
> When pushing contractions kicked in, the mother pushed for about ten minutes, as Carrie recalls, and delivered on her hands and knees while the nurse-midwife caught the baby. The baby stayed with the mother. The placenta came fairly quickly after the birth; when Carrie and the CNM examined it, they could see a five centimeter clot on it—an indication that the placenta had partially detached in that area and had been bleeding from that place for a while. (If a placenta detaches uniformly after the birth, there will not be many clots on it unless it has been sitting in the uterus for quite a while, but if there is a partial separation, there will be clotting or additional clotting at the site of the partial separation.) The mother and baby went home the next morning. After the birth, the doctor told Carrie that she probably could have stayed at home for this one. And Carrie told him, "You have to realize that it's important for me to transport sooner rather than later when I have the option." And he said "You are right—I don't always see it from your side."

In the hospital, a partial placental separation is not cause for major alarm, since facilities for a cesarean are there at hand. But homebirth midwives like Carrie prefer to err on the side of caution—if you see too much bleeding to feel OK about it, you transport. A primary ingredient in Carrie's willingness to transport early rather than late is the excellent relationship she has established over time with this doctor and this particular hospital. She said:

> Since the early years of my practice, over time we have built up a lot of really good rapport, so that we have a lot of unoffficial backup [it can't be official as Carrie's practice is not legal or licensed in Georgia]. We now have a doctor who is providing backup for us in that during the pregnancy he will see the mothers if we need him too—if we need an ultrasound he'll do one in the office. He says he doesn't like homebirth but also he doesn't like the fact that many doctors are refusing to see homebirth mothers. He says everybody deserves good medical care when necessary. And if something comes up in labor, we can call the nurse-midwives who are always in-house. They listen to what we have to say on the phone and have everything set up when we arrive—the operating room ready, the doctor already in-house. So it is a really good situation—there are no animosities or repercussions or "attitudes" toward homebirth mothers. The doctors aren't exactly thrilled—they have said to the CNMs, "I wish you'd quit being so nice to these midwives so they'll quit bringing women in." And the CNMs have answered, "Would you rather leave them at home?" And the hospital is wonderful! It has no newborn nursery—I would consider them mother-baby friendly. The babies are never taken away from the moms unless they are really in trouble and *need* to be in the NICU.

Carrie's experiences point out that *different kinds of articulations can happen in the same location as the actors come to know and develop trust* in each other over time.

In 1978 with the first publication of *Birth in Four Cultures*, Brigitte Jordan issued a call for the replacement of top-down, culturally inappropriate obstetric systems with models of "mutual" or "fruitful" accommodation between biomedical and indigenous systems—a plea that is equally significant for non-indigenous homebirth midwifery systems. Both Paz's earlier story about transferring a patient from an unsupportive hospital to a private clinic with a physician who knew and trusted her, and Carrie's story above, illustrate the positive results of this sort of mutual accommodation. Nurse-midwives are especially well placed to achieve it, as they inherently straddle and bridge (and occasionally fall into the fissures between) biomedicine and homebirth midwifery.

Establishing close relationships with homebirth midwives who are not legal is simultaneously a transgressive and a boundary-spanning act. This prior communication between Carrie, the nurse-midwives, and the supportive physician certainly facilitated the smooth articulation of systems that both of these stories illustrate. Carrie feels that the key to this sort of smooth articulation is mutual respect and a cooperative attitude on the part of all concerned. Carrie's long and safe practice in her community has earned her this kind of respect from the hospital practitioners who know her best. She notes that it can take years to build up this kind of relationship, especially with physicians who start out mistrusting midwives. Once established, though, such relationships tend to last.

Many homebirth midwives, including Carrie, Susan, Dina, Marina, and Paz, do presently enjoy mutually accommodating relationships with one or two supportive physicians that they have worked hard to build over the years. But they note that such smooth articulations are jeopardized when the supportive MD moves away or retires and is replaced by a younger doctor "with an attitude," as Carrie puts it, and then the midwife has to start all over again on the process of building trust. And most of my interviewees cannot always count on the availability of the physicians who support them; thus, even those who have spent years building good reputations and good relations with certain physicians sometimes still have to deal with fractured articulations during transport.

But in Carrie's case, because of her long-term relationship with the nurse-midwives in her local hospital, the articulation between her knowledge system and that of the hospital and its practitioners is so smooth that she is more than willing to transport even for situations that have nothing to do with risk but rather with the mother's comfort alone, as the following short story shows.

> A primapara [mother giving birth for the first time] had pulled a muscle in her back at end of pregnancy and was in a lot of pain as a result; she

called Carrie to her home in the middle of the night. Carrie arrived to find the mother was in very early labor, at two centimeters dilation, but with close to unbearable pain from the back spasms. Carrie spent hours trying to relieve the pain in her back with showers and warm compresses and massage. She said:

> After a while we were running into brick walls as far as pain relief for the spasms, so we decided to go into the hospital where they have Jacuzzis in the labor rooms. By the time we got there, she was six centimeters. The nurse-midwives who received us told her she was doing great. The jets did good counter-pressure on the back pain. They never started an IV and she had no pain medication. The baby's heart tones always sounded great. I was able to catch the baby as "the grandmother" on the chart—the nurse working with us had had her babies at home, and the nurse-midwife was very supportive and felt this mom really deserved the continuity. The baby was fine and the family went home 12 hours after the birth.

As these two stories illustrate, smooth or seamless articulation between knowledge systems proceeds through points of overlap, transition, and communication that facilitate the seamless flow of information and linked, imbricated decision making in which the actions taken by one person or group build on the information supplied by another. The relationships between Carrie and the hospital-based CNMs encompass such points, as do the relationships between the Cuernavaca midwives and their supportive MDs. When this kind of decision making takes place within the top-down biomedical system, such imbrication requires a rejection of its tendency to discount or dismiss as irrelevant other ways of knowing. Such rejections can and do take place at the level of the individual even when the system as a whole remains dismissive.

How Physicians Can Come to Develop Respect for Midwifery Knowledge

What motivates or inspires a physician to reject the top-down system and give credence to homebirth midwifery knowledge? In my experience, the ingredients key to an individual physician's rejection of biomedical hegemony in favor of mutual accommodation include: (1) exposure to midwifery care; (2) exposure to midwives; and (3) attention to the scientific evidence.

Exposure to midwifery care. Some doctors train in hospitals where nurse-midwives practice and thus are able to observe firsthand the benefits of midwifery care. Physicians I have interviewed are often awed by the midwife-attended births they witness, which are usually visually and audibly nothing like previous births they have seen. Women attended by midwives in hospitals are more likely than women attended by physicians to give birth in upright positions, without an episiotomy, and with a great deal of hands-on support. Nurturance and consideration tend to characterize the midwife's approach to the mother; shared decision making takes place in a context of mutual respect. Physicians who do not ordinarily witness this kind of birth can find the experience transformative, can become imbued with a desire to incorporate this kind of respectful, humanistic approach into their own practice, and will be more likely to work with nurse-midwives in the future from a partnership, rather than a hierarchical, perspective. Occasionally a brave physician will venture outside hospital bounds and observe a midwife-attended homebirth—an experience that tends to be emotionally evocative and ideologically transformative (see, for example, Wagner 1997).

More profoundly, it is important to note that clinicians judge other clinicians as individuals, not just as members of a class or category; individual judgments can overcome prejudices based on subcultural differences. Does a practitioner give good care, make good decisions, communicate accurately? Individual practitioners decide the answers on the basis of experience. All clinical practitioners constantly gather experience and information and react differently to a comment, order, or action from someone they trust as opposed to someone whose judgment has been faulty in the past or whom they do not know. Midwives work best with the doctors they have come to trust as a result of experience, and vice versa. But most doctors have little or no experience of working with homebirth midwives; the experience they do have may be skewed if it comes only during emergency transports (see note 5). Lack of experience with working together creates problems that exacerbate and perpetuate lack of experience with working together (Judith Rooks, personal communication).

Exposure to midwives. Postmodern midwives in the US and Mexico, I can say without overstatement, tend to have huge hearts, impressive personalities, a strong sense of commitment and dedication to serving women, a secure sense of their own self- and professional worth, and a large fund of knowledge about parturition that seamlessly permeates their conversation. Simply spending time with them can turn a hospital practitioner from an opponent to a supporter. In US communities where smooth articulation characterizes transport, home and hospital midwives, and sometimes physicians, often participate in periodic potluck dinners where models of mutual accommodation begin to emerge over casseroles and drinks. Hospital midwives who develop respect for and good relationships with homebirth midwives often transmit this trust to the physicians with whom they work, in a kind of spillover effect that paves the way for future smooth articulations during transport. This kind of socializing, facilitated in the US by the middle-class status shared by participants, is far less likely to occur in Cuernavaca, where differences in social status between physicians and traditional midwives are more extreme.

Attention to the scientific evidence. There is increasing emphasis these days on "evidence-based medicine." As we have seen, midwifery offers more evidence-based effective care than obstetrics because midwives are generally less interventive than physicians (Cheyney et al. 2014b; Frye 1995; Davis 1997; Gaskin 1990 [1977]; Rooks 1997), and the scientific evidence (Rooks 1997; MacDorman and Singh 1998; Goer 1999; Enkin et al. 2000) shows that many common interventions do more damage than good. Any doctor who actually looks at the evidence instead of relying solely on what he is taught by biomedical tradition will take note of the benefits of midwifery care, and will thus be less likely to assume the blanket superiority of obstetrics. In recent correspondence (August 2016), Carrie told me, "Things have gotten much better in Atlanta since this story was written. A local perinatologist who felt women's choices were limited decided to go back into OB practice and provide backup for all the homebirth midwives. The hospital has restructured, become Baby-Friendly, and now welcomes homebirth transports along with the midwives."

Cross-Cultural Perspectives on Transport: Biomedicine as the Ultimate Recourse and the Ultimate Enemy

Articulation is the production of identity on top of difference, of unities out of fragments, of structures across practices. Articulation links this practice to that effect, this text to that meaning, this meaning to that reality, this experience to those politics. . . . And these links are themselves articulated into larger structures.
— Lawrence Grossberg

The experience of transport looms large in the minds of midwives because it is so emotionally loaded for them: they transport in hopes of resolving a situation they feel they cannot or should not handle at home, with hopes and prayers for a good reception, most especially for the mother, but also for themselves. A positive reception in the hospital reinforces midwives' sense of themselves as competent practitioners and elicits in them feelings both of pride in their good judgment and of gratitude toward the biomedical system for its efforts; a negative reception can leave the midwife and the mother emotionally scarred. Once burned, twice shy, they may in the future try too hard to avoid another transport, with potentially unfortunate results. Cross-cultural research provides multiple examples (e.g., Allen 2002; Barnes-Josiah et al. 1998; Iskandar et al. 1996; Graham 1999; Kroeger 1996). For one brief example, Deborah Barnes-Josiah and her colleagues (1998) have shown that in Haiti, community midwives who have been badly treated in hospitals, or whose clients have received inadequate care after transport, try in the future to avoid transport by coping with emergencies at home as best they can, often until it is too late to seek help. If disaster befalls, the midwife is handed the blame, with no account taken of the prior experiences that generated her avoidance behavior.

As we have seen in this volume, the solution to the trouble with transport that the governments of low-resource countries have generally sought to implement usually involves the goals of eliminating homebirth and traditional midwifery in favor of hospital or clinic birth attended by physicians and/or professional midwives trained in government-approved courses (Hsu 2001; Jenkins 2001; Sargent 1989). Yet for a variety of reasons, as we have seen in previous chapters, women in many countries continue to choose their traditional attendants (Hunt et al. 2002). Again, as Roger and Patricia Jeffery pointed out in 1993, it is important not to romanticize indigenous midwifery and indigenous midwives; some indigenous customs are beneficial and some are not; some traditional midwives are competent practitioners within their own systems and some are not. Similar notes can be sounded about Western-trained obstetricians: some intervene inappropriately, ignoring the evidence, while others exercise a more balanced and judicious approach. The transport stories I have recounted here should not be simplistically interpreted to indicate that all midwives are good and all biopowerful practitioners are bad or vice versa, but rather as ways of illuminating points of disjuncture and fracture, as well as models of smoothness, in the cross-boundary articulation of disparate knowledge systems.

System-Wide Possibilities for Seamless Articulation

Today in most developed countries, the homebirth rate hovers around 1%. That homebirth might be more widely chosen in the developed world if it were more readily available is indicated by the Netherlands, where the homebirth rate, although it has dropped significantly since 2009, still stands at around 13%; by New Zealand, where in recent years it has risen to 12% as the result of a strong alliance between midwives and consumers that has generated active government support; and by the UK, where it is rising steadily and has recently passed 3%. These three countries stand as models of what I would name *seamless articulation*—their midwives practice and their health care systems generally support birth in all settings, creating ease of choice and continuity of care across what in most other countries can only be seen as the home/hospital divide (DeVries et al. 2001). In Europe as in the US, active movements seek to restore homebirth as a viable option, with variable success. Meanwhile, in the developing world, homebirth rates continue to decline in response to the pressures of modernization, yet millions of women still give birth at home, some because there is no other option, some out of active rejection of their region's biomedical system, and others out of ideological choice.

Homebirth was both normal and normative for most of human history. But with the advent of biomedicine in the industrialized West, hospital birth became normative, and homebirth for most women ceased to exist as a viable or even thinkable option. In the developing world, this process is still untolding; in countries like Mexico, it has already taken root to the extent that while homebirth remains normative in many rural areas, in the cities it has become an alternative and marginalized choice as it is in most of the developed world. Nevertheless, some women still make that choice, and traditional midwives continue to serve them; only now, like American midwives, these urbanized traditional midwives are developing hybrid techniques that reflect the multiple systems of knowledge that intersect in their practices. They value the knowledge systems they are creating *and* the sometimes lifesaving knowledge system of biomedicine; yet the biomedical system, generally speaking, values only itself. Thus for both Mexican and American homebirth midwives, *biomedicine stands at once as the ultimate recourse and the ultimate enemy,* often with no guarantees in any given transport as to which aspect will manifest.

The six transport stories I have recounted and analyzed here are fractals for thousands of others that shed light on the trouble-filled and stress-full interface between the worlds of biomedicine and homebirth midwifery. Spiraling beyond the bounds of the specific situations they recount, they index both the myriad possibilities for tragedy inherent in one knowledge system's closed dismissal of its marginalized competitor, and the enhanced possibilities for more positive outcomes when members of that system open its boundaries to admit the fingers of articulation extended by practitioners from the outside. When parallel fingers reach out from the inside, taking account of midwives' information, acting on their recommendations, and encouraging them to remain with the mother to provide ongoing support, the result can be what Grossberg (1992:57) terms "active structures . . . that cut across domains and planes." Further elaboration of such structures of smooth articulation could extend individualized links and nodes across the hospital/home divide, ending the disarticulations, and mending the fractures, that generate much of the trouble with transport.

The Spectrum of Transport Articulations

Disarticulations
Fractured articulations
Smooth articulations
Seamless articulations

Transport Epilogue 2017: Developing Smooth and Seamless Articulations in the United States

And indeed, there are efforts being made in that direction. Since the original publication of this chapter as an article in 2003, continued discourse on the relationship between midwives and hospital-affiliated physicians has led to some improvements in the US around home-to-hospital transport (see Vedam et al. 2014). Apparently my original article on this topic (from which this chapter is updated) drew attention in medical and midwifery circles; many midwives gave it to their backup hospitals and it helped to generate better communication and smoother and more seamless transports in some cases. Then in 2014 Melissa Cheyney, a practicing CPM and anthropology professor (profiled in Chapter 8), Courtney Everson, a researcher and a doula, and Paul Burcher, an obstetrician, published an article entitled "Homebirth Transfers in the United States: Narratives of Risk, Fear, and Mutual Accommodation." Their article extended mine by focusing on presenting the views of both the receiving physicians and nurse-midwives, and the homebirth midwives who were transporting to their hospitals.

The researchers found that fear—of the unknown, of legal liability, and most particularly of getting criticized during hospital peer review sessions for dealing with homebirth transports—was the primary motivator for medical resistance to smooth articulation during transport, along with the emotional effects of the truly dangerous and traumatic (for all sides) transports. All obstetricians and CNMs interviewed expressed the understanding that the vast majority of transports are not emergencies and turn out well, but in spite of that understanding of the larger context, they were heavily emotionally impacted by the small percentage of transports that happen under truly dangerous conditions. (Please recall that the transport rate for all certified midwives attending out-of-hospital birth is around 10%—in other words, around 90 out of 100 planned, midwife-attended homebirths in the US take place successfully at home; out of the approximately 10 out of 100 that are hospital transfers, only three are in emergency situations.) And that emotional impact makes hospital practitioners react negatively to transports in general. They admit the irrationality, yet emotions are powerful and fear is one of the most powerful. It is rare for anthropology to have an effect on provider behavior and change, yet our two articles in conjunction apparently have had a positive impact that has helped to result in the generation of an actual set of protocols for transport.

In 2011 and 2013 (the Cheyney et al. article was not yet published, but was available in draft form), the US Homebirth Consensus Summit met to generate an "Interprofessional Collaboration and Communication" vision statement. The group was comprised of obstetricians, family medicine physicians, midwives, consumers, women's health advocates, and nurses. This group researched existing standards for universal intrapartum transport, transfer, consultation, and collaboration guidelines for all professionals who are involved when a woman or baby is transferred to a hospital from a planned homebirth. These guidelines, called "Best Practice Guidelines: Transfer from Planned Homebirth to Hospital," were created to improve communication between midwives and hospital staff through policy changes and best practices recommendations.

The guidelines recommend a standard of protocols for both the midwife and the hospital staff. The midwife is advised to prepare the mother prenatally for the possibility of transport should the necessity arise; to identify risks and communicate them to the mother as often as is necessary; to notify the receiving hospital in these instances with a well-documented prenatal history and clear charting, especially of the labor events that led to the transport; and to maintain support of the mother within the midwife's scope of practice at the receiving hospital. In turn, the hospital is advised to be sensitive to the psychosocial needs of the mother that arise from change in birth setting; to communicate directly with the midwife and respond with timely care and direct admission into the labor and delivery or pediatric unit; to accommodate the presence of the midwife if the mother so chooses; and to coordinate follow-up care with the mother and midwife. (Recently [August 2016], I have heard anecdotally from several midwives that these guidelines are indeed having a positive effect. They can be found at www.homebirthsummit.org/wp-content/uploads/2014/03/HomeBirthSummit_BestPracticeTransferGuidelines.pdf.) To date there are no actual studies on the effects of these guidelines, yet at the very least they exist and could, if applied in both countries and around the world, eliminate much of the trouble with transport.

Questions for Thought and Discussion

1. Home to hospital transport was not an original focus of Davis-Floyd's midwifery research. Why did she then choose to write an article on the topic?
2. What are the four kinds of articulation between home- and hospital-birth and knowledge systems that Davis-Floyd identifies?
3. What are the primary differences between obstetric knowledge about birth and midwifery knowledge?
4. Is transport during labor a common, or rare, phenomenon? Why or why not?

Recommended Films

The British TV series ***Call the Midwife*** shows many successful homebirths and a number of transports characterized by smooth articulation, as during the 1950s and early 1960s, homebirth was still normative in many British cities and towns. This historically accurate TV series, based on the memoirs of midwife Jennifer Worth, has generated a boom in the number of young British women applying to midwifery schools, as it depicts true community-based midwifery, the kind of inspiring and committed midwifery that many young women now aspire to practice. In one episode, the community doctor fights to keep his small birth center, which he opened for women in the Poplar district (a poor section of London) whose homes were inappropriate for giving birth. He is sternly informed by a government official that such places are now "things of the past," as the "march of progress" is now toward moving birth into fully equipped and modern hospitals. As the show clearly demonstrates, women want care close to home and do not appreciate having to travel long distances to obtain it.

Why Not Home? The Surprising Birth Choices of Doctors and Nurses: producer/director Jessica Moore. This film focuses on hospital birth providers who choose homebirth with the goal of moving toward improvements to maternity care in hospitals and at home. http://www.whynothome.com/

ACKNOWLEDGMENTS

For their invaluable assistance in analyzing the transport stories, I wish to thank Sara Wickham RM, a homebirth midwife and midwifery instructor in the UK and New Zealand; Richard Jennings CNM, Clinical Director of Midwifery at Yale University; Debbie Pulley CPM, a homebirth midwife in Georgia and NARM board member; William Camann MD, an obstetric anesthesiologist in Boston; and Judith Rooks CNM, an epidemiologist and expert on midwifery who also provided extremely helpful general editorial assistance, as did Melissa Cheyney PhD, CPM, a homebirth midwife, associate professor of anthropology, and director of MANA's Division of Research. Many thanks also to Brigitte Jordan (now deceased), Gwynne Jenkins, Marcia Inhorn, and three anonymous reviewers for their excellent editorial assistance, and to Heaven Handley and Christina Weis for help updating the references for this chapter. I also wish to express my appreciation to the Wenner-Gren Foundation for Anthropological Research for its support of this research through grants #6015 and #6427.

11

The Midwifery Model of Care

Anthropological Perspectives

During my observations [of nurse-midwifery care in a community hospital], I took note of common characteristics among the midwives—the care and concern provided to clients; the intimacy and emotional connection between the mother and individual nurse-midwives; the time given for education and individualized care; the fight by midwives to provide the patience and time needed for patients to successfully give birth vaginally. These professional characteristics . . . all go to the heart of the culture of nurse-midwifery. I had expected that many mothers would express satisfaction with the care given to them, but was surprised by what I can only describe as overwhelming satisfaction with nurse-midwifery care.

— Maureen May, *Epiduralized Childbirth and Nurse-Midwifery*

The Importance of Ideology: What's in a Name?

The "medical model" shows us pregnancy and birth through the perspective of technological society, and from men's eyes. Birthing women are thus objects upon whom certain procedures must be done. The alternative model . . . which I will call "the midwifery model" . . . is a woman's perspective on birth, in which women are the subjects, the doers, the givers of birth.

— Barbara Katz Rothman

This chapter is revised, adapted, and expanded from the "Conclusion" to *Birth Models That Work*, R. Davis-Floyd, L. Barclay, B. Daviss, and J. Tritten (eds.). (2009). Berkeley and London: University of California Press.

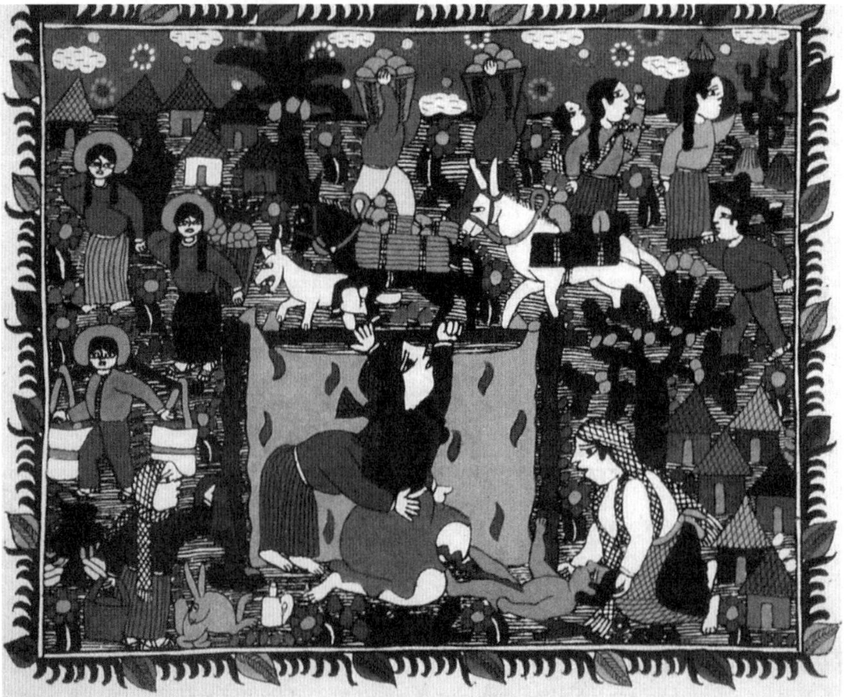

A traditional Mexican folk bark painting showing a woman at the center, holding up the world, as she gives birth upright with another woman supporting her and her midwife receiving the baby.

My coedited volume *Birth Models That Work* (Davis-Floyd et al. 2009) offers an educated tour of functional birth models whose practitioners are providing optimal maternity care; my description in this chapter of the midwifery model of care (MMOC) is largely based on the depictions provided in that book of how that model is practiced around the world. All of the models presented in *Birth Models That Work* share a common ideology based on the fundamental notions that birth is normal and women are its protagonists. This shared ideology has received various names over time. It was first described in print by sociologist Barbara Katz Rothman in 1982 as the "midwifery model of care"; this label has since become internationally recognized as a useful signature by which to differentiate the philosophy and ideology of midwifery from that of obstetrics. Recognition of the difference between the two professions—midwives focus on normalcy, obstetricians on pathology—goes back centuries; serious discussions about the implications of those differences have been taking place since that time.

Because midwives are the most numerous primary maternity care practitioners in the world and have long engaged in discussion and reflection with each other and with social scientists about what they do that works and doesn't work, they have continued to articulate and refine the midwifery model of care (e.g., Rooks 1999a). In many midwifery educational programs around the globe, this model is held out as an ideal for midwifery practice, while in others it is actively taught as the standard for care. Others have suggested other names for this model, in part to avoid identifying it with a particular profession and to acknowledge that many midwives overmedicalize their treatment of birth, while some physicians work very hard to practice the "midwifery model." To date there is no international consensus on the most appropriate name for the ideology and practice of supporting normal birth.

In *Birth as an American Rite of Passage* (2003 [1992]), I expanded on Rothman's discussion of the differences between the medical and midwifery models of care, using the labels "the technocratic model of birth" and "the holistic model of birth" to name these contrasting paradigms. Some years later, I further expanded my understanding of the dominant paradigms operative in global maternity care to include a third paradigm, the humanistic model, which stretches across the divide between the technocratic and holistic models. As I noted in Chapter 1, humanists wish simply to humanize technomedicine—that is, to make it relational, partnership-oriented, individually responsive, and compassionate. The humanistic model of birth places supreme importance on mind–body connection (the influence of mental and emotional states on the body, and vice versa), defines the body as an organism, and most essentially, stresses the importance of the caregiver–patient relationship. The essence of a humanistic approach to birth is relationship, communication, and caring between patient and practitioner—a supervaluation of the needs of the individual instead of those of the institution or its practitioners.

Birth activists in all Spanish- and Portuguese-speaking countries appear to have reached consensus around the term "humanization"—they speak of *la humanizacion del parto y nacimiento* (the humanization of birth), *parto humanizado* (humanized birth), and so forth. But to focus reform efforts on the humanization of birth can be a relevant strategy where birth is almost totally *dehumanized* but not, generally speaking, in many hospitals in countries such as in the US, Canada, the UK, the Scandinavian countries, Switzerland, and New Zealand. In these places, the interventionist technocratic approach still usually prevails in hospitals, yet women are often treated humanistically—that is, with compassion and respect, and with support from companions they choose: these are the essential ingredients of a humanistic approach. And therein lies the rub: as I emphasized in Chapter 1, the humanistic paradigm is highly co-optable—I have witnessed some Latin American hospitals suddenly start calling their maternity care "humanistic" simply because they decided to allow a partner to accompany the mother during labor or to allow mothers to stay with their babies in the freshly painted postpartum ward while many unnecessary interventions are still routinely and unkindly, sometimes violently, performed.

If *humanistic* is to become as widely used in other countries as it is in Latin America, we must be careful to distinguish the *superficial humanism* of the respectful and caring unnecessary cesarean from the *deep humanism* that acknowledges and facilitates the deep physiology and emotionality of birth, for example, through freedom of movement, upright positions for birth, and full emotional and physical support. *Superficial humanism* involves beautifying the birth environment, making the mother more comfortable, and treating her kindly and respectfully—but this approach can easily include the respectful and caring administration of multiple unnecessary technological interventions. *Deep humanism* goes much further, involving a profound understanding of the normal physiology of birth and how to facilitate it and including an understanding of the power of the mother's emotions to affect the progress of labor.

The *holistic model of birth* goes beyond the definition of the body as an organism to viewing it as an energy field in interaction with other energy fields. In the holistic view—one adopted by many midwives and some obstetricians (see Chapter 5)—practitioners can preclude the need for technological interventions by intervening at the level of energy, changing or focusing the "energy of birth" to facilitate optimal outcomes. For one very entertaining example of how energy can affect the birth process, Ina May Gaskin tells a story of a homebirth at the Farm in which, although the labor had gone very rapidly and smoothly, the mother seemed stalled in the pushing phase. Ina May asked if anyone in the room might be holding back anything, and the laboring woman's husband, on whose lap she had been sitting during pushing, replied that he had a desperate need to pee! Once that was accomplished, he resumed his supportive position and the baby was quickly born. *Change the energy, change the outcome.*

Descriptions of other models exist. For example, in *Pursuing the Birth Machine* (1994), Marsden Wagner contrasted the medical model with the "social model" of birth—a terminology followed by Lesley Barclay (2009) in her discussions of midwives in Samoa. Of course, the social model is one that emphasizes the sociality of birth. Dutch midwives speak of the "physiologic" model because their focus is on understanding and facilitating the deep physiology of birth (DeVries et al. 2009). Yet a focus on physiology can appear to minimize birth's social aspects, while a focus on sociality can seem to minimize the importance of physiology. Spreading out from France via the work of Bernard Bel and others is the term *naissance respectée* (respected childbirth)—a term that reflects a deeply humanistic focus. American birth activists struggle with "natural" vs. "normal" birth as their conceptual standard because both of these terms are problematic: nearly all human births are culturally shaped, and "normal" is hard to define, especially when interventions are "the norm" in hospitals. Anthropologist Brigitte Jordan (1993) utilized a "biocultural" approach to her analysis of birth in four cultures—and yet birth is more than a combination of biology and culture. It is therefore difficult to find terminology that communicates the full spectrum of essential values.

Other nomenclature abounds in areas where individuals or organizations are aiming to improve care models. An international collaboration between WHO and UNICEF resulted in the creation of the highly successful *Baby-friendly* Hospital Initiative (BFHI), primarily to facilitate successful breast-feeding. In 1995, the Coalition for Improving Maternity Care (CIMS) in the US developed a national initiative based on a *mother-friendly* model of care. And the International MotherBaby Childbirth Organization (IMBCO), a CIMS spin-off, in 2008 launched the *International MotherBaby Childbirth Initiative (IMBCI): 10 Steps to Optimal MotherBaby Maternity Services* (www.imbci.org and Chapter 14). This Initiative is organized around what its proponents have labeled the *MotherBaby Model of Care,* acknowledging its basis in the midwifery model. Its creators (including myself) chose the term MotherBaby to emphasize the integrity of this dyad. Two of its principles state:

- The MotherBaby Model of Care promotes the health and wellbeing of all women and babies during pregnancy, birth, and breastfeeding, setting the gold standard for excellence and superior outcomes in maternity care. All maternity service providers should be educated in, provide, and support the MotherBaby Model of Care.
- Midwives, who are the primary care providers for millions of birthing women in most countries, have developed a model of care based on the normal physiology, sociology, and psychology of pregnancy, labour, birth, and the postpartum period. The International MotherBaby Childbirth Initiative draws on the midwifery model of care and affirms that midwifery knowledge, skills, and behavior are essential for optimal MotherBaby care. (IMBCI 2008:3)

As the International MotherBaby Childbirth Initiative (IMBCI) grows in influence and spreads over time (see Chapter 14), perhaps the term MotherBaby Model of Care will gain international popularity. Yet for now, wishing to name and describe the model that underlies optimal birth practices, I note that *by definition midwives are or should be the primary guides and guardians of normal pregnancy and birth, while obstetricians, by definition, are or should be the backup providers dealing with conditions of actual danger or risk.*

Midwives are indeed primary practitioners in all the models described in *Birth Models That Work*, and "the midwifery model" seems to me at this point to be the most appropriate term to utilize. (It is difficult to translate into Spanish or Portuguese, so the English version is often used in those countries). The midwifery model as I define it here combines all elements of humanism with many elements of holism. Although the midwives in the models described in *Birth Models That Work* do practice according to this midwifery model, many thousands of midwives around the world are technocratically trained and do not. Nurses serve as primary birth attendants in some places, with disparate results, and "skilled birth attendants" with widely varying types of training are now internationally promoted (e.g., by WHO). In almost every country one can find committed obstetricians who apply the "midwifery model" daily in their practices. Thus I use the term "MMOC practitioners" (Midwifery Model of Care practitioners) to index those care providers who practice according to the ideology I describe in the following section.

The Midwifery (Humanistic-Holistic) Model of Care

Those last moments of sweat and struggle, and the ensuing immeasurable reward—the slippery sweetness of the brand-new being on bare skin, the first time those eyes open to search for the face that goes with that familiar voice, the ecstatic murmurings of the parents, grandparents, and even midwives, and that first latch when the baby finds its way home—these are the moments that we treasure, and for which we hold the space in a way no other profession can match.

— Mdiri Breen Rothman CNM, Region II Update, *ACNM Newsletter*, Fall 2016

The midwifery model of care comes from a woman-centered perspective, defines women as active agents in pregnancy and birth, and sees the female body as normal in its own terms and pregnancy and birth as healthy, normal parts of women's lives. It takes a holistic, integrative approach, defining the body not as a machine but as an organism and an energy field in constant interaction with other energy fields. It views mind and body as one and mother and baby as an inseparable unit; the use of the term "MotherBaby" in the International MotherBaby Childbirth Initiative indicates its authors' understanding of how profoundly the treatment of one affects the other. The safety and emotional needs of the mother and baby are the same; *what is good for the mother is good for the child.* As Rothman put it:

> The medical model dichotomizes not only mind and body, but also mother and infant. Mother/fetus are seen in the medical model as a conflicting dyad rather than an integral unit. In the midwifery model, mother and fetus are genuinely one, and what meets the needs of the one meets the needs of the other. Emotional, physical, maternal and infant needs are not, in the midwifery model, at odds. (1982:48)

The family, not the institution, constitutes the most significant social unit, and the mother, not the practitioner, is the most significant birthing agent.

Birth as Normal

I was on the birth stool, and as I got into the pushing, I could feel her coming down. It really burned and was intense, but I welcomed it because at that point I wanted to see her so badly. It was so hard. I pushed harder than I ever thought I could have . . . but I loved it. I felt so strong, so unstoppable. . . . I can see why someone might want drugs—it does hurt—but I wouldn't want to be numbed for the good, no

great, amazing feeling that comes with the hurt. I can still call on my experience when I need to and re-experience all that love and power. It was all so very, very worth it.
— quoted in a working draft of Cheyney 2011

Fundamentally, birth has evolved to work well the vast majority of the time—birth outcomes are better when labor and birth are nurtured and supported but not interfered with. MMOC practitioners understand the deep physiology of birth. They know that labor, when allowed to flow, has its own rhythms—it can start and stop, speed up or slow down, take a few hours or a few days as the uterus tones and prepares and the mother works through her emotions. Facilitation is appropriate; intervention is usually inappropriate. MMOC practitioners use specific technologies (e.g., artifacts that facilitate upright positions like birthing balls, wall ladders, ropes, and chairs) and modalities (e.g., massage, acupressure, and visualization) that work to support normal birth and minimize medical interventions, relying on a physiologically and emotionally supportive range of strategies and watchful vigilance.

They read and understand the scientific evidence showing that laboring women should be encouraged to do as they please—to eat, drink, move about, rest. The first line of care for minor delays and complications is with low-tech interventions such as position changes, emotional support, massage, immersion in warm water, aromatherapy, herbs, homeopathy, hand maneuvers, and most fundamentally "changing the energy" by working to create a more positive and trust-based atmosphere; higher-tech interventions are reserved for cases of true need. It is time that such modalities move into the mainstream.

MMOC practitioners see labor pain as normal and understand that a woman's ability to bear it can be greatly increased by nurturant care and a supportive, calmly energetic and environmental ambience permeating what obstetrician and MMOC practitioner Ricardo Jones (2009) calls the "psychosphere" of labor and birth. *Patience* is the most essential attribute of the MMOC practitioner—what some call the "tincture of time" (Melissa Cheyney, personal correspondence, August 2016). In their chapter on Japanese maternity homes in *Birth Models That Work*, Matsuoka and Hinokuma (2009:223–226) explain midwives' emphasis on "the importance of waiting": "Waiting does not mean so much time wasted or the time of just enduring pain for a birthing woman. It is a meaningful time, shared by the birthing woman, her family and the midwife together." As described in Chapter 8, these midwives consider labor pain to be "metamorphic": "a necessary process for a birthing woman as she grows into motherhood—to face her own self through the experience of pain." They believe that the comforting presence of the midwife and family members is enough to support the woman to experience this pain in a positive way; they see the pain as in fact positive because it is *productive* of the baby's birth and the *woman's* birth as a mother. They also see it as a way for the family and friends attending the birth to bond, and thus they recognize the actual benefit of long hours of labor.

MMOC practitioners are not afraid of labor pain or of watching women experience it; they know that their own calmness facilitates the woman's ability to move through the pain without the anxiety and fear that increases it. Midwives often work to master "the critical art of doing nothing well"—a watchful vigilance that can include simply knitting during a labor, as many women say that if they see their midwife knitting, they are sure everything is OK, because she wouldn't be just sitting there knitting if something were wrong (Kennedy 2009:421).

High Values on Emotions, Intuition, and Listening

I had a hard time letting go of the fact that people don't necessarily feel like giving birth is something that should be a challenge. They say, "I want an epidural. Why should anyone want to go through that kind of pain?" . . . So I've had to give up some of that thinking, you know, that this is the right way—you should want to feel that pain and feel proud of yourself after you give birth. . . . [I've been working on] being able to support people in their choices, though they may not have been my choices.

— CNM (quoted in Kennedy 2009)

The uterus responds to the mother's emotional state; thus the best care is based not only on measurements and information but also on body knowledge and intuition (see Chapter 7). In the midwifery model, experiential and emotional knowledge count as much as or more than technical knowledge. Essential attributes of maternity care include empathy, compassion, caring, and loving touch. MMOC practitioners know the importance of "*presence*: the ability to *be* fully with another person, completely attentive and focused, listening with an open heart" (Houston et al. n.d.). In a study of midwives in Austin, Texas, Brazilian midwife Gabrielle Carleto (2016) found when she asked which skill seemed most important to them, that most of her interviewees replied "listening to women"—which in fact is ACNM's motto, beautifully emblazoned on a rhinestone pin.

Reflective Practice, Knowledge Preservation, and Holistic Risk Assessment

Optimal health of the woman and infant is clearly the summit for both the obstetrical and midwifery models, but [under the midwifery model] during the journey other outcomes are achieved by the woman, including trust, power, satisfaction, as well as growth and pride for the midwife.

— Holly Kennedy, "'Orchestrating Normal': The Conduct of Midwifery in the United States" in *Birth Models That Work*, 2009, Chapter 15

MMOC practitioners value and work hard to achieve cultural appropriateness and sensitivity, treating women as they wish to be treated and upholding their rights. They rely on introspection and case reviews with colleagues to reflect on how they are practicing and make efforts at improvement on an ongoing basis. They are aware of the de-skilling of obstetricians—who are increasingly taught simply to perform a cesarean for most complications—so they consciously work to learn and to preserve the myriad skills that some midwives and obstetricians have learned and recorded over time that can keep birth normal, including massage, external cephalic version, positions and hand maneuvers for breech and twin delivery, variations on upright positions, stair-climbing or using a rebozo (shawl) to shake loose a stuck baby, and nonmedical means of stopping hemorrhage (since drugs are not always available—see Chapter 8, pp. 235–236 and 256 on "the postmodern midwife" for a description of those techniques). Such skills, and more, have long been part of the repertoire of traditional midwives in many regions and are consciously sought out by MMOC practitioners.

The midwifery model entails a two-way exchange—each group (e.g., midwives and obstetricians, or professional midwives and traditional midwives) learns from and teaches the other, with mutual attitudes of respect. What Cheyney, Everson, and Burcher (2014c) call "holistic and co-negotiated risk assessment" was considered by all the midwives they interviewed for their study on home to hospital transfer to be one of the core values of the midwifery model of care; it is also one of the primary skills Holly Kennedy CNM (2009) includes in her concept of "orchestrating normal," by which she means "the conduct of the midwife's work with the woman to meet her needs within the existing health care system"—which midwives must constantly negotiate to get those needs met. One of the participants in the Cheyney, Everson, and Burcher (2014c:449) study said:

> The midwifery model of care is about acknowledging more than just clinical risk. It's about the whole person. . . . There are other kinds of risk. There is psychosocial risk, the risk of unnecessary procedures, the risk of having to parent from a position of victimization and regret [from a traumatic hospital birth]. Does that matter? We think it should.

Relationships among Midwives and Obstetricians: Collaboration as Key

As I noted above, the midwifery model positions the midwife as the guide and guardian of the normal birth process; her skills should be used to keep birth normal in the vast majority of cases and to identify and treat complications herself if she is qualified, or to seek appropriate medical help when she is not. MMOC obstetricians work respectfully and collaboratively with midwives and provide appropriate services for high-risk and emergency births. In her ethnography of nurse-midwifery practice in a community hospital in the US, Maureen May (2017) describes extreme variations in physician–midwife "collaboration"—some OBs do collaborate in egalitarian ways, while others assume and maintain a distinct hierarchy. Regarding the latter, the midwives she observed and interviewed developed a range of strategies for dealing with OB "interference," from sweet-talking to outright confrontation. The positive side was that as these OBs grew more familiar with the benefits of CNM practice and came to respect and trust the midwives, they tended over time to interfere less. Yet, as May (2017:245) cogently notes:

> Nurse-midwives, when practicing in a hospital maternity service that is not truly midwifery-led, are impeded from practicing the midwifery model of care that has been shown by numerous studies to improve maternal and child outcomes. . . . Nurse-midwifery is easily subsumed into a culture of medicalization. Its ideal is a belief in physiologic birth, but the promotion of physiologic birth is difficult in the context of a subordinated midwifery. Collaboration in the context of a hierarchical relationship with obstetrics is an illusion. There can be no genuine collaborative relationship when an obstetrician has the right to ultimate decision-making. . . . Reliance on a beneficent, friendly obstetrician is not true independence.

If obstetricians who practice according to the midwifery model, such as some of those in the Netherlands, and the Brazilian "good guys and girls" described in Chapter 5, receive a client referred by a midwife due to a risk or complication that later resolves, they will then reclassify the client as normal and *refer her back* to midwifery care because they understand that normal birth is the midwife's specialty, while complicated conditions are theirs. As Dahlen (quoted in May 2017:239) observed:

> To build a bridge . . . you need pylons at each end of equal strength . . . until we are equals the bridge will not be built. The stronger we become as midwives, the better we will collaborate with our medical colleagues. Strength invites respect, and respect gives strength. . . . We need to do some serious work . . . on the notion that we are not a second-rate option, we are a first-rate choice.

Community-Based, Caseload, and One-to-One Midwifery: The Importance of Continuity of Care

The relationship between the midwife and the woman is foundational and mutual . . . it is through this relationship that the midwife works to create an environment conducive to meeting the needs of the woman and her family.

— Holly Kennedy CNM

MMOC practitioners are likely to be community-based, even if they use hospitals for birth. Their woman-centered ideology is reflected in the priority they place on continuity of care. When continuity of care is incorporated into employment models, these may be described as "team," "caseload," or "one-to-one" midwifery. The caseload model of care entails several midwives seeing the mother prenatally, getting to know her, and guaranteeing one of them will be present throughout her labor and birth (Reed and Walton 2009). The more common practice of hospital-based "shift midwifery" interferes with full provision of humanistic care—midwives leave after 8–12 hours no matter where the mother is in labor, a situation that can feel disruptive to the laboring woman. This situation can also produce anxiety for the midwife, especially when the midwife who is leaving is providing the MMOC and knows that the midwife replacing her will not, and that the mother will find the sudden switch to technocratic care an unpleasant shock that may interfere with her ability to give birth successfully. But even shift midwifery can constitute a model that works when *all* staff midwives practice the MMOC, as is demonstrated at the Lichfield Maternity Unit in the UK described by Walsh (2009) in *Birth Models That Work*, where the departing midwife knows that her client will continue to receive the same kind of nurturant care that she was providing.

As at St. George hospital in Sydney, Australia (Brodie and Homer 2009), a number of midwives have found that caseload midwifery is better not only for the mother but also for the midwife—there is less burnout than is found in the "team" model of care in which a group of midwives share the care of a large number of women. Pregnant women in the team system are less likely to build close, continuous relationships with a particular midwife and are more likely to have midwives they do not know at their birth. The team model provides less continuity of care and is associated with high levels of burnout for midwives.

"One-to-one" midwifery care means that the same midwife attends a pregnant woman throughout her prenatal, labor, and postpartum care. This ideal, however, is very difficult to achieve—midwives have families and busy lives and cannot always be present to one mother; caseload midwifery is the next best thing.

The phrase "the midwife follows the mother" means that the mother is free to choose her place of birth—home, freestanding birth center, or hospital—and the midwife will attend her there. This principle represents an evidence-based ideal that has long been the norm in the Netherlands and was one of the founding principles of the midwifery renaissance in New Zealand (Hendry 2009) and Ontario, Canada (MacDonald and Bourgeault 2009). Homes and freestanding birth centers are the places where the MMOC can be most fully applied, yet it is clear that the humanistic midwifery approach can thrive in highly biomedical environments as well. Again, as Hodnett (2002a, b) showed, *it is the ideology of the practitioner, not of the society or the institution, that has the greatest effect on an individual birth.*

Practitioner Education

Health care practitioners tend to practice as they were taught, so much so that when new information is presented, many longtime practitioners refuse to integrate or implement it because they are so habituated to doing things the way their teachers did (see Chapter 4). A primary key to instilling the MMOC in nascent practitioners is the reform of professional education so that instead of being educated exclusively in the technology- and pathology-oriented biomedical approach to birth, student doctors, nurses, and midwives would also be educated in the humanistic- and normality-oriented midwifery model of care. Such education is exemplified in medical, midwifery, and nursing training in the Netherlands (DeVries et al. 2009), in midwifery education in New Zealand (Hendry 2009), Ontario, Canada (MacDonald and Bourgeault 2009), the CASA School in Mexico (Mills and Davis-Floyd 2009), many US nurse- and direct-entry midwifery programs (Kennedy 2009), and Samoa (Barclay 2009), where the best of both traditional and professional midwifery are incorporated into an integrated university-based degree that involves traditional midwives as teachers in the program.

Following is an example (which I have taken from my article "The Ups, Downs, and Interlinkages of Nurse- and Direct-Entry Midwifery: Status, Practice, and Education" [Davis-Floyd 2010:66]) of how *the kind of education a student midwife receives can affect her ability in the future to practice the midwifery model.* The excerpted commentary, which is highly revelatory of the differences between the medical and midwifery models of care, comes from a student nurse-midwife (SNM) I interviewed, who had previously been what was called a "lay" midwife attending homebirths in the early 1980s. She was sent in to attend a hospital birth with a mother whom she had never met. She said:

> By the time I got to this woman, her labor was kind of stalled and she was just wild, writhing around, pulling out her IV. I didn't know what to do with her; I simply didn't know what to do. So I called in the OB, who pitted her [administered pitocin via her IV] and got her contractions stabilized, got her under control and her labor back on track. Once she was back on track and pushing, I felt like I could handle the birth.
>
> Q. You say you didn't know what to do with her. What would you have done if you had been at home with no OB to call?
>
> Oh, I would have done everything differently! I would have put my arms around her and asked her what she was feeling. I would have gotten her up, given her something to drink, helped her take a shower or walk around. We would have gotten to the bottom of her emotional issues before we tried anything else.
>
> Q. So it sounds like you did know what to do with her! Why didn't you do that, instead of calling the OB?
>
> Because the circumstances didn't allow it. There was no space for me to connect with her at that level.

This SNM was reporting on her exposure to the dual models of medicine and midwifery. In this case, as she does, we can attribute her decision to turn over control to a physician and to follow the medical approach to the fact that she was still a student and had not yet matured into a sense of autonomy. Trained and capable of operating in both models, she preferred the midwifery approach as she would be free to apply it at home. But, constrained by her environment, she was practicing (and thus internalizing) the medical way. Calling in the doctor or "pitting" a stalled labor can get her out of a difficult situation once, twice, three times without affecting her too much. But by the time she has taken this approach 40 or 50 times, will she even remember that she once knew another way? A poignant commentary on this SNM's experience was provided by CNM Fran Ventre. She wrote:

> After practicing as a "lay midwife" for several years, I had the same experience in nurse-midwifery school at DC General Hospital as the student quoted above. The difference was a nurturing caring faculty person who, when I was at sea, asked me the same question, "What would you do at a homebirth?" After easily rattling off the same things the student said, my teacher replied, "Well, why don't you just do that now?" (Personal communication 1998)

This faculty member created an ideologically safe space inside the hospital in which Fran could practice the MMOC as she would have done at a homebirth. The contrast between Fran's experience and the experience of my student-interviewee provides an excellent example of the individual variations in nurse-midwifery training and SNMs exposure to and ability to practice the MMOC. While some nurse-midwifery programs and some preceptors stress this more holistic approach, and the students are encouraged by their preceptors to apply it, in other programs students may find that approach difficult or impossible to apply because there is no one who can or will "hold that space" for them.

MMOC Leadership: A Postmodern, Flexible Style

In all of the models described in *Birth Models That Work*, effective leadership is noted as essential in promoting and maintaining the MMOC—what Denis Walsh (2009) describes in his chapter as "a postmodern leadership style":

> Prior to [Helen's] coming, the staff structure was very hierarchical and relationships with both women and each other were formal and deferential. Helen . . . addressed staff by their first names . . . introduced informal visits for women considering booking at the centre. . . She relaxed the institutional feel of the centre by deregulating visiting times. . . and morning routines like bed-making. She brought in midwifery-led care by negotiating the withdrawal of General Practitioners from intrapartum care and the setting up of an antenatal clinic at the unit, run by the midwives. She continued the refurbishment of the unit and deregulated staff work patterns.

> In all of these initiatives, she used a variety of methods in bringing about change. She worked with a supportive GP who mediated the changes in GP practice. With clinical changes, she used a combination of explaining her rationale and leading by example. Other staff were especially interested in upgrading the décor, and she gave them the freedom to lead this initiative. She built a team ethos by organizing regular social outings and shared fund-raising activities. She eschewed role demarcations by encouraging all staff to be involved in the upkeep and cleanliness of the facility. . . . She would never say to us, "Could you make them a cup of tea?" She would clean the kitchen out just like the rest of us.

Walsh notes that characteristics of this postmodern leadership style include flexibility, an integrated and team-based approach, a value on diversity, the aim to empower others, change as a constant, and a focus on people and relationships instead of places and things. His findings resonate with my own description of the "postmodern midwife" in Chapter 8.

Postmodern midwifery and postmodern leadership as Walsh and I describe them are profoundly characteristic of MMOC practitioners. This brand of postmodernism, eschewing hierarchy in favor of relationship and rigidity in favor of flexibility, encourages the levels of creativity, generativity, and out-of-box thinking that are essential to transcending the limits of the technocratic medical model in favor of what really works. In such efforts, the participation of consumers is extraordinarily important.

Conclusion: The Model behind the Model

You have to want to be there and you have to listen to the woman . . . as the midwife I'm there almost as a life-preserver, as a safety person to watch but not to do unless it is necessary to do. If it's safe, I'm happy with whatever she wants to do. . . . I also feel like it's the woman's responsibility to work with me and if I think that is not safe, I'm going to tell her and I'm going to tell her why and then comes the question of "If it's still not safe, then what?" So then it's kind of a little negotiation that goes on, I guess. And in the end, it's not my birth.

— Mary Ann, American midwife

In conclusion, I return to Ellen Hodnett's systematic review of reports on factors influencing women's evaluations of their childbirth experiences, which concluded that "the influences of pain, pain relief, and intrapartum medical interventions on subsequent satisfaction are neither as obvious, as direct, nor as powerful as the influences of the attitudes and behaviors of the caregivers." Attitudes and behaviors stem from ideologies that form the template for the caregiver's beliefs about birth. In other words, again, it's the *model behind the model of practice that most determines the kind of care a practitioner will provide.*

The midwifery model of care, when fully implemented, improves the physiological, psychological, and social outcomes of pregnancy and birth and saves money for systems and families, exposing the need for the total reform of existing dysfunctional yet hegemonic models. The MMOC issues a clarion call to health organizations and individuals to replace technocratic models that don't work with midwifery models that do, at local, regional, and global levels, in order to reduce maternal and perinatal mortality and morbidity, empower women and their families, and facilitate healthy birth and breastfeeding. The end game of this much-needed ideological shift is healthy mothers and babies who can generate a more conscious and sustainable future for our human family.

Questions for Thought and Discussion

1. What is the "midwifery model of care" and how does it relate to the technocratic, humanistic, and holistic paradigms Davis-Floyd describes in Chapter 1?
2. Can only midwives practice this model of care?
3. What are some of the primary characteristics of the MMOC as described in this chapter?
4. Would you like your birth practitioner to practice the MMOC, or would you prefer a more technocratic approach? Why?

Recommended Films

Giving Birth, Unveiling Birth: The Wisdom, Science, and Heart: conceived and created by Suzanne Berthiaume and Suzanne Arms and produced by Amy Guilliland. Shows fully natural birth and bonding under a midwifery model of care. To order, go to SuzanneArmsPresents.com. Running time: 36 minutes plus 60 minutes bonus viewing material.

Newborn Exam for the Student Midwife: produced by Birth Joy Consultants. Shows the basic skills needed for student midwives to assess the newborn baby. 5 hours long. Available at midwiferytoday.com

Birth Emergency Skills Training: produced by Bonnie U. Gruenbert. Shows the interface between the world of midwifery and the world of medicine, available at midwiferytoday.com

Microbirth: a 60-minute documentary exploring the latest scientific research into the microscopic events that occur during childbirth and strongly affect the baby's "microbiome"—the bacteria that colonize its gut and body as it travels through the birth canal and that can have life-long consequences for the baby's health and potentially impact the future of mankind. Winner of the Grand Prix award at the Life Sciences Film Festival in 2014, the film features leading world-experts including Martin Blazer and Maria Gloria Dominguez Bello. Available at https://vimeo.com/ondemand/microbirthfilm

12

Renegade Midwives
Assets or Liabilities?

with Christine Barbara Johnson

> *Scratch any midwife, and you'll find a renegade.*
> — Richard Jennings CNM, Clinical Director of Midwifery, Yale University

Renegade Midwives' Stories

Story 1: A Post-Dates Birth

A homebirth midwife in Massachusetts received a knock on the door in the middle of the afternoon. She opened it to find a woman she had never met before in early labor and in tears. She had planned to give birth in a birth center run by nurse-midwives, but was refused at the last minute because she was two days past the 42-week deadline, after which the nurse-midwives, by state regulation, are obliged to refer her to obstetric and hospital care for her birth. They officially transferred her to the hospital, but instead she drove to the home of this particular midwife because she was known as a "renegade" who would sometimes ignore protocols in the interests of serving the woman. The homebirth midwife conducted an exam, concluded that the baby and mother were fine, and proceeded to assist the mother to give birth in the midwife's home, with an excellent outcome.

This chapter was first published in *Mainstreaming Midwives: The Politics of Change,* eds. Robbie Davis-Floyd and Christine Barbara Johnson. New York: Routledge, pp. 447–468. This revised and updated version is published here with permission.

Story 2: Illegal Attendance at Homebirths

A nurse-midwife in California attended homebirths in her community for many years; in so doing, she was practicing outside the protocols of nurse-midwifery in the state because she had no official physician backup. She was honored and revered by the women she served and by many California midwives, who saw her as a courageous, skilled, and compassionate midwifery pioneer. One day she had a mother with an obstetric emergency and transported her to the hospital appropriately. Both mother and baby were fine, and the birth turned out well. But the hospital and the state prosecuted the nurse-midwife for illegally attending births at home, and she was not supported by the local or national nurse-midwifery associations, some of whose members had long considered her a renegade. She was forced to stop practicing. A few years later, she died both of cancer and of grief. Her name was June Whitson.

Story 3: A Baby Death after Transport

A young nurse-midwife in Washington State opened a highly successful homebirth practice. One day she made an appropriate transport for an emergency; the baby died in the hospital. She experienced immediate ostracism from the hospital-based nurse-midwives but was supported during the trial by the homebirth midwives of her community. Her license was revoked; nevertheless, she continued to practice as a "renegade."

Story 4: Too Many Births Too Far Out of Protocol

A highly experienced direct-entry midwife in Southern California, who had been in practice for 20 years and had trained many of the younger homebirth midwives in her community, was attending over ten homebirths a month, a huge stress factor in itself; when the births happened back to back, she was going without sleep for days at a time. And she was taking on cases that even the midwives she had trained as apprentices felt were "way too far out of protocol." (At the time, all of the midwives in California were practicing illegally, but they had formed a state association and created their own set of protocols and their own peer review process.) Several peer reviews of this particular midwife's practice resulted in censure, but she paid no heed. Then she was approached by a woman with two previous cesareans who asked her to attend a VBAC (vaginal birth after cesarean) at home. The midwife went to the library and did some research, and warned the couple that there was an approximately 3% risk that the woman's uterus would rupture. The couple declared their willingness to accept this risk. In early labor, the woman's uterus did rupture. The midwife transported her immediately, but the baby died. On this and several other counts, the midwife was prosecuted by the state. None of the midwives in her community would testify on her behalf. Even though they loved her and many of them had been trained by her, they were angry that she had not heeded their warnings, which they had repeated over four years. She was convicted and spent four years in prison. The letters she sent from prison to her supporters and friends were published in newsletters and widely distributed. They revealed her enormous courage, strength of will, compassion for other prisoners, and her openness to learning and growing as much as she could from the often devastating things she experienced during her imprisonment (from leg chains to extreme verbal abuse). Finally she was released, returned home to her family and friends, and to our knowledge has not gone back to attending births.

Story 5: A Footling Breech and a Failed Resuscitation

A couple in Illinois, deeply committed to homebirth, received their prenatal care from a direct-entry midwife. Toward the end of the pregnancy, the midwife diagnosed the position of the baby as footling breech, meaning that feet were coming first rather than the head. This condition can be dangerous, however breeches sometimes change their position from footling to frank (bottom presenting) at the end of pregnancy or during the delivery. Frank breeches generally carry lower risk than footling breeches. The client insisted that she did not want to go to the hospital or have a cesarean. About 3% of babies are in a breech position at term, and most medical practitioners consider breech a significant risk factor. In states where they are licensed and regulated, homebirth midwives are usually prohibited from attending any kind of breech birth. In this particular state, homebirth direct-entry midwives are illegal anyway, and so their practice is entirely unregulated and autonomous. This midwife felt that she had the skills to handle a footling breech birth, so she agreed to go ahead and attend the birth at home. She successfully delivered the baby's feet, but there was a significant delay between the emergence of the feet and the emergence of the baby's head. The baby did not breathe upon birth. The midwife attempted resuscitation, which failed. The baby died. The couple remained supportive of the midwife, but she was put on trial by the state. At the time she attended this birth, she was already on probation because the state had discovered that she was attending homebirths illegally. Her attendance at this birth constituted a tremendous risk for her, for the parents, for the baby, and for the efforts of the direct-entry midwives in her state who were pushing for legalization in that state. The birth had been filmed, and the video was viewed by some midwives for legal purposes.

Some months later, Robbie attended a meeting of highly experienced midwives involved in the national midwifery movement. This case came up for discussion. Some of these midwives had seen the video and had concluded that the midwife was guilty of irresponsible practice: (1) She should not have taken on the birth in the first place, given the risks of footling breech and her own already probationary status. (2) She waited too long between the delivery of the feet and the head, when she could and should have intervened to make the birth happen faster. (3) They believed her neonatal resuscitation skills were not up to par, as her efforts as recorded on the video seemed to them to be inadequate and inappropriate. There was general agreement at the meeting that her care had been substandard and that not only had she been responsible for the baby's death but also had enormously impeded the legalization efforts of the midwives in her state. The discussion did not focus on the issue of footling breech in itself.

So, ever the anthropologist, Robbie asked these experienced midwives how many of them had attended footling breech births at home. About half of the hands in the room went up. Then she asked, "Have any of you experienced a bad outcome as a result?" No one had. Her next question was, "How many of you would do it again?" and the same midwives raised their hands. For them, the issue was not attendance at a footling breech per se, but the particular instances of this particular birth: a challenging delivery position, known about in advance, and attended by a midwife already on probation in a state currently in the midst of legislative procedures involving midwifery in general. "Too many tensions and risks all in one basket," one midwife noted.

A bit shocked that footling breech, considered an immediate indicator for a cesarean in the hospital, was not per se the issue for this group of experienced midwives, Robbie was forced once again to realize how much these midwives' philosophy, practice, and experience differed from American norms, how deeply reliant and confident they were in their hands-on skills, and how willing some of them were to take what any obstetrician, most nurse-midwives, and about half of all homebirth midwives would consider a totally unacceptable risk. Further questioning revealed that the midwives who had raised their hands both times had attended, over 20 to 30 years of practice, dozens and sometimes over 100 breech births, footling and otherwise, and considered themselves the preservers and guardians of this skill, which, they pointed out, the vast majority of American obstetricians do not have because they are taught simply to do a cesarean for any type of breech. (See Daviss and Biskits forthcoming for a description of recent international efforts to "bring back breech.")

Stories from Women Who Chose to Give Birth with Renegade Midwives

Mary's Story

Mary's first birth by cesarean section had taken place years before, but she still lived with the deep psychological scarring that she sustained as a result of this experience. In fact for close to a year after the birth she was deeply depressed and unable to function, a recluse in her home. Before this birth, she had been vibrant, active, and professionally and personally successful. Eventually, she began to sense that she had mostly put this traumatic birth experience behind her and was feeling more and more like her old self. Then Mary discovered that she was pregnant again. She did not feel ready to handle a hospital birth, as she was still in the final stages of completing her recovery from the first one. A number of midwives she approached declined to attend her, due to her VBAC status (VBAC attendance was outside of their state-regulated protocols). Finally, she located a willing "renegade" midwife in her state. This homebirth was transformative and nurturing for her; afterward, she felt that all the scars from the first birth had healed. She emerged from this second birth with an enthusiasm and strength that she "had never experienced before."

Celene's Story

Celene was pregnant and planning to give birth at home when she and her midwife determined that she was carrying twins, which made her ineligible for a homebirth, since her midwife was unwilling to jeopardize her professional standing in the community by attending what most would consider a risky birth. Celene was beside herself; she was terrified of hospitals and believed that if she were to be forced into this option, she would have a very difficult birth and an even more difficult time recovering. She called midwife after midwife, but they all said the same thing: "It's not worth the risk."

Finally, some midwives referred Celene to a midwife from another state willing to fly in to attend her. Ultimately, two midwives came. The birth of the first twin went smoothly but the second one was stuck. They transported; the second baby was delivered by cesarean and emerged healthy and well. The hospital staff was aghast and gave Celene many severe looks and lectures. But Celene herself was ecstatic that she had been able to labor and birth the first baby at home. She was sorry about the hospital birth but was grateful that she had her midwife there to support her through it. She felt very empowered and was most grateful that this alternative was available to her, certain that had she been forced to start out in the hospital she would have been discounted and disempowered in ways that would have been difficult to recover from and would adversely affect her parenting.

Cynthia's Story

Cynthia attempted to have her first baby at home, but transport was required and she ended up with a CS. She was so emotionally traumatized by this birth that no midwife in her state would agree to attend her second birth at home. Cynthia was a highly respected professional with a demanding career, a commitment to social activism, and an enthusiastic attitude for life, but the scars from her first birth ran deep. This emotional baggage, coupled with a VBAC at home, seemed "just too risky" for the midwives in her state. Some were willing to assist at the birth but refused to be the primary midwife in charge. They found instead another midwife from out of state who would fly in and attend her; the result was a successful homebirth. This birth was deeply healing, and in the aftermath Cynthia noted that her parenting improved immensely as well as her overall emotional well-being. She stressed that if had been forced to enter the hospital, she was sure she would not have been able to achieve this state of wellness.

Lauren's Story

Lauren was diagnosed with severe schizophrenia and depression. She believed that part of the cause lay in the highly medicalized hospital birth she had endured a few years earlier. She was pregnant again and desired a homebirth because she believed it would help her to heal. No homebirth midwife in her state would take her on because they all considered her "crazy" and therefore high risk. Finally she found a doula in another state who was willing to fly to her city to assist her, and the doula found a midwife who was also willing to fly in from another state. She successfully gave birth at home to twins, and her psychological health improved enormously. She became a birth activist, organizing various conferences and meetings in her community, and advocating for midwives to expand their definitions of "normal."

Teresa's Story (told by Robbie)

After I completed a talk on humanistic childbirth at a university in Michigan, I was approached by a student/mother with tears behind her eyes, who spoke of the trauma of the cesarean birth of her first baby. Pregnant with her second child, this woman deeply desired a homebirth, but had been told that no midwife in Michigan would attend a VBAC at home. Certain this was not the case, I made a few calls to various homebirth midwives and was assured that some of them would attend home VBACs. I gave their phone numbers to the mother, who went away radiant with the hope that her dreams of an empowering birth might yet be achieved. I was close to tears myself: my certainty had been reaffirmed that these professional Michigan midwives, although prohibited by protocols from attending VBACs at home, would not deny this option to this mother who so deeply desired it and had nowhere else to turn.

Normalizing Uniqueness: How Far Should It Go?

I think being a midwife makes you a renegade, in our society, since such a small percentage of the population is born outside of the hospital with midwives. That itself does, and I also think as a midwife, standing up for women's rights again makes you a renegade. But I also think that you are not a renegade in that what you are doing is completely normal and natural and going with human nature. Maybe being a renegade is going against society's structure, but you are still going with human nature.

— CPM in Austin, Texas

All midwives can be considered renegades to some extent. As previously noted, just to be a midwife, any kind of midwife in the US, is to constitute a radical critique of the dominant obstetric system, in which physicians attend around 88% of all births. But there is a special category of "renegade midwives," illustrated in the above stories, which we specifically addressed in this chapter because they are very important to American midwifery in both positive and negative ways. The term "renegade midwife" is used by midwives themselves. Sometimes they use it pejoratively, as a criticism of the midwife who practices, in the majority peer opinion, too far outside the protocols of her peer group or state regulations. Some midwives proudly apply the term to themselves, using it to acknowledge the fact that they often practice outside of protocols and to emphasize that their doing so constitutes a very conscious critique of those protocols, which they consider too restrictive to fully reflect the full range of what they consider their appropriate scope of practice.

Renegade Midwives as Both Assets and Liabilities

The midwife who calls herself "renegade" believes that other midwives adhere too strictly to protocols and standards of care and do not go far enough to serve the birthing woman. She believes that a woman's desire to give birth naturally, even in conditions that others would regard as prohibitive to homebirth, should be primary and that the midwife should serve the client and not the regulatory system. Thus "renegades" are often highly skilled and experienced midwives who feel confident in their abilities to handle such conditions as VBACs, breeches, and sometimes even twins at home. Unless there are signs of fetal distress or insufficient amniotic fluid, they are often willing to let a woman go two or three weeks past her due date and still attend her at home (most protocols state that women should be induced after 42 weeks). As the above stories illustrate, they will take on women whom other midwives might screen out because of the mother's psychological characteristics or even for complications as extreme as footling breech. These midwives believe they are placing the desires of the client first, and that doing so is appropriate. When there is a condition that they truly believe they cannot handle, even renegade midwives refer the woman to a physician in advance or transport her if the condition develops during labor. What makes them "renegade" is usually not ignorance, arrogance, or lack of training, but rather the fact that they will take on women whom most other midwives would reject for homebirth, or assist only as one member of a larger team in a planned hospital birth. Thus such midwives constitute both a liability to other midwives, and an asset.

The asset has to do with the services renegade midwives provide. Licensed professional midwives who are not renegade, who do practice within agreed-upon peer protocols or established state regulations, often feel conflicted when confronted with a woman who deeply desires an out-of-hospital birth but should, according to protocols, be screened out in advance. As we have seen in earlier chapters, homebirth midwifery itself began as a renegade social movement in which midwives and mothers together agreed to flout obstetric norms and to jointly take responsibility for conducting births in radically alternative ways. Many homebirth midwives are still loyal to the flavor and force of this movement and feel a strong pull to place the interests of the client first, as "lay" midwives in the beginning tended almost always to do. But those were the days (the early 1970s) when lay midwives had little experience with birth complications and risk management. Since homebirths attended by midwives turn out fine for the vast majority of the women who plan them, it took years for some of the early homebirth midwifery pioneers to encounter enough complications and dangers to begin to take more seriously their responsibility to acknowledge and deal with risk. Herein lies the liability: in spite of the fact that babies die in the hospital, too, because homebirth is so culturally marginal, all it takes is one death at home that would most likely have been prevented in the hospital, or one "botched transport," to end years of goodwill.

Professional vs. "Plain" Midwives

As the battle for legality and licensure in various states got underway during the 1970s and 1980s, the homebirth midwifery movement in some states became deeply divided over the issue of the renegade midwife. On one side were the professionalizing midwives who were willing to accept regulations (such as prohibition from attending VBACs, breeches, and twins) in return for legality and the benefits of not having to live in terror of arrest or prosecution and of opportunities to serve many more women. On the other side were midwives who refused to accept any restrictions on their practice and preferred to remain illegal or a-legal, completely outside the system, because as long as they were not regulated they were fully autonomous and able to practice in any way they pleased. In Pennsylvania and a few other states, such midwives refer to themselves as "plain midwives." This rhetoric constitutes a deep critique of labels such as "direct-entry midwife" or "nurse-midwife," which these plain midwives perceive as restrictive. For the sake of clarity, in this chapter we use the term "plain midwife" to refer to any midwives who reject legalization, licensure, and the usually resultant restrictions on practice.

In *The Rhetoric of Midwifery: Gender, Knowledge, and Power* (2000), Mary Lay thoroughly described this divide as it occurred in Minnesota, where the professionalizing midwives developed a rhetorical strategy that stressed accountability, protocols, and regulation, and the plain midwives stuck to their insistence on keeping the woman central and not being restricted in any way. This rhetorical strategy on the part of the professionalizing midwives impressed state legislators and won legalization for the professionally oriented midwives; at the same time, it clarified and magnified the gap between the "professionals" and the "plains."

Some plain midwives are so because of religious reasons. There are hundreds of Christian midwives practicing in various states completely outside the law and the health care system; their belief system revolves around the concept that "God is the real midwife," that God's will should and will prevail, and that any complications that develop during birth can be resolved through prayer and openness to the Holy Spirit, should that be God's will. Christine has interviewed a number of these midwives who are deeply committed and can recount story after story about the practical results of relying on divine intervention at birth. (See Klassen 2001 for a cogent analysis of the various types of spirituality that influence the choices of homebirthers and the midwives who serve them.)

Many professional midwives do believe in God and do pray during birth, but tend to take the more pragmatic approach that "God helps those who help themselves." Thus they transport to the hospital when they believe they do not possess the necessary knowledge and skills to handle complications at home. Such homebirth midwives are the ones who worked hard to help create CPM certification and to lobby for legalization and licensure of the CPM (achieving it in 30 states to date—see Chapter 6). Their nurse-midwifery counterparts worked hard in earlier decades to achieve the same thing for the CNM.

It would be easy to say that the plain midwives are the renegades while the professionally oriented midwives, most of whom are CNMs or CPMs, are not. But reality is not that simple. As we noted above, renegade midwives are often highly skilled and experienced. Many of them practice outside of protocols because they believe that they can handle the complications the protocols would instruct them to avoid better than OBs. They observe that such protocols are often set by state legislators or regulatory boards who understand little about the knowledge base of homebirth midwives. And they know from statistics and from long experience that their services are the only ways women with complications defined obstetrically as "high risk" can avoid a cesarean. (As previously noted, most obstetricians will automatically do a cesarean for breeches or twins, and often for VBACs; many younger OBs have little or *no* experience with vaginal delivery in such situations.)

Many such midwives achieve CNM or CPM certification and state licensure; in the process, they fight for regulations that will allow them the broadest possible scope of practice. But if they lose the regulatory battle and are forced to accept narrow protocols, they deal with this failure by occasionally flouting the state regulations that they resisted in the first place. In this way, they distinguish themselves from midwives who stick carefully to such regulations. Such midwives place a higher priority on protecting the profession of midwifery in their state than on putting the desires of the client first. They believe that protecting midwifery is essential to keeping out-of-hospital birth as an option, at least for women who do meet protocols, and that endangering it by taking obvious risks is irresponsible. They are often angry and resentful of renegade midwives who threaten the status of professional homebirth midwifery.

But these same professionally oriented midwives are simultaneously often grateful for the existence of the renegades (who are often also licensed or certified), because when a professionally oriented midwife is confronted with a potential client whom she has to screen out, she does not have to let the woman down utterly by telling her that her only option is the hospital birth she dreads. Instead, she can refer the mother to the renegade midwife who lives down the road or perhaps many miles away, who is more likely to go out on a limb to honor the mother's wishes.

Hospital Midwives as Renegades

It is important to note that even hospital midwives have a whole myriad of strategies for subverting the system: they fudge charts to keep the laboring woman off of Friedman's curve and thus give her more time, let her family members slip in food and drink even when the hospital prohibits it, avoid the monitor when they can, break amniotic sacs covertly (and/or stretch the cervix) with their fingers to speed labor when the threat of pitocin looms, and sometimes even lock the door to the labor room to give the couple the privacy they need to make love and thus strengthen labor through nipple and clitoral stimulation (which naturally increases oxytocin levels) instead of through a pitocin drip. As the quote from Richard Jennings with which we began this chapter was intended to express, many hospital-based midwives are *closet renegades*; they just do subtly what homebirth midwives do much more overtly. As a CNM in Austin, Texas recently noted:

> The 25% [of me that is] renegade would get people out of bed and the stuff like "If you want to bring snacks to eat during labor, just don't tell me about it"; that kind of thing. One of the famous, very famous, renegade things is the very common hospital midwifery practice of doing a cervical exam saying that the woman is 8cm when in fact she is 10cm, because you don't want the doctors to start looking at the clocks saying, "How long has she been pushing?" So I have done a lot of that, and I'm not necessarily proud of that, but in the circumstance where you know that the doctors are going to be "How long? How long again?" and especially when there are guidelines or protocols that say "No, if it's a primip [a woman delivering for the first time], after two hours you have to consult; if it's a multip [a woman who has previously given birth] you have to consult after an hour"—Hello, an hour?! So, those consultations often meant that the doctor was then going to be taking over the situation and you just didn't want that, so you told a little white lie, but I think we all do that, because we have to. It shouldn't be necessary and maybe someday soon it won't be but it certainly has been. (quoted in Carleto 2016:24)

For this CNM, being a renegade means, "I guess being willing to step outside the comfort and [regulatory] safety of the guidelines and do what you think is right and evidence-based."

As previously emphasized in this anthology, the great myth about themselves that nurse-midwives have created is that they only attend low-risk, normal births, an area in which they are the experts. In truth, from the beginning of their entry into hospitals in the mid-1950s, CNMs have been attending the births of poor, inner-city, malnourished and therefore high-risk women. And they have been doing an excellent job. But their attendance of these high-risk women is in contrast to the public image of themselves they have sought to create, an image they hope makes them appear to be less of a threat to physicians and safe practitioners for normal women. Their frequent attendance of low-income, relatively high-risk women, in tandem with the many subversive strategies they develop in-hospital, reinforces our point that CNMs are often closet renegades, flouting the system while appearing to comply with it, and expanding the choices for their clients while appearing to normatively conform to medical protocols and state regulations.

Robbie's Story and the Renegade Dilemma

We acknowledge that Robbie's take on homebirth renegade midwives is necessarily influenced by her own experience of a home VBAC at 43 weeks with a three-day labor, a ten-pound baby, a short period of fetal heart rate decelerations during pushing, meconium staining, and a brief shoulder dystocia. This birth would not have been allowed to take place naturally in any hospital in the US. In her written birth stories (Davis-Floyd n.d.), Robbie notes that the pain was stunning but the accomplishment was far more so. Her deep intuition that her choice was right and that the baby was safe all the way through seemed to Robbie and to her midwives to be far more meaningful than "risk factors." Robbie's experience of pushing through the pain to give birth with her own psychological strength and physical power was utterly life-transforming. Had she not been able to find two renegade midwives in Austin, Texas, in 1984 who were willing to attend her VBAC at home even though their state regulations made that illegal, she could not have experienced the empowerment of that birth, but would have had to relive the devastating disempowerment of her previous cesarean (and most certainly would not be writing this book today).

Is the price of the risk worth the value of the reward? Robbie in effect is in the same dilemma as the midwives she studies. She supports and has actively aided the development and implementation of national certification for direct-entry midwives and national recognition for direct-entry schools, which perforce has entailed some degree of standardization of skills and care.

At the same time, she is also keenly aware (through her own experience and her interviews with over 140 women about their birth experiences) of the importance of "normalizing uniqueness" though individualized, intuitive care—the kind of care that sometimes can only fully be offered by those midwives who proudly claim the term "renegade."

Renegade midwives acknowledge that their existence and praxis threaten the tenuous toehold in the technocracy that their professional compatriots, and often they themselves, are working so hard to establish. They are also aware that their existence and praxis help to keep the spirit of the homebirth midwifery movement alive and the full range of options open to American women. Here again the differences between plain and professional midwives come into play. Plain midwives make it clear that they prefer to practice completely outside the law; they desire neither national certification nor state licensure. Thus plain midwives who are renegades can at least be rhetorically excluded (Lay 2000) from the professionally oriented CNMs, CPMs, and LMs, who have worked for the creation of, and themselves obtained, national certification and/or state licensure. But when one of these professional midwives practices as a renegade, she cannot be rhetorically excluded or differentiated from licensed or certified midwives who do (usually) stick to protocols (or at least try to appear to) in the interests of protecting their profession. Thus the overtly renegade professional midwife constitutes the greater liability. And yet the fact that she has achieved licensure or certification at least demonstrates she has obtained the requisite knowledge, skills, and experience to practice safely, and presumably to trust her own judgment, and thus is perhaps more qualified to be a renegade that the plain midwife who has not been tested in any way.

Many midwives have noted that "the CPMs remind the CNMs about the dangers of overmedicalizing, and renegades remind both groups of the same danger." One very experienced CPM reaffirmed this perception: "I'm glad there are people out there pushing the envelope—if they didn't, people like us would be on the edge." Another longtime midwife, who had been somewhat of a renegade in her early years, responded, "I don't want to go out on a limb anymore. My heart can only handle so much stress. You end up on the edge often enough without knowingly, premeditatedly going there."

Results and Consequences: The Renegade Spectrum

Our awareness of the existence of various renegade CPMs in the US is the reason we waited with baited breath for the outcomes of the first CPM statistical outcome study (Johnson and Daviss 2005). When those data became available, our fears were allayed. To recap from Chapter 6, in that first study, 88 out of every 100 women who planned a homebirth with a CPM did give birth at home successfully and safely. CPMs exhibited their caution by transporting 12 out of every 100 women to the hospital during labor; most of these transfers were preventative, and only 3.6% of the time were they considered urgent, emergency situations. The cesarean rate for CPM clients was 3.7%, and the perinatal mortality rate was 2/1,000—equivalent to what it is for CNMs attending out-of-hospital births and for physicians attending low-risk women in hospitals (in other words, exactly what it should be given optimal care).

The outcome data submitted by 350 CPMs for this first study, which was required by NARM to include *all* the births they had attended for the year 2000, were confirmed by the follow-up (Cheyney et al. 2014b) study on CPM-attended births from 2004 to 2009. Both studies included data from a number of known "renegades." And we are grateful that their willingness to practice outside of regulations and protocols does not statistically generate negative data but rather reinforces the point that CPMs attending homebirths have outcomes as good as, and often better than, other kinds of birth practitioners. But homebirth is still such a marginal practice that *one* bad outcome from a CPM-attended birth still has the detrimental effect of reinforcing cultural stereotypes and making all midwives of all types appear incompetent to the general public. Such stereotypes constitute part of the reason why these midwives, after decades of practice, still attend less than 2% of US births. Combating such stereotypes through an emphasis on professionalization and professionalism has been a dominant ethos of nurse-midwifery from its inception; such an emphasis only became important to the former lay midwives in the 1990s. Now they, too, wish to change the cultural image of midwifery, but at what price? This is a question many nurse-midwives also pose to themselves.

And so we repeat at the end of this section the thought with which we began this chapter: *All midwives to some extent are renegades*—most especially those who truly practice the MMOC. Yet there is a spectrum of "renegadeness," and those at the further end of it threaten the cultural acceptance of professional midwifery. Every midwife must decide for herself to what extent and under which circumstances she will adhere to regulations and protocols, and to what extent and under which circumstances she will flout those protocols in what she believes are the best interests not of her profession but of her individual client.

The Role of the Stranger

The stranger does not share the local assumption and so becomes essentially the one who has to place in question nearly everything that seems to be unquestionable to members of the approached group.

— Zygmunt Baumann

Renegade midwives are to professional midwives what midwifery is to biomedicine—challengers to everything that appears evident and beyond question. This is the role the "stranger" has played from time immemorial. Without exception all societies produce strangers, and most subgroups in society produce their own unique set of strangers. Knowledge systems appear to be self-evident as long as no one from a contesting ideology is around to ask questions "about their grounds and reasons, point out the discrepancies, lay bare their arbitrariness. This is why the arrival of the stranger [can have] the impact of an earthquake. The stranger shatters the rock on which the security of daily life rests" (Bauman 1997:9). Encounters with the stranger stir things up and produce uncertainty, anxiety, and questions about boundaries. One of the most exasperating things about this state of affairs is the difficulty in creating definitive guidelines for action when "the stranger exhales uncertainty where certainty and clarity should have ruled" (Bauman 1997:18).

In confrontations with the stranger, one of two options is usually chosen: assimilation or banishment. In the case of the renegade, no matter how many are assimilated, there will always be more who refuse and resist this assimilation. Is banishment a viable alternative? With banishment, the lines of communication are broken and there is precious little chance to develop shared meanings leading to constructive dialogue and transformation (as Robbie points out in Chapter 10 on home-to-hospital transport). The third and most radical alternative is remaining in dialogue and keeping the channels of communication open. Nothing meaningful can be accomplished if trust is not established. Midwives have the opportunity to chart new territory in today's world, not only with respect to their systems of knowledge but also with respect to innovating new typologies for collegial conduct. They have the chance to pioneer ground-breaking forms for staying in discourse despite ferocious disagreements with one another. This effort will take tremendous commitment time and energy, but what is the alternative? Keeping these lines of communication open can only add to the rich heritage and contemporary viability of midwifery.

We see three possible paths for relations between protocol-oriented and renegade midwives. The first path involves co-option, which is akin to assimilation; the second is remaining isolated from one another, with minimal contact and in which hostility and competition prevail. The third alternative calls for a convergence of views in which the best of both are combined into a unified whole. While renegade midwives and protocol-oriented midwives will continue to reside in separate domains, a great deal more convergence between the two ideologies (protecting the profession vs. putting the woman's desires first) can be accomplished. This convergence can only add to the vitality of the midwifery knowledge system. The renegade's very existence can contribute to clarifying the boundaries and parameters of the midwifery knowledge system. As mentioned earlier, homebirth midwifery itself arose as a renegade movement that captured society's attention with regard to the need for reforms in technomedical birth practices. At her best, the renegade can serve as check and balance that professional homebirth midwives do not stray too far from the heart of their commitment to women.

During one of Christine's conversations with a CNM, the nurse-midwife explained that she remained in continuous contact with a renegade midwife to keep herself from straying too far from her midwifery origins. Plain and renegade midwives can sharpen the edges of midwifery social change by imploring careful consideration of the compromises that are made in the bid for cultural legitimacy. In addition, renegade midwives serve as keepers of alternative knowledge that thereby remains available to both protocol-oriented midwives and their clients to provide alternatives that formal regulations deem unacceptable. Given enough evidence over time, VBAC, breech, and perhaps even twin births may become acknowledged as variants of "normal" and thereby become viable candidates for both homebirth and natural births in the hospital.

The potential for radical change in institutional views about midwifery with respect to issues such as breech birth became evident in a California court case in which a renegade licensed midwife (LM) was sued by the Medical Board for attending a vaginal delivery of a breech baby at home. The court brief noted that "the medical 'standard of care' for breech birth is to do a cesarean section in most cases"; however, the court also emphasized that "*the medical model's applicability to midwifery is inappropriate and summarily dismissed*" (Department of Consumer Affairs, State of California 1999:3,11). The tribunal hearing the case allotted the midwifery model the same level of authority as the medical model:

> Midwives employ a midwifery model of practice distinct from the medical model of practice. . . . Unlike physicians, physician's assistants, physician assistant midwives, registered nurses, or certified nurse midwives who practice within the context of a medical model, licensed midwives practice within the context of a midwifery model. Complainant contends that the medical model should function to define the scope of a midwife's practice. This issue arises because the ACT provides that a licensed midwife is authorized by his or her license, "under the supervision of a licensed physician and surgeon to attend cases of normal childbirth." . . . "Normal" within the context of the medical model specifically excludes, inter alia, breech presentation because of the risk for complications. *Within the context of the midwifery model, breech presentation is merely a variant of normal childbirth.* (Department of Consumer Affairs, State of California 1999:11, 14, [italics added])

This case is noteworthy and instructive in that it dramatically illustrates how important renegade midwifery can be for mainstreaming midwifery practices often sacrificed in the name of state prohibition.

At her worst, the renegade midwife can go too far with resultant bad outcomes either at home or in a hospital transport. These incidents do considerable damage by spoiling the reputation of midwifery and requiring years to reestablish its legitimacy in a given community. In a tit-for-tat way, protocol-oriented midwives can provide a check and balance for renegade midwives by reminding them of the larger context in which they practice. Much as the renegade would prefer the luxury of only considering the needs of the individual woman she is attending, the renegade acts in a larger context and is responsible for the reputation of the profession at large, whether or not she chooses to acknowledge it. Ongoing dialogue with professionally oriented midwifery groups will give the renegade midwife a stronger sense of orientation.

Living into the Answers

Trust is not something "out there" but rather a social process that is constructed for and by people and a matter of the choices and actions of individuated subjects.
— Christine Garsten

At the 2001 MANA conference in Albuquerque, New Mexico, Robbie was asked to moderate a panel entitled "When Clients' Wishes Conflict with Midwifery Protocols." The room was packed—obviously this was an issue of great import to MANA members, because, as we mentioned above, it places the social movement of midwifery in direct conflict with the professionalization process (see Daviss 2006), leaving many midwives in a quandary that they are often unable to philosophically resolve. If they refuse care in "high-risk" cases, they are letting the woman down. If they grant care, they are endangering the profession they have worked so hard to build. Quite a dilemma!

On the panel was a mother who had had two previous cesareans and wanted a home VBAC, her husband (who had fully supported her choice), the midwife whom she had originally approached but who had refused to take her case because it was out of protocol, and an obstetrician who is very supportive of homebirth. The mother described how devastated she was when the professional midwife refused to take her on for a homebirth, and how relieved she was when that same midwife provided her with the option of going to an illegal, unlicensed (and therefore unregulated) midwife who lived over 100 miles away, in an adjacent state. The woman and her husband went to talk with that renegade midwife, who agreed to take them on. The result was a "fantastic" birth experience for the couple, who had such faith in their choice that they gave birth in a remote desert location.

The CPM who had originally refused homebirth care keenly felt her responsibility to her profession and did not regret making this responsibility her priority. At the same time, she was thrilled that the renegade midwife had been able to provide the birth experience the woman had so deeply desired. (The alternative would have been giving birth completely unassisted. Some women do choose this option [Moran 1981; Shanley 1994], but since our focus is on midwives, we do not address such choices here.) Again paradoxically, the gratitude of the professional midwife to the renegade "plain midwife" was accompanied by the fear that the renegade would eventually have bad outcomes that would then endanger the status of midwives everywhere.

The obstetrician on the panel at first spoke about the importance of "risk management" and of appropriate referral. She noted with regret that this would mean that women like the mother on the panel might not be able to have the birth experience she and her husband longed for, but felt that this was the price that had to be paid for assuring safety in birth. The obstetrician was challenged by several homebirth midwives in the audience and, toward the end of the discussion, did a complete about-face. In essence, she acknowledged her fears as inappropriate and reflective of her socialization as an obstetrician; she apologized to all the midwives present for forgetting that "trusting birth and a woman's ability to give birth is the most important ingredient in a successful birth outcome."

Near the end of the scheduled time for this session, Robbie as moderator noticed that the audience was about to be left with an irreconcilable conceptual split between sticking to protocols for the sake of the profession and flouting them for the sake of the woman. Seeking to provide the midwives on the panel and in the audience with another way of thinking about this opposition, Robbie attempted to provide a deeper, less oppositional approach. She reminded the audience of her study of midwives' use of intuition during prenatal care and birth (Chapter 7, this volume), noting that midwives themselves had told her that one of their greatest skills is listening to the inner voice that can inform them which woman is truly at risk and which woman can actually achieve the homebirth she wants. She spoke of the importance of individualization, as opposed to standardization, of care, reminding them that whereas obstetricians are taught to standardize, midwives ideally are taught to individualize, to *normalize uniqueness*.

As an anthropologist who had studied midwives for a decade at that time, Robbie was able to speak a truth that every midwife in the audience recognized. Almost all homebirth midwives, and many nurse-midwives, will respond to the individual beliefs, desires, and circumstances of an individual woman in individual ways. The standards and protocols of midwifery care and of "evidence-based medicine" are there in front of them. But for midwives, standards are only "standard" (in other words, representative and expressive of the hegemonic obstetrical system), and research that compares two groups within a hospital can be irrelevant and often actually misleading and detrimental to homebirth practice.

For example, the infamous "Friedman's curve," which has for many years set the standard for how long women should be allowed to labor, was based not on normal, natural childbirths but on women drugged on scopolamine and whose labors were often augmented with pitocin. In spite of this extreme deficiency, obstetricians still utilize Friedman's curve to justify radical interventions to speed up labor (from pitocin to episiotomy to forceps to cesareans). Midwives' experiences of homebirths teach them that Friedman's curve is not a reliable standard but rather a detriment to successful homebirth outcomes, because labors with no medical intervention can vary in time from a few hours to a few days without danger to mother or baby. I cannot stress enough that the latent phase of labor can take a very long time, while the active phase (defined as starting at 6 cm) usually goes much faster. If there must be a clock, it should not start ticking till 6 cm; Friedman's curve does not recognize the difference between latent and active labor in the ways that MMOC practitioners do. A recent study (Dekker 2017) showed that a hospital in Italy that stopped using Friedman's curve dropped their low-risk Cesarean rate fairly quickly, from 22.2% to 10.3%.

Thus every midwife who practices out of hospital has good reasons to ignore, even to scorn, obstetric standards that many midwives who practice in hospital are obliged to heed. In some cases, their scorn results from the inadequacy or misuse of medical "evidence." In other cases, such as VBACs, breeches, and twins, homebirth midwives do acknowledge that the evidence does indicate increased risk. But they also note the risks are small and hospital birth entails its own set of risks, which include unnecessary cesareans and iatrogenic damage to mother and/or child.

Thus, homebirth midwives who look carefully at the data come to understand that negative outcomes can occur as much or more from inappropriate obstetric interventions as from deficiencies of nature. When confronted with specific women with specific complications, their only viable option becomes individualization of care. Sometimes a homebirth midwife's intuition tells her that *in this particular case, this particular woman needs and can achieve natural birth* even if her condition does not meet protocols, and consequently the midwife will accept the risk of attending the woman at home. Conversely, when everything seems normal and totally within protocol, that same homebirth midwife may transport simply because she intuits that something is wrong (see for potent examples Roncalli 1997). In other words, midwifery care under the midwifery model of care is individualized, not standardized, and some of that individualization comes from the deep reliance many midwives come to develop on their inner knowing and that of their clients.

As Robbie spoke, every midwife in the audience nodded her head; some were sobbing. What we noted at the beginning of this chapter was displayed in that moment—the spirit of the renegade lives in every midwife, whether she acts on it or not. And in fact, every midwife either Robbie or Christine has ever interviewed (over 400 practicing midwives of all types) admits or is overtly proud of the fact that she will sometimes practice out of protocols in any setting in order to protect a woman from unnecessary intervention.

Battles between professionally oriented and renegade midwives over the proper domain of midwifery invoke larger philosophical issues of choice and responsibility. Creativity comes through the courage to engage the tension of opposites until a new synthesis can be fashioned. In ending this chapter we propose that each midwife ask herself the following questions: What is my responsibility to the "other" midwife? What is the best way to address this issue from a position of higher rather than lower consciousness? The answers to these questions cannot be intellectually crafted or analytically developed but must be "lived into." How each midwife decides to answer these questions involves nothing less than the quality and integrity of the legacy contemporary midwives bequeath to the future.

Questions for Thought and Discussion

1. What is a renegade midwife?
2. What do the authors see as the role of the renegade midwife in the larger context of American midwifery?
3. Are all midwives renegades? Why or why not?
4. Why do the authors suggest that renegade midwives are both an asset and a liability to the profession of midwifery? Which side of that argument resonates most with you?
5. Do you believe that midwives' primary responsibility is to serve the wishes of the mother or to protect the reputation of the profession when those two responsibilities come into conflict in potentially high-risk births?

Recommended Films

Birth Story: Ina May Gaskin and the Farm Midwives: produced by Kate Roughan and Zachary Mortenson, 2012. This feature-length documentary tells the story of counterculture heroine Ina May Gaskin and her spirited friends, who began delivering each other's babies in 1970, on a caravan of hippie school buses, headed to a patch of rural Tennessee land. With Ina May as their leader, the women taught themselves midwifery from the ground up and, with their families, founded a communal, agricultural society called the Farm. They grew their own food, built their own houses, published their own books and, as word of their social experiment spread, created a model of care for women and babies that changed a generation's approach to childbirth. Available at: http://birthstorymovie.com/the-film/

Guerilla Midwife: produced by Robin Lim and Deja Burnhardt, 2011. This film features midwife Robin Lim, who was voted CNN Hero of the Year for 2011, showing her work in Bali where she owns and operates a world-famous birth center called Bumi Sehat Bali, as well as her disaster-relief work and later construction of a Bumi Sehat Aceh in Aceh, Indonesia, after the tsunami. Available at http://www.guerrillamidwife.com/

ACKNOWLEDGMENTS

Our thanks to Betty-Anne Daviss, Barbara Katz Rothman, and Raymond DeVries for their careful reading of and corrections on the original version of this chapter.

PART THREE

Anthropology and Birth Activism

13

Anthropology and Birth Activism

What Do We Know?

Penny's Toast

One night some years ago at a dinner for birth activists and scholars held in Seattle in the home of Penny Simkin, the most revered of American doulas and doula trainers, the 15 or so women (and one man) gathered there held our glasses aloft as Penny made the last toast—"*for all the women who don't know.*" My reactions trembled on the existential brink. As both an anthropologist and a birth activist, I am trained to honor and respect women's choices and the knowledge systems on which they base those choices, but also to deeply question the cultural conditioning underlying all "choice." And in both roles, I heard just as deeply the pity in Penny's voice, the regret, the sadness—this was not a toast of celebration made *to* these women but rather one of longing, a hope *for* these women (who constitute over 85% of the US childbearing population) that they may come to "know"—to see the light and truth of what birth activists are sure such women are missing—the deeply embodied, tremendously empowering experience of giving birth on one's own, without the artificial aids of drugs and technologies.

The only obstetrician at the table, Ricardo Jones, whom we met in Chapter 5 and who (accompanied by a nurse-midwife and a doula) attended both home- and hospital births in Brazil for over 30 years, used the following

This chapter was first published as a short article in *Anthropology News* 46(5):37–38, 2005. This version is greatly updated and expanded.

analogy for self-actualized birth: "Would you choose to take a taxi to the finish line halfway through the marathon?" In an immediate sense, this analogy seems to work—*of course* anyone who starts out to run a marathon would rather complete it than cop out in the middle. But, as all of us at the table were extremely aware, most US women plan on taking that taxi (via having an epidural) at some point during the race. Birthing is not a marathon for them—a hard and painful physical task that they train for, work toward, and strive to achieve for that glowing sense of accomplishment that comes on the other side of the finish line. Birth is just something that has to be done in order to have a baby. The gain is the baby; technology promises that pain should not be part of the picture.

The Fault Line

The sadness, the pity, that birth activists feel for women who "miss out on birth" is unwanted, unappreciated, and largely unnoticed by the vast majority of women who give birth in the US. The 100 interviews I conducted with American women in the late 1980s and early 1990s clearly showed that only about 25% of them even wanted a fully natural childbirth. Seventy-five percent either desired or were relatively content with their highly technologized birth experiences. These data were greatly amplified by a 2002 Harris poll survey designed by the Maternity Center Association (later renamed Childbirth Connection), which showed that 63% of survey respondents received epidurals, 93% received electronic fetal monitoring and many other forms of technological intervention during labor, and over 90% expressed general satisfaction with their birth experiences (www.childbirthconnection.org).

It was not always so. During the scopolamine era (the 1940s–1960s), laboring women were strapped down and left to scream for hours or days until their babies came out, on the assumption that they wouldn't remember. But they often did remember, and reaction to such abuses sparked the natural childbirth movement of the late 1960s and 1970s, during which thousands of women became birth activists and practitioners—childbirth educators, midwives, and later, doulas—and thousands of women were grateful for the natural childbirths they actually, for a while, wanted, and which these activists helped them achieve. But without high levels of emotional and physical support in the hospital environment, "natural" (intervention-free) childbirth is extremely difficult to accomplish, so the advent of the epidural was widely welcomed by women who wanted to be "awake and aware" during birth but did not want the pain or to fight the hospital system for a natural childbirth. Today, over 60% of women have epidurals, attendance at childbirth education classes is decreasing (many doctors tell women, "you don't need childbirth education if you have an epidural"), and both the older and the newer generations of birth activists find themselves generally ignored by the women for whom they are "activizing"—a daunting reality in the face of which, inspired by occasional striking successes, they carry on.

The endless dialogues birth activists engage in about how to effect changes in childbirth center around the need for education: if women "only understood" the disadvantages, indeed dangers, to their bodies and their babies from drugs and technologies, then surely they would be asking for better births. They would seek out midwives who can offer these better births and who presently attend only around 13% of US births because doctors don't want the competition (and because their numbers are very small compared to the 35,000 or so OBs in practice). They would give birth at home and in birth centers, where a holistic/midwifery model of birth prevails and the focus is on facilitating women to give birth on their own and on avoiding unnecessary interventions. As we have seen in previous chapters, homebirth midwives have created a national certification—the Certified Professional Midwife (CPM)—achieved legalization and licensure in 30 states, carried out two large-scale studies demonstrating their excellent outcomes (Johnson and Daviss 2005; Cheyney et al. 2014b), generated numerous websites, articles, books, blogs, and brochures—and rates of homebirth have indeed risen in some communities. But in spite of the demonstrated safety of out-of-hospital birth and the fact that it has doubled in recent years from .006 to around 1.5% of US births, homebirthers and those who choose birth centers are still in the tiny minority.

Evidence vs. Practice

Birth activists have scientific data on their side, but this data has made little difference in the praxis of birth. Routine electronic fetal monitoring remains pervasive, even though it does not improve outcomes but does raise the incidence of unnecessary cesareans. Induction of labor increases prematurity and labor complications, but its use has skyrocketed in the past decade. Epidurals can slow labor, generate fevers, and necessitate further interventions for mother and baby (who will end up in the NICU if the mother does develop a fever). Cesareans generate higher rates of infection and other complications (including death) than vaginal birth, but the cesarean rate in the US is at an all-time high of 32%. The cesarean rates in many low-resource countries, from Turkey to Brazil to Greece, range from 40% to 70%. Cesarean rates in low-resource countries in rural areas "underserved" by modern medicine are generally (often dangerously) low; they are much higher in urban areas, especially in private hospitals, where they often range between 70% and 90%. This normative use of the cesarean means that whole generations of women in such countries do not experience vaginal birth, giving new depth to the anthropological saying, "We're all cyborgs now."

Given that much of what I have long called "technocratic birth" emerged and was transmitted around the world from the American technocracy, it is ironic that the US cesarean rate is lower than that of various low-resource countries. Birth activists claim the credit for this fact, noting there have been few large and organized activist networks in the countries with the highest cesarean rates to protest every percentage point increase, as US birth activists have done. They believe their outcries against unnecessary interventions were what held obstetricians back from raising the US cesarean rate beyond 23–25% for 23 years (from 1979 until 2002). Then there was a big increase resulting in part from studies generating a decline in the once-popular VBAC and the growing number of women choosing elective cesareans, which the American College of Obstetricians and Gynecologists (2007) declared to be an ethical choice that doctors should provide. (Although they do not recommend it, they feel that if a woman truly wants a CS, she has the right to have it—she cannot be forced to have a vaginal birth.) Yet, as previously mentioned in this volume, the US CS rate has been holding at 32% since 2012, and birth activists are claiming some of the credit for that apparent miracle, as they have worked hard to educate doctors about the dangers of placenta accreta

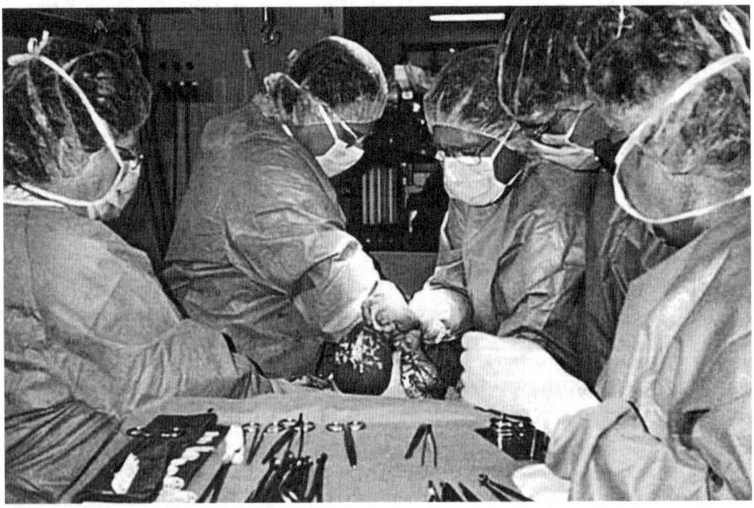

A cesarean birth. In Brazil I watched the performance of one cesarean, standing right at the foot of the bed and staying out of the way of the OBs and nurses. I was a bit shocked by the violence of the operation—the OBs position large clamps on the cut abdominal skin on each side and pull it back quite forcefully. What the mother, who has an epidural, is feeling is a lot of pulling and tugging, sort of like a boot placed on your stomach and someone pulling up your skin for laces. I relived those feelings from my own cesarean birth in 1979 as I watched this cesarean in 2016, and found myself clutching my stomach as if to protect it. Cellular memories run deep!

during future births after cesareans and many other risks (again, including infection and, rarely, death), and it appears the OBs are listening.

Ethnography as Activism

Most birth activists come to be such because they experienced the joys and rewards of natural birth and they want at the very least to ensure that this option remains available to women; thus their buzz words include "informed consent and refusal" and most especially, "informed choice." Others come to birth activism because of traumatic hospital experiences that inspire them to fight in the future for their own better births and for those of others. A common sequence among birth activists is a first "horrible" birth in a hospital, with future births in a birth center or at home. Once women "know" the difference, it's hard to resist wanting other women to want to "know" it too.

In the interests of alternative socialization, birth activists have created a culture of intentional difference from normative and hegemonic biomedical birth culture. The names of the authors of myriad studies supporting normal birth roll easily off our tongues, as do the studies most often cited by obstetricians to justify their practices, which we criticize with a perverse pleasure tinged with bitterness. We learn what obstetricians learn because we read what they read, but we know better than they do the lurking flaws in methodology and interpretation in those studies—such as the infamous "Wax et al.," a study often cited by homebirth opponents that purported to demonstrate that homebirth is dangerous, but was seriously flawed as it excluded the Dutch data from its analysis of neonatal mortality (see De Jonge et al. 2015 for a thorough critique) and *failed to distinguish between planned, midwife-attended homebirths and unplanned, unattended, accidental homebirths*, which carry a much higher risk. And so we know that those who cite that study as proof that homebirth is dangerous are wrong—it has been formally discredited by various epidemiologists for its multiple flaws.

Ours is a culture of reference-sharing. "Have you seen the latest NEJM study supposedly showing that epidurals don't slow labor? It compares drugged women with drugged women—can you believe that? There was no drug-free control group! So now all they know is that one drug slows labor less than another drug. How pathetic is that?" we exclaim in mock horror that is actually real horror—but we lighten it up because you can't live well if you spend most of your time feeling horrified.

I think most of all we want women to understand, as Liza noted in Chapter 2, that contractions only last about 45–60 seconds, and that anyone can get through them if they interpret that pain as productive of the baby's birth and metamorphic for them, as it transforms them into capable and confident mothers—a process researcher and midwife Denis Walsh calls *matres-*

ence. We want them to *know* that if they fight the pain, it will hurt more, but if they surrender to it, they can become one with it and find actual pleasure in the process, what one of our members, Debra Pascali-Bonaro, has called "orgasmic birth." In fact, some women do experience orgasms during birth—OK, perhaps only a few, but still, it's all in your attitude, we say, because we know that those women who want a painless vaginal birth will have that epidural at 1 or 2 cm. And thereby they set themselves up for that "cascade of interventions," which Maureen May, in *Epiduralized Birth* (2017), describes as an integrated system of interconnected procedures that cannot be stopped once started and are very likely to lead to a cesarean birth. And also we know, again, that the pity we feel for those women is unwelcome and unwanted when *a painless birth is their informed choice*, no matter how many more interventions that choice may entail. We just want that choice to be *truly* informed—as May notes in a quote in a previous chapter, there is no true choice without full knowledge.

So we want women planning hospital birth to know that it helps greatly to avoid interventions to stay at home until they reach 6 cm of cervical dilation—the onset of active labor. Yet it can take days to get there, and the contractions of latent labor can be painful, and more and more so as time goes on. That pain sends most women racing to the hospital way too early in labor; we want them instead to have a doula with them at home who can support them through that pain and the sometimes long hours of waiting, and let them know when it's time to go.

And so in a sense *we are asking women to choose to suffer*, for their own good and for the good of their babies, and for the glow of accomplishment they feel when that last push gets the baby out and they can both bask in the afterglow of the rush of hormones that accompany natural birth and help to easily establish breastfeeding. (Labor interventions stop that hormonal flow, thereby interfering with the woman's ability to push, to bond with her baby, and to breastfeed.) And women who want what we want for them will do as we ask, while those for whom *no pain is the real gain* may regard us as the Gestapo of normal birth and mightily resent our advice and encouragement, especially when we get self-righteous about it because we *know* we are right! As Lina insisted in Chapter 3:

> I read all this stuff that told me I would be a complete asshole to have an epidural and I revolted. [The books said that] I would be able to see that it's much better for the baby and it's a natural experience, and there's just all this pressure. . . . I quit smoking, ate meat, drank milk for months and months—I had been such a good girl. A couple of hours of whatever an epidural was going to do to me, tough. You can put up with it, kid.

Yet we know that it's going to be a lot more than a couple of hours that those potent drugs of bipuvicaine (an anesthetic), and fentanyl (a narcotic), along with pitocin are going to be flowing into their bodies and straight into the baby via the placenta, and that in addition to the above issues, epidurals often result in “floppy” babies unable to latch on, or can give the mother a fever that entails assessing the baby for sepsis and possibly putting him or her in the NICU . . . and so it goes. We just want them to know those risks, which we also know are often not fully explained to them, making a mockery of the concept of “informed choice.” Lina assumed her doctor would keep her baby safe from harm, while we keep wondering, if he had told her about all of the very real risks, would she still have made the same choice? So we try, via childbirth education in advance or on the spot, to tell them about those risks. Yet fewer and fewer women seem to want to be “educated”—they just want that epidural and to feel no pain. It’s a cultural privilege that just a few decades ago was available only to those who could pay extra for it; now that it’s available to everyone, the poor, who have a lot of historical memory, want it even more (May 2017).

And our culture doesn’t value or celebrate the mighty accomplishment of pushing out a baby on one’s own, without drugs or interventions—instead, people tell us we are crazy to want to do so—why suffer when it’s so easily avoidable? And that’s just the point—epidurals and all the technologies that accompany them are so readily available in high-resource countries, and using them is such a culturally sensical act, that not using them appears non-sensical, even irresponsible, especially when a woman makes the radical choice not only to choose to experience pain, but also to give birth outside the culturally perceived safety of the institution. That’s precisely why birth activists often appear to be the Gestapo of normal birth—no one in a techno-cratic society has to fight to have a technocratic birth—including a scheduled CS—so there is no need for us to advocate for women’s right to choose that kind of birth. What must be fought for are those marginal options that our cultural trends seek to deny us—that’s why we advocate so fiercely for out-of-hospital and midwife-attended births—because *those are the marginal choices that will cease to exist if not fought for*, and because the scientific evidence tells us that those marginalized choices are in fact the healthiest and safest ones.

High Art to Birth Activists

Our culture of intentional difference values being present at normal births and/or at least watching countless slide shows and videos of them. Huge photos of women whose facial expressions indicate an altered state of consciousness as a baby’s head crowns through their beautiful bulging vaginas are high art to us, as are photos of women breastfeeding and of couples glowing together as they hold their baby after (what we perceive as) a gorgeous homebirth.

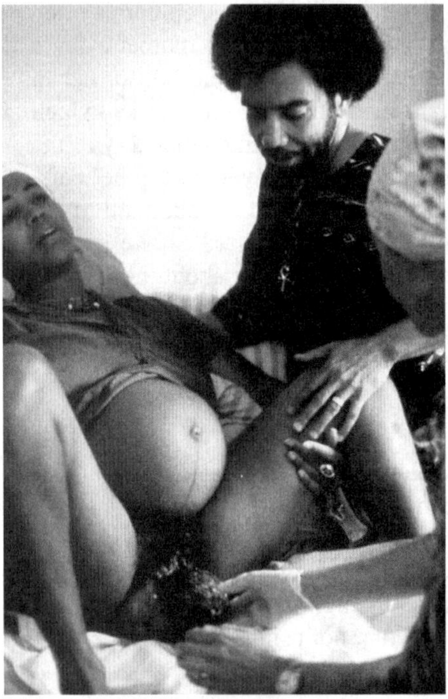
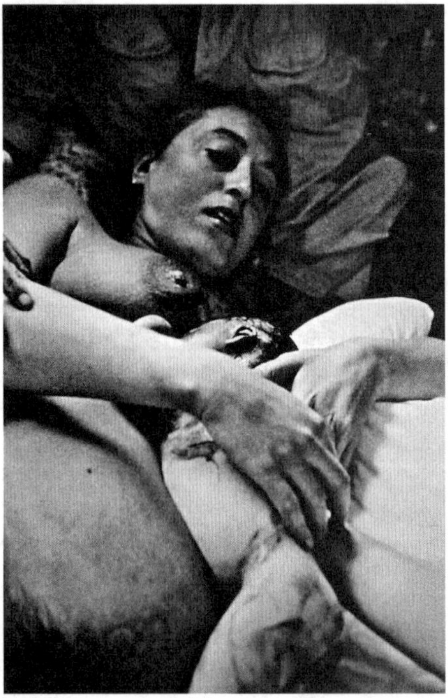

High art to birth activists, who love to display such photos in their offices and birth centers. Left photo by Faith Gibson; right photo by Mayri Sagady Leslie

Activist-practitioners adorn the walls of their birth centers and offices, their childbirth education and doula training classrooms, with this kind of birth art because they want the women who pass through these spaces to come to see such pictures—and the experiences they represent—as normative and beautiful—and to want what the women in those photos have achieved.

A quick side story: Once I was on a plane to somewhere in the aisle seat next to my dear friend Ina May Gaskin, who was in the window seat. I had my laptop open on the tray table so I could go over the PowerPoint presentations I was planning to give at the conference where we both were speaking, which contained many images such as those shown here. Before long, the flight attendant approached and asked me to turn my computer off, as the "pornographic" images I was showing were offending some of the other passengers who could see them! The experience made me realize just how radical and counter-cultural the values birth activists hold appear to the wider public.

We birth activists and MMOC practitioners wince and grab our necks when we see a video of a baby's neck being pulled and twisted during a manual or forceps delivery; we shudder at photos of scissors cutting vaginas; we cringe at the image of the woman wrapped by huge belts whose gaze is trans-

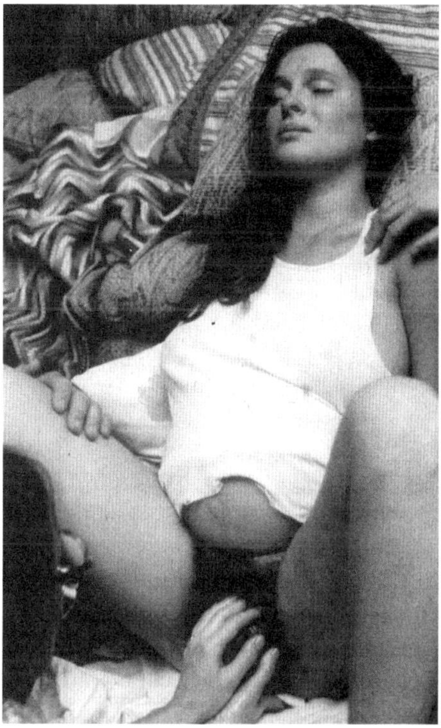

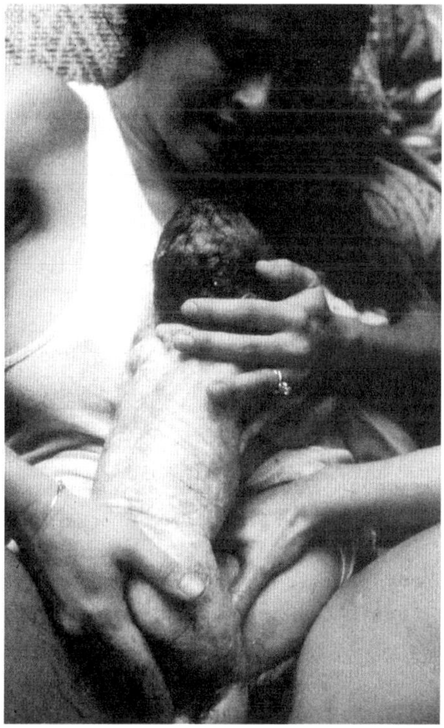

You may note that the midwife is not wearing gloves; this birth occurred during the very early days of homebirth midwifery, when "lay" midwives were profoundly countercultural. Today all US midwives wear gloves to attend births. Photos by Harriette Hartigan

fixed by the tracings on the fetal monitor, because we know that her experience of birth and what she and her attendants "know" about birth will be utterly shaped and largely controlled by the information produced by this machine, and we know (because the studies show it and our experience confirms it) that what her body really needs to birth that baby is to be up and moving, to be eating and drinking if she is hungry or thirsty, to be rocking and swaying with the contractions, uttering deep guttural moans that help her throat and her cervix to *open, open. . . .* [1] We rejoice at every birth that happens that way, and mourn for those that don't. We celebrate the increasing cultural acceptance of breastfeeding, but we know that a major impediment to successful breastfeeding is the very birth interventions we protest: drugs administered during and after labor impede the flow of hormones and phero-

[1] American homebirth midwives tend to believe that there is an energetic connection between the throat and the cervix; as the throat opens through the woman making low guttural sounds, the cervix will stretch and open as well, whereas if the throat is tight and constricted (exemplified by high squeaky sounds), the cervix will be too.

mones that enable the baby to find the nipple and latch on fully (see *The Impact of Birth Practices on Breastfeeding*, by Linda Smith 2010).

Holding Spaces for Informed Choice

The vast discrepancy between what we know and what the culture practices (and thus what women do) makes us crazy, but every now and then, someone really listens to us speak or reads one of our books or articles and has a wonderful birth that changes her life, and we know that our work is helping to create small, intentionally different cultural spaces in which others might come to personal transformation, as most of us did. And so we keep building and holding these spaces, in case even one pregnant woman wants to climb in. Birth has become mundane for many women, but we *know* it can be magnificent, and we want every woman to know that too.

Interestingly enough, although many feminists suspect and sometimes accuse birth activists of essentialism, the large and growing body of anthropological ethnography about birth supports birth activist positions, often from feminist perspectives. As often previously noted in this volume, and to recap here, from the 1960s to the present, anthropologists have reported similar responses to biomedical birthways from women in developing countries around the globe: "They shave you, they expose you, they cut you, they leave you alone to suffer and don't let your family members be with you, they give you nothing to eat or drink, and sometimes they yell at you and slap you." In the remotest rural clinics and the biggest urban hospitals, impoverished laboring women lie on narrow cots as (sometimes reused) IV needles drip pitocin into their veins. The pain from pitocin-induced contractions can be terrible, and there are no doulas to mitigate it or epidurals to take it away.

Not surprisingly, many rural women resist hospital birth, leaving development planners to shake their heads over this unaccountable unwillingness to use modern facilities, attributing it to ignorance and close-mindedness. But birthing at home with a traditional midwife is often a considered decision that women make after weighing the risks and benefits of their options. To recap from Chapter 9, Soheir Morsy (1995) notes that in the Nile Delta, such a choice is "not a result of reified 'cultural attitudes' but a measured judgment about the inadequate health care extended to peasants and the urban poor in modern-health care settings."

Like anthropologists, birth activists (who are sometimes also social scientists) support traditional midwives and work to help them remain viable in the contemporary world, and react with extreme outrage to the biomedical abuses so often inflicted on women in low-resource countries that occur when these women are urged or forced into unsafe medical institutions to give birth. In contrast to these women's lack of choices, US women seem to have all the choice and agency in the world. These choices and agencies are the result of real struggles (by early feminist activists in the 1920s and beyond who demanded medical rights to drugs during labor and bottle-feeding after birth, and by later ones demanding humanistic rights to food, water, family, friends, doulas, and more comfortable environments for labor and birth, not to mention breastfeeding support). And indeed birth activists succeeded in getting these options to be offered in most US hospitals. The current generation of US birthing women takes them for granted, right along with the epidural and the fetal monitor, which has served to ensure that US mothers will use their choice and agency to reinforce biomedical hegemony and the increasing technologization of birth (see Chapter 3).

The choice for drugs and technology in the US during the 1920s was first made by upper- and middle-class women (Wertz and Wertz 1989). Such choices were for decades denied to the poor, the minorities—the underserved, who then turned around to demand all the technology they could get as soon as they won the right to have it (Fraser 1995). Because the privileged women had it, poor and minority women "knew" it was the best. Now that "knowledge" blankets the planet, convincing women that they should want technobirth and justifying its infliction if they don't. What is choice and privilege in one setting becomes an almost invisible coercion in another. What obstetricians *know* is that many women are choosing drugs and technology, so forcing drugs and technology on women who *don't* choose them can be easily coded as "giving women what they want" and "respecting women's choice"; birth activists in contrast code such practices as "obstetric violence," which takes many forms, from subtle persuasion to overt cruelty. (See Sadler et al. 2016, "Moving beyond Disrespect and Abuse: Addressing the Structural Dimensions of Obstetric Violence," and Chapter 2, this volume.)

In *Birth as an American Rite of Passage* (2003 [1992]), I analyzed the intensely technocratic socialization process that underlies American women's birth choices. Here I seek to highlight how "choice" in the "First" World—the world of the resource-rich in every country—actually obscures and mystifies coercion in the "Third" World of the resource-poor in every country (see *Birthing Justice: Black Women, Pregnancy, and Childbirth*, edited by Julia C. Oparah and Alicia D. Bonaparte 2016). Seeing ultimate agency in birth as the ability to choose the ultimately biomedical birth reconfigures (reasonable) choice in biomedical terms and renders alternative choices unreasonable. It is in the shadow of the women who schedule elective cesareans, making them appear to be "the best care," that the "other" women suffer the abuse of forced choice. Birth activists "know" that what the rich women "choose" is too often a travesty of what birth can be. Doctors "know" they are giving women "the best care," and "what they want." Anthropologists only know what the women they study show and tell them. It is our job to specify, contextualize, and render meaningful the choices these women make, so we can tell the world what *women* know.

Questions for Thought and Discussion

1. Why did Davis-Floyd "tremble on the existential brink" in response to Penny Simkin's toast to the "women who don't know"?
2. What do you think is the role of the social scientist in the study of birth? Should social scientists be activists too?
3. Throughout this book, Davis-Floyd has made clear her advocacy of midwifery and normal physiological birth, including homebirth. Do you think her biases have obscured her anthropological objectivity?
4. Should anthropologists and other social scientists be objective, or should they become advocates and activists as well regarding the issues confronting the cultures and groups they study?

14

Working with Anthropology in Policy and Practice

An Activist's Experiences

Introduction: My Choices to Study Birth and Midwives, and to Become a Birth Activist and Midwifery Advocate

Question from me to famed birth activist Diony Young, long-time editor of the prestigious journal Birth: Issues in Perinatal Care, *at the very first birth conference I ever attended, in 1983, held by the International Childbirth Education Association (ICEA):*

"What can an anthropologist do to aid and participate in the birth movement?"

Answer: "I have no idea!"

So I had to find my own way, carve out my own path—one that, I am delighted to say—others have since followed. I did not start out intending to do "applied anthropology," but birth drew me in! Before I even completed my dissertation in 1986, I was being asked to give talks at childbirth conferences because of some articles I had published. I was aware from very early on of the confusion felt by birth practitioners over the apparent irrationality of childbirth in the technocracy. As we have so often seen in the preceding chapters of this anthology, most standard procedures performed on most

This chapter, which has been updated and expanded, originally appeared as an article in *Anthropology in Action,* edited by Chris McCourt, 18(2): 3–8, 2011. © Berghahn Books and the Association for Anthropology in Action.

American women as they give birth often cause more problems than they solve, yet are routinely applied anyway. Because US medicine claims to be based on science, the unscientific nature of hospital birth begs for explanation. My analysis, as the readers of this volume will know by now, holds that routine hospital procedures, in addition to their instrumental ends, serve as rituals that generate a sense of human control over natural processes and enact the core values and beliefs of technocratic culture—most especially the supervaluation of high technology—thereby working to ensure the perpetuation of those values and beliefs.

In other words, hospital procedures do not make scientific sense, but they do make cultural sense. This finding of mine has been appreciated in the alternative birth community as a useful insight into why the problem exists and is so very difficult to resolve. Ritual change requires—and can generate—cultural change, not an easy thing to achieve. For the past 33 years, I have been giving talks at universities and at childbirth, obstetric, and midwifery conferences in many countries on a multitude of topics, including obstetric procedures as rituals and what I have identified as the three major paradigms influencing birth and health care around the world—the technocratic, humanistic, and holistic models (Chapter 1). Practitioners especially appreciate my explication of these paradigms because it gives them clear ways of understanding the ideological pressures they experience: hospitals push them to technocratize birth—to apply multiple technological interventions, while patients ask for humanistic treatment, and science supports a more holistic approach based on the normal physiology of birth (which works best in upright positions and with minimal intervention) and attention to women's emotional needs through the kind of one-on-one care provided by midwives and doulas.

From 1991 on, my birth activism increasingly came to focus on helping American midwives widen the toeholds they were establishing in the technocracy. Supporting midwives in general has always been for me a matter of both the heart and the head. Midwives perform fewer interventions and give more nurturant care than doctors, they offer a wider range of choices and more fully informed consent, their perinatal mortality rates are the same as those for doctors attending low-risk births, and their rates of iatrogenic damage are much lower.

After an unnecessary cesarean for my first birth in 1979, in 1984 I gave birth to my second child at home. The power of that experience committed me to help preserve that choice for women who want it. Because I am an anthropologist, and was totally confused about why I ended up with a cesarean during Peyton's birth, I started asking other women about their birth experiences and realized I was not alone in my confusion. And then I understood that there was something really curious about American birth, and my eventual primary research question became: "Given that birth is so unique and individual to every woman who experiences it, why is it so standardized in the American obstetrical system?"

Yet even before I was able to formulate that fundamental question, I went to lunch with my dissertation supervisor, Barbara Kirshenblatt, to pick a topic for my PhD dissertation. I told her all about my years of research on myth, ritual, and shamanism in Mexico, and then, hesitantly, I mentioned that I had also recently become very interested in American women's experiences of birth. Without hesitation, and with a downward wave of her hand, she said, quite dismissively, "Shamanism, shamanism, shamanism—everybody and their dog is doing shamanism! You do women's things, you do birth!!!!" And, following the upward wave of her hand, my heart and my head said "YES, OK, I will do women's things—I will do birth!"

Participant-Observation and Activism in the American Midwifery Movement: Conducting Political Ethnography

I want to provide here a sample of the feel and flavor my anthropological activism has taken as my exposure to midwifery politics over the years has increasingly informed my perceptions. In 1991, I was invited to be a keynote speaker at the annual conference of the Midwives' Alliance of North America (MANA), an organization formed by "lay" (the term used at the time) and nurse-midwives attending homebirths. Of course I accepted—I was already a huge fan of homebirth midwives because after that unnecessary cesarean for Peyton's birth in 1979, I gave birth to my 10-pound son Jason at home with the help of "lay midwives"—to date that remains the most transformative experience of my life. At that first MANA conference I attended in El Paso, Texas, in 1991, a very informal tally was taken of how many births those midwives had attended, and it was over 80,000! Yes, homebirth midwives at the time attended only about .6% of American births per year, but still, those 450 midwives in that big conference hall had given around 80,000 mothers the chance to achieve a normal birth at home. That moment was when my ongoing fascination and dedication to midwives took hold and has never let me go.

My 15 Years of Service on the NARM Board

In the end, isn't it probable that all ethnographers ultimately become an insider, even if they began their research as an outsider?
— Maureen May

To explore avenues for professionalizing, MANA created the North American Registry of Midwives (NARM). In 1994, I was invited to sit on the NARM board in the position of Consumer Representative. I was thrilled! I had extensively interviewed consumers of birth services and was already planning a research project on these homebirth midwives' professionalizing efforts. I made clear to the NARM board my desire both to participate in and to study their process, and they accepted me on those terms. I promised them that before I published anything about them, I would run it by them; I have always been careful to abide by that agreement.

Participating in Choosing the Name for NARM's New Direct-Entry Certification: Influencing the Process I Was Studying (Yikes!)

By the time I came on the NARM board, it was clear to the board members that their primary purpose was to create a national certification process that would preserve multiple routes to midwifery, including apprenticeship. The potential names for this new direct-entry certification were up on the flip chart: Certified Midwife, and Certified Professional Midwife (this latter title had been suggested the day before by Debbie Pulley, a NARM board member).

As we were going around the large table with each person speaking about their preference for either of these titles, I realized with dismay that most of them seemed to want "Certified Midwife" because it seemed simple and straightforward to them, while I thought it would be a huge mistake. But I didn't want to try to influence their process under my aegis alone, so I rushed to a pay phone (this was before the age of cell phones) to call well-known sociologist Barbara Katz Rothman, who was the only other social scientist in the US at the time who understood our midwifery problems and issues as fully as I did, and probably more so, as she had been engaged in midwifery research much longer than I. She was firm that they very much needed to include the word "professional" in their title, in order to help them surpass the negative stereotype of "lay" midwife.

Vastly relieved to have her support, when it came my turn to speak, I told them all that Barbara and I both agreed strongly that they should choose "CPM" to overcome the "lay" stereotype. There was a short, kind of stunned silence, and then Ina May Gaskin said, "Well, if the two most important social scientists studying us feel the same about this, and for the same reasons, I really think we should reconsider CPM instead of CM. I *am* a professional midwife, and I wish to be recognized as such." The two midwives who spoke after me, including Marimikel Potter of Austin, agreed. So those who had been happy with the simpler "CM" suddenly changed their votes, and chose unanimously to name this new certification the "Certified Professional Midwife" (CPM)—again, in an effort to remove the appellation "lay" from public understanding of their considerable professional expertise (see Davis-Floyd 2006 for a full description of the creation of the CPM, and Chapter 8, this volume, for a short story about it).

I was a bit shocked to have had such an influence on this process, but years later I found that the midwives present at that Certification Task Force (CTF) meeting barely remembered I had said a thing, claiming the choice as theirs—a great relief to me, as there were some negative repercussions:

Helen Varney, Director of Midwifery at Yale, author of the popular text *Varney's Nurse-Midwifery* (later changed to *Varney's Midwifery*), had wanted to call ACNM's new direct-entry certification the CPM, and had written an article or two using that appellation. It was circumstantial happenstance that the CTF meeting in which we chose the name of our new direct-entry certification fell two months before ACNM was to meet to choose its name (in other words, nobody planned it that way on purpose). Because CPM was taken, the ACNM committee was left with CM, which Helen was not happy about for quite some time—she seemed to feel it was a personal "slap in the face" to her—but it was not. It had nothing to do with ACNM and everything to do with the professionalization of lay midwifery. Anyway as time passed, the ACNM members came to prefer "CM" for their new title, because if they had called their new direct-entry midwives "Certified Professional Midwives," then it might imply that Certified Nurse-Midwives were not professionals. So in the end the name choices worked out well for everyone—phew!

Writing NARM's Mission Statement, and Other Contributions

During this CTF meeting, NARM decided they needed a Mission Statement, and because of my anthropological interviewing skills, they asked me to produce it. With tape recorder in hand, I asked every member of the board, "Why do midwives matter?" "What's important about midwifery education?" and "What do you want this CPM certification to achieve?" Then I wove their passionate replies into a strong Mission Statement that guided and informed their work until 2009, the year of my retirement from the board after 15 years of participation. By then we had realized that the mission statement I had created was more of a philosophical vision than an actual mission statement, so my final act on the NARM board was to separate out the philosophy as a principle on its own and to create a simpler and fully pragmatic mission statement. Full circle!

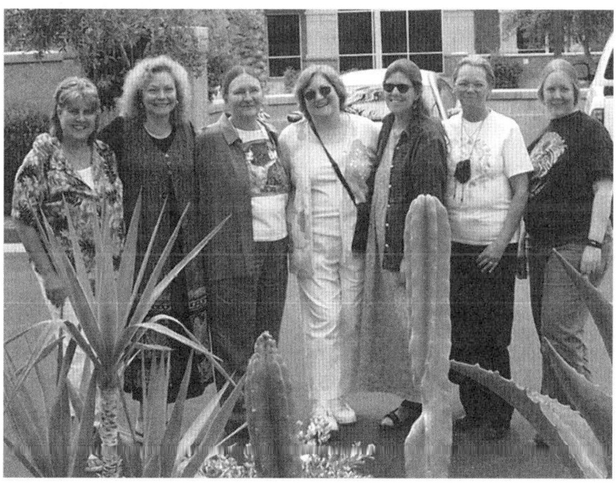

NARM board members in 2004. From left to right: Debbie Pulley CPM, Robbie Davis-Floyd PhD, and CPMs Carol Nelson, Ida Darragh (NARM board chair), Joanne Gottschall, Sharon Evans, and Shannon Anton. Photo by a passerby

Anthropology gave me the skills to (1) realize the importance of including the NARM board members' individual visions and words; (2) ask the right questions so that they could give me the answers that mattered most to them; and (3) refract their individual values back to them in a clear and unified way—many colors making one beam of light. My other contributions to NARM included helping craft their *How to Become a CPM* manual and other documents, copyediting official documents and letters, participating in visioning sessions and philosophical discussions aimed at ensuring that CPM certification remained true to its original intent, and participating in trips to Mexico with board members to support the incipient professional midwifery movement there. I even got to name their apprenticeship route—one NARM board member was wanting to call it the Portfolio Education Evaluation Process, which would have had the not-so-great acronym "PEEP." A frantic late-night call to me asking for a better name led me to suggest simply PEP—Portfolio Evaluation Process—which it is still called today.

Mediation Work: Trying to Resolve Disputes and Help Midwives Work Together

I augmented my usefulness as a NARM board member by immersion in national and international midwifery communities and conferences at which I was asked to be a speaker—from the platform, I could point out the advances and successes, the barriers, the cultural meanings of their efforts, and suggest ways forward. This intense participant-observation within the midwifery community facilitated my research on midwifery politics and professionalization and my ability to advocate effectively. My more distanced role and status (I am not a midwife) also enabled me to act as a mediator in challenging situations over these years as midwives attempted to advance their position and negotiate their mutual roles with other maternity care providers.

In the US, homebirth midwives had operated outside mainstream health services, and as they changed their identity from "lay" to "certified professional" midwives, conflicts arose between MANA, whose members primarily attend out-of-hospital birth, and the American College of Nurse-Midwives (ACNM), which represents CNMs and CMs who primarily attend births in hospitals. These two organizations, which represented widely disparate views of appropriate standards for midwifery education, often engaged at the time in various forms of quite destructive internecine warfare, often over legal issues. My anthropologically gained ability to see the world from all sides was of great service in all my "applied" midwifery mediation work as I attempted to translate the intentions of each organization to the other and to smooth relationships between them as best I could.

For one brief example, one evening at a midwifery conference somewhere, I was having dinner with the then-president of ACNM. She mentioned to me in irritation that she had sent a letter to Ina May Gaskin, then-president of MANA, some months ago and had not received a reply, which she took as just another example of how disorganized those pesky "lay" midwives could be. I excused myself to go to the bathroom and immediately called Ina May to ask her about the letter. She told me she had replied as soon as she had received it, and had sent her reply to ACNM headquarters in DC. Upon returning to the table, I gave the ACNM president this information. She looked rather embarrassed and said, "Well, I guess the board will give me the letter at our meeting next week."

For another example, at a midwifery conference I became aware that two wonderful, big-hearted CNMs, whom we shall call Francis and Zeda, were at extreme odds with each other because of events that occurred when Francis went to Africa to help Zeda and the other midwives working in a small rural birth clinic attend to the needs of the local community women. They had previously been good friends, and I thought it a shame that they were now avoiding each other and speaking badly about each other to friends. So I made it a point to have lengthy conversations with each to try to get to the heart of the matter. I learned from each that when a laboring woman was brought into the clinic in a state of extreme emergency, Zeda and another midwife had pitched right into to try to save her and her baby while Francis simply stood there watching, which infuriated Zeda. From that moment on, Zeda had treated Francis with scorn and displeasure throughout the rest of her stay, and Francis did not understand why, so she started to think that Zeda was just a mean person, ungrateful for her efforts and expenses to get to Africa to help out.

It turned out that the misunderstanding was a cultural one. Francis, used to hierarchies in other clinics, was desperate to jump in but thought that she should wait for a request from Zeda, whom she saw as the higher authority. Zeda had no tolerance for such hierarchies and could not understand why Francis just stood there, so she started to think of Francis as lazy, fearful, and unwilling to help. Once I explained each midwife's perspective to the other, they started to laugh at the silliness of this simple misunderstanding and became fast friends once again.

It was my experience, during all my years of intensive immersion in midwifery culture, that so very many misunderstandings and conflicts could be avoided if the aggrieved party would only talk directly to the person who had aggrieved her, instead of telling everyone else how irresponsible or whatever said person was. So whenever possible, if the midwives themselves were unwilling to do so, I made that direct contact for them, solving many issues and disputes in the process. This task was self-appointed and not easy—there were times when each organization accused me of supporting the other more—even of "spying" for the other—yet I did this mediation work because, since I was studying both organizations, I had a pretty good perspective on the motivations and stereotyped perceptions of each and knew when I could solve a given problem or misunderstanding. I hope my published works have clearly demonstrated that I support both organizations equally and have sought only to help, and never to harm, either one. (Occasionally, CNM leaders would accuse me of "bias" because of my work with NARM; I always pointed out to them that NARM had invited me onto their board whereas no CNM group had ever asked for my participation, which I would have been happy to provide.)

My Greatest Challenge as a Midwifery Ethnographer

In that endeavor of telling the truth as the members of each organization perceived it, one of my greatest challenges as an applied anthropologist came from an invitation from Jan Tritten, founder and editor of the magazine *Midwifery Today*, to write a chapter for a book called *Paths to Becoming a Midwife: Getting an Education*—I was to write a "brief overview" of American midwifery, comparing and contrasting the various types of midwives. I had been studying US midwives for four years at that point (see Davis-Floyd and Johnson 2006) and felt keenly the anthropologist's responsibility to publish not only for ourselves but also for the people we study. So I accepted. I was very busy, and I didn't want to spend much time on this assignment, so I dashed off a nine-page first draft and sent it to one nurse-midwife and one direct-entry midwife, not thinking to specifically request confidentiality—which is assumed among scholars but apparently not among midwives. I should have known better—midwives do almost everything in groups—as my friend Alan Huber used to say, "telephone, telegraph, tell-a-midwife"! They circulated those drafts and I received irate phone calls from both nurse- and direct-entry midwives who did not appreciate my generalized portrayals. None of these women saw reflected in my "brief overview" the midwives they believed themselves and their compatriots to be. And I wasn't even in some exotic place struggling with a language I didn't understand. These were mostly white middle-class women, just like me!

I took this as a gut-level challenge to get my description both factually correct and "thick"[1] enough to encapsulate the meanings both groups of mid-

[1] The influential anthropologists Clifford Geertz (2000 [1973]) and George Marcus (1998) made a strong point of distinguishing between "thin" and "thick" ethnographic description. In "thin" description, the anthropologist describes only what he sees, without interpretation; in "thick" description, the anthropologist layers in the meaning behind the behaviors and events he describes. For example, my colleague Charles Laughlin observed and participated in a ritual performed by the So tribe of Uganda in which everyone lined up at a clay pit and got swabbed with a line of gray goop across their chests. Charlie was thrilled to participate in his first So ritual, and wrote down in detail what had occurred (thin description). Yet he was humbled when he realized he had no idea what it meant. It took him a year to figure out that the gray goop was considered protection against demons who caused the major drought under which the So had been suffering (thick description—layering in the meaning).

wives find in their experiences. I realized that the core dividing issue was education—CPMs believed in a homebirth apprenticeship model or private vocational schools, CNMs only accepted university-based training. I realized that I did not fully understand these educational models or the motivations of the students who chose one track or the other. So I asked Jan for more time and a lot more pages, and embarked on a six-month study of midwifery education, eventually interviewing 75 midwifery students of all types.

The original nine-page article turned into 45 pages full of discussion of the core educational issues and multiple quotes from both students and practicing midwives. Eventually, I had a draft that I thought was reasonably close to representing reality as I and my subjects—*all* my subjects—understood it. I sent it off to equal numbers of nurse- and direct-entry midwives for review and had long dialogues with each responder that deepened my understanding of the issues involved. I revised draft after draft and ultimately, to my enormous delight and everlasting relief, succeeded in capturing in print the disparate realities of each group, the sources of their often-bitter conflicts, the meanings they attributed to the circumstances of their education and practice, and their intense interlinkages. (The last two reviewers, one CNM and one CPM, said that the article "rings like crystal"—whew!) That article, entitled "The Ups, Downs, and Interlinkages of Nurse- and Direct-Entry Midwifery" (Davis-Floyd 2010) became required reading in many midwifery educational programs and helped students and practicing midwives to understand the issues that divide and those that link the two major midwifery organizations in the US. I am told it has also helped many students choose the right educational route for them.

Applying Anthropology: Creating Positive Change in a Nurse-Midwifery Educational Program

During my ethnographic research on nurse-midwifery education, I interviewed all the student nurse-midwives (SNMs) at a particular university midwifery program in the US Northeast and also gave them a questionnaire asking them to rate this program in terms of clinical and didactic excellence. They gave the program a 10 in terms of clinical experience gained, a 3 in terms of didactic (they didn't feel that their professors actually spent much time teaching them didactically), and they *all* added in a third category—emotional and spiritual quality, which they all rated at a –2. They explained that their professors were often emotionally abusive, encouraging them in discussion sessions to open up and share their feelings, then later using what the students shared against them to criticize their clinical performance. ("Oh, your sister died, right—no wonder you made a big diagnostic error during that exam! You've got to learn to separate your professional life from your personal emotions!" Or, "You are distracted by your fight with your boyfriend—you need to focus!") In addition, the students hated being forced, sometimes without their consent, to perform vaginal exams on each other (to learn how to do them) in a cold sterile room with no spiritual context, no sense of being taught to honor each other's bodies as sacred, holy temples of the soul (something Elizabeth Davis often stresses in her introductory midwifery "Heart and Hands" seminars).

These students clearly were feeling a deep sense of emotional and spiritual, not to mention physical, violation—what was an anthropologist to do? I called the current director of the program, who was about to retire, and gently told her my findings; her response was, "Oh, we get to the spiritual part in the last semester." Unsatisfied, I met with the students and asked them if they wanted me to take this information to the new program director. They did; so I did. His response was to fire several faculty members (the ones the students had named as the most emotionally abusive), revamp the program, and to completely change the flavor and context, the "energy" of the vaginal exams, making them voluntary and performed with attitudes of honoring and valuing the student's body they were, softly and respectfully, penetrating. When I checked in with the students in that program a couple of years later, they reported they loved the program and gave it a "10" on all three scales; of course, I was delighted to have been able to play a role in those improvements.

Participant-Observation and Activism in the Birth Movement at the International Level

In 1995, members of various national alternative birth and breastfeeding organizations came together to create the Coalition for Improving Maternity Services (CIMS). Our first action was to create the *Mother-Friendly Childbirth Initiative* (*MFCI*): *Ten Steps to Mother-Friendly Hospitals, Birth Centers, and Home Birth Services* (see www.motherfriendly.org). I served as the chair of the Editorial Committee for the MFCI, so it was on my computer for months as my other committee members (Henci Goer and Roberta Scaer) and myself dealt with suggestions and feedback from dozens of US birth activists—we worked hard for about four months and finally produced the final document, still extant today. The MFCI is an excellent initiative but is solely focused on the United States. By 2004, many birth activists and professionals from other countries were attending the CIMS annual conferences and asking us to develop an international initiative that would be appropriate in all countries. We did not want to become "American imperialists" telling other countries what to do, so we encouraged these international activists to start with the MFCI and adapt it to their own countries or regions. But they kept pressuring us to do it, as we already had an organization in place and the experience of creating the MFCI. So CIMS created an International Committee, of which I was a founding member. In 2006, that committee became the International MotherBaby Childbirth Organization (IMBCO) and created the *International MotherBaby Childbirth Initiative (IMBCI): 10 Steps to Optimal Maternity Care*, for which I also serve as editorial chair. In that capacity I spent almost an entire year taking feedback on various iterations of the IMBCI and wordsmithing them into a viable and polished document, assisted greatly by the other members of the IMBCO board. My activist efforts are currently focused on promotion of this groundbreaking international initiative, which is designed to set a global gold standard for optimal maternity care (see www.imbci.org and the following chapter).

My Role as an International Speaker in the Movement for the Humanization of Birth

The Initial Pivot Points: My First Book, Gitti's "Mantle," and Midwifery Today

Although I had started giving talks at birth-related conferences in 1983, and was sort of becoming the "public face of anthropology" to the birth movement in the US, prior to 1993, the most internationally recognized spokesperson for the anthropology of birth had been my mentor and friend Brigitte Jordan (now deceased), author of *Birth in Four Cultures* and founding mother of the anthropology of birth. Yet she changed fields (to corporate anthropology) and quite directly passed her birth "mantle" to me, partly by referring others who asked her to write or speak about birth or midwifery directly to me, and largely by asking me to revise and update that book for her as its 4th edition (the 3rd edition had come out in 1983), which I was only too delighted to do. (Funny side story: Gitti told me later that to give herself the courage to knock on my hotel room door to ask me to update the book, she had fortified herself with two glasses of Glenlivet, her favorite Scotch. I burst out laughing—how could she not know that I would have gotten on my knees and begged for that privilege?)

After my first book, *Birth as an American Rite of Passage*, came out in 1992, and then my update and revision of *Birth in Four Cultures* was published in 1993, I suddenly seemed to become the international spokesperson for the anthropology of birth, just as Gitti had been. As my reputation grew, Jan Tritten increasingly began to invite me to speak at her many national and international Midwifery Today conferences, and these talks led in turn to invitations from birth activists, midwives, midwifery schools, and universities in many other countries (Gitti's mantle often seems to enfold me as I speak)—it was and remains a perfect fieldwork feedback circle. In every country, I learn as much as I can about the cultural context and the conditions of birth there, so I am able to incorporate the knowledge gained into my PowerPoint presentations, keeping them fresh and relevant, and to find new topics for research and publication.

The Next Pivot Point: An International Conference in Brazil and Where It Led Me

The second major turning point in my speaking career was when I was invited to be one of only five international speakers at the huge first International Congress on the Humanization of Childbirth, held in Fortaleza, Ceara, Brazil, in November 2000. We expected around 600 attendees, yet more kept arriving until the auditorium was packed beyond capacity, and I realized that I was witnessing the birth of the social movement for the humanization of birth in Latin America! I delivered my keynote speech, titled "Three Paradigms of Birth Care: The Technocratic, Humanistic, and Holistic Models," in front of 2,000 people, with simultaneous translation (which can be really funny when you tell a joke that the English-speakers laugh at right away, while it takes about 45 seconds for the translation to sink in and the waves of laughter to spread around the auditorium—a lovely and heart-warming experience!). I want to share with my readers the devastating fact that my 20-year-old daughter Peyton had died in a car accident only three months before, and so it took every ounce of professionalism I had to pull off that talk and get that standing ovation. I think women are amazing—so many of us are suffering yet are able to put aside that suffering to do our work in the world.[2]

These two events—my being included as a Midwifery Today speaker at so many conferences around the world, for which I am deeply grateful to Jan Tritten, and this overwhelmingly well-received speech in Brazil—truly launched my career as an international speaker—and in my mind, always an anthropologist first. The Fortaleza conference was the spark and the inspiration for many others, so in the subsequent four years I found myself privileged to speak at the very first conferences on the humanization of birth held in 10 Latin American countries. In these talks, I did my best to warn practitioners about the profound differences between what I call "superficial" and "deep" humanism: in *superficial humanism,* you can simply invite fathers into the delivery room or just paint it in pretty colors and call your site "humanistic," whereas *deep humanism* honors the deep physiology of birth, avoids the use of unnecessary interventions, and lets women eat, drink, move about fluidly, and labor and give birth in upright positions. I am very proud to say that for this work and others, at the III International Congress on the Humanization of Childbirth, held in Brasilia in 2010, I was awarded an *Homenagem* for my work—a lovely framed certificate handed to me onstage personally by the Brazilian minister of health—a peak moment!

[2] At Diony Young's request, I wrote about my experiences of Peyton's death in my 2003 article "Windows in Space/Time: A Personal Perspective on Birth and Death," which Diony published in *Birth: Issues in Perinatal Care*. Writing that article was excruciating yet worth it—Diony later told me that it became the most-read article they had published to that date, so I can hope that it has helped others through their own grief processes. It is freely available at www.davis-floyd.com.

The social movement for humanistic maternity care under a true midwifery model is in process around the world. I described what I learned about how people are creating that movement in many countries via 21 essential steps in "Changing Childbirth: The Latin American Example" (Davis-Floyd 2007). In any particular country, the movement may start with midwives themselves (as in Latvia and particularly New Zealand, which after almost losing midwifery completely by the 1980s, now has one of the best midwifery models in the world),[3] or with doulas, childbirth/breastfeeding educators, and engaged consumers who are outraged or simply damaged by the intense overmedicalization of their births. I have had the honor of speaking multiple times at the International Congress of Midwives (ICM). This conference is held every three years and is attended by thousands of professional midwives from all over the world. At the ICM Glasgow conference in 2007, I was beyond delighted that my session on "Birth Models That Work" was one of only two that were so in demand—so many people were turned away at the door—that ICM asked me to offer it a second time, in a huge and very full ballroom. I think the popularity of that talk and of the book on which it is based speaks volumes to midwives' deep desires to find, create, replicate, and sustain birth models that truly do work to produce excellent statistical outcomes and high quality care, and to the value of anthropological perspectives on how those models were created and what makes them work.

Out of deep gratitude, I should also mention that MANA honored myself and Barbara Katz Rothman at their 2012 conference in Asilomar, California. In a surprise ceremony during a general session, they presented us, separately, with beautiful framed certificates that read:

> Beloved Midwife to the Movement, for years of visioning, researching, and communicating the essence of midwifery to the larger world and unending advocacy for midwives, the midwifery model of care, and the Midwives Alliance.

Barbara was speechless during her standing ovation, and I was in tears during mine.

I taught anthropology at various universities for over 25 years, have published in a number of anthropological journals, reviewed for many more, organized and chaired panels at the Annual Meetings of the American Anthropological Association for 10 years straight, mentored a generation of students in the anthropology of reproduction, still serve as senior advisor to the Council on Anthropology and Reproduction (CAR), and have and will always con-

[3] New Zealand's outstanding midwifery system is the result of a midwifery renaissance that took place there during the 1980s and 1990s (see Hendry 2009; Guilliland forthcoming). On my most recent speaking tour there, I was asked to meet with the faculty members of various midwifery educational programs. Their primary questions to me were, "How can we preserve the wonderful system we have? What dangers should we watch out for?" It was extremely encouraging to be asked those sorts of questions, rather than the usual "What must we do to make it better?"

sider myself an anthropologist first. Yet my path has turned far more to activism than to "pure anthropology." My presentations to the birth community are and have to be theoretically based, as I am not a practitioner. Yet I've interviewed literally hundreds of practitioners and have worked to internalize their realities and to be able to see the world from their points of view, so that I can present both theoretical and practical perspectives in my talks.

Forging My Path and Passing on Gitti's Mantle: An Ongoing Journey

I've never been the kind of activist who carries placards or lobbies in legislatures, but my writings and public presentations, I am told, have inspired and given fresh impetus to those who do. I am a better activist because I'm an anthropologist, and I can therefore take the broader view, explain the other side, and make the invisible seen. And I'm a better anthropologist because my activism makes me care deeply and passionately about getting it right and keeps me engaged in childbirth research for the long term, so that I can track changes and trends, note the nuances, and detect the implications of events as they unfold.

I no longer teach at university, but I do still travel to give talks and have several books in process—via two of them I am beginning to slowly pass on Gitti's "birth mantle" to Melissa (Missy) Cheyney, who is both a tenured professor of anthropology and a practicing CPM. (She is profiled in Chapter 8.) Together we will coedit a replacement for Jordan's *Birth in Four Cultures*, which I had revised and updated in 1993 and is still being used for teaching. The working title is *Birth in Eight Cultures*. Missy will also be my coauthor for the complete update and revision of my first book, *Birth as an American Rite of Passage*.

With internationally renowned Canadian midwife Betty-Anne Daviss as lead editor, and myself as her happy sidekick, we are nearing completion of *Speaking Truth to Power: Birth Models on the Human Rights Frontier.* Betty-Anne and I are also both coeditors for *Sustainable Birth*, lead-edited by anthropologist Kim Gutshow. And I'm slowly putting together a book of short stories I've been working on for years about certain episodes in my life, to be called (tentatively), *Robbie's Reader: Vignettes of My Magical Life*.

I also take in student interns who wish to live and study with me for various periods of time, perhaps to work on their dissertations with my assistance, or simply to learn about a particular aspect of reproductive anthropology that interests them. (I can be reached at davis-floyd@austin.utexas.edu.) As I hope my readers will agree, I did indeed find my answer—well, many answers—to the question I asked Diony Young so many years ago, quoted at the beginning of this chapter. It has been a great adventure, and the journey is ongoing! And I hope my anthropologist-as-activist story will inspire budding social scientists to remember that paths to activism via applied anthropology—using anthropology to help others and create positive change—can be, and indeed usually are, forged where there is no prior path to follow. As my Mexican friends would sing:

> *Caminante no hay camino (Walker, there is no road)*
> *Se hace el camino al andar (The path is made as you walk)*

Questions for Thought and Discussion

1. What do you think about Davis-Floyd's combination of anthropology and activism?
2. Should anthropology be confined to the arena of scholarship, or should anthropologists try to make a difference in the cultural arenas they explore?

15

Creating the International MotherBaby Childbirth Initiative (IMBCI)

Anthropologically Informed Activism

This chapter tells the story of the creation of an international initiative designed to improve childbirth care and childbirth and breastfeeding outcomes for all women and my role in that process—a role that I felt very privileged to play and that was specifically informed by my anthropological perspective.

The Role of CIMS and the Creation of the IMBCI

The Coalition for Improving Maternity Services (CIMS) was founded in 1996 in the US with a mission to promote a wellness model of maternity care to improve birth outcomes. The founders of CIMS (including myself),

This chapter is adapted (revised and updated) from "The International MotherBaby Childbirth Initiative: Working to Achieve Optimal Maternity Care Worldwide" by Robbie Davis-Floyd, Debra Pascali-Bonaro, Mayri Sagady-Leslie, Helene Vadeboncoeur, Rae Davies, and Rodolfo Gomez Ponce de Leon. *International Journal of Childbirth* 1(3): 196–212, 2011. Used here by permission of the other authors and the journal.

created the *Mother-Friendly Childbirth Initiative (MFCI): 10 Steps to Mother-Friendly Hospitals, Birth Centers, and Home Birth Services* for the US. In 2005, in response to multiple requests from around the world to create a global initiative that would work for all countries, CIMS created an International Committee. It later evolved into the International MotherBaby Childbirth Organization (IMBCO), with the internationally renowned childbirth educator, doula trainer, and film producer Debra Pascali-Bonaro as chair and myself and five other birth activist leaders as members. We created an international network of regional and country representatives and, with help from the Center for Women's Health Research at the University of North Carolina, conducted a global survey of the MFCI 10 Steps. This survey assured us that there was indeed strong international support for the MFCI 10 Steps, which gave us a sound basis for creating what we eventually called the *International MotherBaby Childbirth Initiative* (IMBCI).

The survey also gave us a clear mandate on what Step 1 of the IMBCI should be: Treat every woman with respect and dignity, fully informing and involving her in decision making about care for herself and her baby in language that she understands, and providing her the right to informed consent and refusal. Every organization we contacted around the world insisted that this is the most essential mandate to stress in Step 1, as respect and dignity during labor and birth are so often ignored in favor of disrespect and outright obstetric (or midwifery) violence and abuse.

Our next steps were to create a technical advisory group (TAG) consisting of representatives from all the major international agencies involved with maternity care, obtain funding, and hold a meeting in Geneva in June 2006 to develop the initial draft of the initiative. (See Box below for a list of the agencies that sent representatives.) We spent hours refining the wording of

TAG Participants

- WHO
- UNICEF
- UNFPA
- International Confederation of Midwives (ICM)
- International Pediatric Association (IPA)
- International Council of Nurses (ICN)
- Partnership for Maternal, Newborn, and Child Health
- Childbirth Connection
- Alliance for Breastfeeding Action
- DONA International
- Lamaz International
- LaLeche League
- Academy of Breastfeeding Medicine
- University of North Carolina Women's Health Research
- Save the Children
- White Ribbon Alliance for Safe Motherhood

the document in an exhausting yet rewarding group consensus process. As designated editor (I had been the lead editor for the MFCI back in 1995, so it made sense for me to be lead editor this next time around), I had a preliminary draft up on PowerPoint, and for two afternoons I took verbal suggestions from the TAG representatives, sometimes shouted out with much discussion around every word. Each night I sat up late incorporating all the verbal suggestions, to present it all again the next day, while the rest of our committee worked on strategy.

Serendipitously, right after this TAG meeting, I was headed to give some talks at the Hecvsante Nursing and Midwifery School in Switzerland. My IMBCO colleague Rae Davies had accompanied me, and together we convinced the entire faculty of the school to review the just-created IMBCI, which we had up on PowerPoint. Many of its steps regarding humane care had long been implemented in Switzerland, so the faculty went beyond those to encourage us to include a whole step on collaborative care—a major issue for Swiss midwives, as obstetricians there, as in many other countries, often took a top-down approach and did not bother to collaborate with the professional midwives. The Swiss midwives' suggestion became Step 9: "Provide a continuum of collaborative care with all relevant health care providers, institutions, and organizations."

In my role as lead editor, over the next year I gathered international input on the IMBCI 10 Steps, Philosophy, and Principles from representatives of all the relevant international organizations and around 100 childbirth experts, practitioners, and grassroots activists from many countries. I cannot begin to describe the intensity of this process! In the end, the final crafting of the IMBCI narrowed down to our five IMBCO board members at the time—Debra Pascali-Bonaro, Maureen Corry, Rae Davies, Mayri Sagady Leslie, and myself. We struggled over every single word, because we were writing an initiative intended to be applicable to the entire world, and we were just "five white girls" keenly aware that the needs and resources of low-, middle-, and high-income countries differ widely. (As we have expanded, our board has become much more diverse.) Our awareness of those differences led to many difficult yet rewarding conversations—for example, should we say that an optimal MotherBaby facility should offer both drug- and drug-free pain relief options? Clearly, the epidural is experienced by many women as a humanistic pain-relieving option during labor. Yet it carries risks and complications, especially if given too early in labor. Anthropology helped us realize that to insist on pain-relieving drugs would be to ask low-resource countries that cannot afford such drugs to provide them, which would be most unrealistic and unfair. On the other hand, drug-free pain-relieving interventions cost almost nothing, can be provided in any setting in any country, and are evidence-based as helping to relieve pain while causing no harm. So Step 4 reads:

> Provide drug-free comfort and pain-relieving methods during labour, explaining their benefits for facilitating normal birth and avoiding unnecessary harm, and showing women and their companions how to use these methods, including touch, holding, massage, laboring in water (where resources allow), and coping/relaxation techniques. Respect women's preferences and choices.

We finalized the wording of the IMBCI and launched it at the CIMS Annual Meeting in Florida on International Women's Day in March 2008 to much celebration and acclaim!

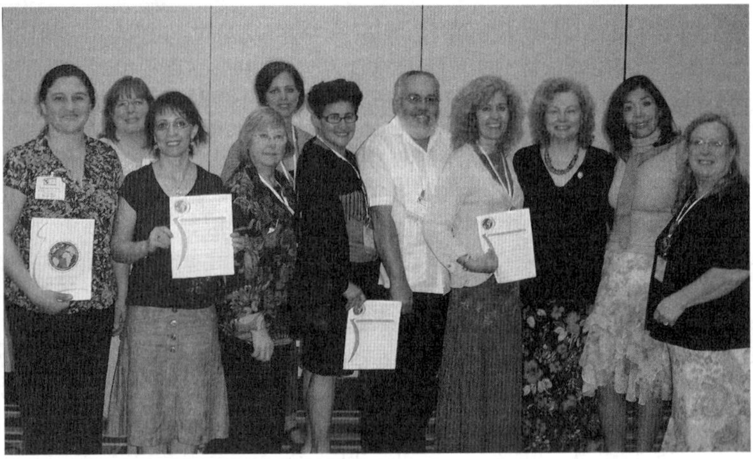

The IMBCO board and some of our regional representatives collectively launching the IMBCI at a CIMS conference in Florida, March 2008. Photo by Jay Hathaway

The MotherBaby, and Women's Rights as Human Rights

We value the mother and her baby as an inseparable and interdependent whole.
— Excerpt from the MANA Statement of Values and Ethics

An important contribution of the IMBCI is the "MotherBaby" model of care. "MotherBaby" is a term first used by Audrey Naylor MD, DrPH (Doctor of Public Health), a pediatrician and CEO of Wellstart International, who sees mothers and babies as a single, interdependent unit, inseparable throughout the continuum of care. Another critical component of the IMBCI is its insistence that "women's and children's rights are human rights" and that "access to humane and effective health care is a basic human right." This assertion is consonant with several recent initiatives. In June 2009, the United Nations Human Rights Council passed a landmark resolution that recognizes "preventable maternal mortality and morbidity as a pressing human-rights issue that violates a woman's rights to health, life, education, dignity and information." In 2010, Amnesty International released *Deadly Delivery: The Maternal Health Care Crisis in the US*, which frames the issue of maternal health care as a human rights issue. While a public health focus on maternal mortality is not new in the global arena, this focus has been virtually invisible in the US. The large, international Women Deliver conferences of 2007, 2010, and 2013, which we attended and which brought together thousands of experts and advocates from around the world, also focused on human rights. To support these efforts, we at IMBCO extrapolated the MotherBaby rights inherent in the IMBCI (found at www.imbci.org).

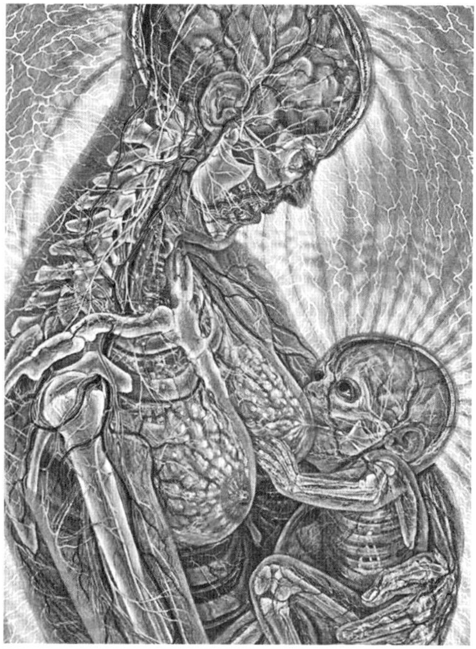

A holistic depiction of the MotherBaby as united in one energy field. Image courtesy of Mary Kroeger

IMBCO's Ongoing Work

Seeking to document the results of implementation of the IMBCI 10 Steps, our board is working with three pilot/demonstration sites: Hôpital Brome Missisquoi Perkins in Quebec; Community Hospital Feldbach, Austria; and Hospital Sofia Feldman, Belo Horizonte, Brazil (see Chapter 5 for photos of this hospital). We are still seeking funding for the research components—all funds obtained will be granted to the demonstration sites for trainings and statistical documentation of the results. *IMBCO would also welcome researchers to study the process of implementation and document both the barriers these sites and others may face and the outcomes we hope they achieve.*

The IMBCI has now been translated into over 20 languages; a number of independent practices have taken it as their chartering document and are working to implement it in their countries on their own. We call them MotherBaby networks (MBnets), and are always open to receiving applications from more (see www.imbci.org). One of our MBnets is Mercy in Action, whose staff members undertook disaster relief efforts after Super-Typhoon Haiyan/Yolanda, which struck the Philippines in November 2013. In a tent, with no running water and no electricity, they attended 165 births with successful outcomes, and provided pre- and postnatal care to thousands of women, managing to implement all of the IMBCI 10 Steps (which they had translated into the local dialect and posted everywhere) in every case of care. Their success in this endeavor showed us that, indeed, the IMBCI 10 Steps can be implemented almost anywhere, from a tertiary-care hospital to a disaster zone.

The FIGO Initiative and a Possible Merger with the IMBCI

One of our initial thoughts as we created the IMBCI was to seek formal endorsement for it from all of the organizations included in our initial TAG group (see box above). But their boards usually only meet once a year, and we knew that it might take years and lots of negotiated wording changes to accomplish that goal. So we simply proceeded to disseminate the IMBCI worldwide via our birth networks, yet always with the hope that someday such international endorsement might be achieved and perhaps we could turn the dissemination and implementation of the IMBCI over to a much larger and more stable organization such as WHO. The IMBCO board members work on a voluntary basis, and while we are quite stable and functional for the foreseeable future, again, we have no funding to allow us to evaluate the results of the IMBCI's implementation in the sites that choose to use the IMBCI 10 Steps as their practice guidelines.

In 2014, the International Federation of Gynecology and Obstetrics (known as FIGO, the acronym for its name in French), published an article called "FIGO Guidelines: Mother-Baby Friendly Birthing Facilities," in conjunction with ICM, WRA, IPA, and WHO. This global initiative is focused on improving quality of care in birthing facilities worldwide, as is the IMBCI. Like the IMBCI, it stresses the overuse of technological interventions in birth, and, going beyond the IMBCI, states firmly that simply moving birth away from home and into facilities in developing countries is not working to lower mortality and morbidity rates because the care in many of those hospitals and clinics is so dehumanizing. The FIGO initiative calls for the complete elimination of "obstetric violence" (Sadler et al. 2016) and of non-evidence-based interventions around the world. We had tried to be included in the process of their creating this initiative, but they had their own committee, yet they did include much that was already in the IMBCI, so there is plenty of common ground between the two.

Noting the many similarities in these two global initiatives, we at IMBCO have been in dialogue with FIGO about merging the two. FIGO representative Dr. Andre Lalonde and I have already begun to work on the first draft of this proposed merger, combining our Principles, Steps, and Global Context sections. Should I, my board, and the FIGO committee charged with working on this merger manage to produce a viable merged document that contains the best of both initiatives, and should it then be endorsed by all or most of the TAG organizations and others, then we at IMBCO will have realized our dream of scaling up our efforts to a more global and sustainable level. This process has just begun and will take some time to accomplish. Stay posted for the results, which will be reported at www.imbci.org.

Completion of this merger may mean that the final document will be a bit more medicalized than the IMBCI itself—for example, to the Step on pain relief we might have to add something like "Offer non-pharmacological pain relief measures during labour as safe first options. When requested or needed, provide pharmacological pain relief options, explaining their benefits and risks. Respect women's choices." So for those organizations, like Mercy in Action, whose members have worked hard to implement and disseminate the IMBCI 10 Steps, they can rest assured that we will not "disappear" the IMBCI—it will still stand as its own separate document for many years to come, available as the excellent template it is for fully humanistic and holistic maternity care practice.

Conclusion: The Educational and Instrumental Goals of the IMBCI

Rising cesarean rates around the world, the increasing overuse of obstetric technologies, and failure to implement the scientific evidence in favor of normal, physiologic birth have created the need for clear guidelines for providing optimal maternity care. The purpose of the IMBCI 10 Steps, like the purpose of the FIGO initiative, is to improve care throughout the childbearing continuum in order to save lives, prevent illness and harm from the overuse of obstetric technologies, and promote health for mothers and babies. The IMBCI addresses the needs of all nations and birthing women for evidence-based and humanistic improvements in the quality of maternity care. The educational purpose of the IMBCI is to call global attention to the importance of the quality of the mother's birth experience and its impact on the outcome, the risks to mother and baby from inappropriate medical interventions, and the scientific evidence showing the benefits of MotherBaby-centered care based on the normal physiology of pregnancy, birth, and breastfeeding and on attention to women's individual needs. The instrumental purpose of the IMBCI is to put into worldwide awareness and practice the MotherBaby model of care—a woman-centered, noninterventive approach that promotes the health and well-being of all women and babies, setting the gold standard for excellence and superior outcomes in maternity care. The full text of the IMBCI is available at www.imbci.org. Individuals and organizations can sign on as supporters of the IMBCI, adopt it as a focal point for their work, and use it as an educational template and guide to help hospitals and other practices to improve their maternity care. We welcome your support!

Questions for Thought and Discussion

1. Why was the IMBCI created?
2. What is Step 1 and why is it needed?
3. What are the instrumental and educational goals of the IMBCI?
4. What were some of the global challenges the IMBCO board faced as we tried to create an initiative that could apply in all settings?
5. If you have interest in birth, how can you and others support and utilize the IMBCI 10 Steps and spread the word about their existence?

Recommended Films

Violência Obstétrica—A voz das brasileiras (Obstetric Violence: The Voice of Brazilian Women): (2012). Available at https://www.youtube.com/watch?v=eg0uvonF25M (A subtitled version in English is available.)

Five Countries, Six Births, Seven Babies: Mother Nature's Design for Birth: produced by Love Delivers. Showcases homebirths in Guatemala, Costa Rica, France, the USA, and Bermuda. The individual chapters in the film make it easy to use in classes, conferences, and lectures. Available at www.midwiferytoday.com

The Time Is Now/Birth and the Primal Period: The Path to Full Human Potential, Volume 1: producer/director Suzanne Arms, 2012. Features perspectives from Kenya, Brazil, the Peruvian Amazon, the Canary Islands, Spain, and the USA. 1 hr 45 min.

The Time Is Now/Birth and the Primal Period: The Path to Full Human Potential, Volume 2: producer/director Suzanne Arms, 2013. Features perspectives from Israel, Egypt, England, Sri Lanka, Mexico, Appalachia, and California.

The Time Is Now/Birth and the Primal Period: The Path to Full Human Potential, Volume 3: producer/director Suzanne Arms, 2014. Features perspectives from Mexico, Canada, Sudan, Venezuela, and the USA.

Epilogue

Inner Space and Outer Space as Cyberspace? Technocratizing Womb and World

The Myth of Technological Transcendence

> *We're getting the first peeks at a bouquet of technologies that could vastly improve the lives of most people on the planet and solve some of our hardest problems—even climate change. Just consider for a moment how much everyday life has been transformed since 2007, when smartphones, social networks, and cloud computing took off at about the same time. What we're going to experience in the next decade, from 2017 to 2027, will make that stuff seem as ho-hum as a wall socket. Artificial intelligence . . . is going to take civilization on a great leap forward. . . . AI is how we're going to find a cure for cancer in the next decade. It's how we're going to build livable cities. It's how we'll stop terrorists before they strike. . . . Humanity is now entering a period of radical transformation in which technology has the potential to significantly raise the basic standards of living for every man, woman, and child on the planet.*
>
> — Diamantis and Kotler, in *Abundance: The Future Is Better Than You Think*

> *Future people will envy us, wishing they could have witnessed the birth we saw.*
>
> — Kevin Kelly, *The Inevitable*

In her pioneering and influential "Cyborg Manifesto," Donna Haraway (1991) presented a paradigm of cyborgification that balances irony with posi-

This chapter was originally a paper presented at the Annual Meetings of the American Anthropological Association, December 1994, Atlanta. I have revised, expanded, and updated it for this book.

tivism, skepticism with hopefulness. Rejecting both the mind-focused patriarchy of old and the body-focused new feminisms, she eschews God and Goddess in favor of the "dangerous possibilities," the infinite expansions allowed and potentiated by transgressing the boundaries between organisms and machines. Haraway takes the notion of the cyborg—"an ultimate self untied at last from all dependency"—from prosthetized humans (e.g., artificial limbs or hearts), through science fiction characters, all the way to "a man in space." Looking at objects and persons as integrated systems, she sees no "natural" architectural constraints on system design, noting that in a cybernetic world "the entire universe of objects that can be known scientifically [can] be formulated as problems in communications engineering" (Haraway 1991:163).

This Epilogue is a think-piece that addresses both macro- and microcosmic versions of systemic issues in communications engineering, in remembrance of that ancient Hermetic phrase that was at one time supposed to encapsulate universal truth—*as above, so below.* In the past, that phrase evoked Mystery—the miracle and wonder of seeing the universe in a grain of sand, or the human life cycle writ large in the stars. Unwilling to remain in the mystery, Western culture has probed and penetrated the natural world, both stellar and cellular, and is now engaged in the technological transformation of that world on all levels. I want to speak here about cybernetic transformations on two of those levels—the part of outer space most contiguous to the planet (once the domain of myth, and now the domain of satellites), and the fetus in the womb (once the domain of woman and of nature, and now, increasingly, the domain of technology and of culture). The cyborgian transformations we are wringing on each of these levels parallel each other and speak in their own expressive ways of our massive technological incursions into all organic domains. The picture they paint is clear enough to me—it shows what I have long called "the myth of technological transcendence"—the story we tell ourselves about how all the problems we are creating with technology can be solved with more technology. I hope in this brief essay to paint that picture for you as well. Its outlines are just now being drawn. Whether they are all filled in is still a matter of human choice.

A Vision for Commercializing Outer Space: The SATWG Story

As above, so below—so let's begin with the cyborgification of the planet. For four years during the 1990s, I attended (and sometimes gave presentations on human evolution, or on the results of my oral history interviews with early NASA pioneers at) the meetings of a NASA/aerospace industry group then called the Strategic Avionics Technology Working Group (acronymically known as SATWG). I did so because at the time I was teaching a course at Rice University in Houston, and I was invited by then-Chair George Marcus to participate in an edited collection he was organizing called *Late Editions VII: Para-Sites,* which was largely focused on technologies. One of the leaders of SATWG, Kenneth J. Cox, had heard me give a talk on human evolution at a conference and subsequently invited me to attend SATWG meetings because he thought I would be interested in their evolutionary work—and indeed I was, as I thought attending the meetings might spark some ideas for a chapter I could write for Marcus' collection. (I had originally thought I might write about the development and rapid spread of the electronic fetal monitor, but it's good to change the subject sometimes and explore new horizons!)

The participants in the SATWG forums included avionics experts from NASA headquarters and field centers, aerospace engineering prime contractors, leading avionics systems suppliers, small businesses that supported NASA programs, professional societies, and selected universities. SATWG (later renamed ATWG) held meetings twice a year, usually hosted by major aerospace corporations at hotels near their corporate headquarters. The host companies, which over the period of my research included Boeing, Rockwell, Hughes, Lockheed, McDonnell Douglas, and Motorola, offered SATWG participants guided tours of their plants and offices as well as demonstrations of new products and technologies. Such companies were looking for an end to the painful layoffs and "downsizings" they were forced to undergo by government budget cuts in the late 1980s. They found some of that end in the development of new commercial products such as Boeing's 777, and they hoped to find a great deal more of it in the commercial development and exploitation of outer space.

My interest in this group was originally sparked by the oxymoronic nature of its major charter—to develop a "shared vision for the commercialization of outer space." The juxtaposition of "vision" with "commercialization" that took me aback turned out to quite accurately express a set of tensions and paradoxes in their collaborative work between the simple capitalist desire to make a buck, and the unavoidable sense that efforts to fulfill this desire in outer space intrinsically carry a transcendent meaning and purpose—perhaps the next evolutionary jump for the human species. (See Davis-Floyd 2000a, "Commercializing Outer Space: The SATWG Stories" for a full accounting of my ethnographic work with SATWG, and *Space Stories: Oral Histories from the Pioneers of the American Space Program*, eds. Davis-Floyd, Cox, and White 2012 for more of its results.)

One of the major areas of concern for these NASA and aerospace industry leaders was at the time of my fieldwork and remains today the enormously lucrative satellite market—a commercial venture that can be seen as a step toward the stars, but itself remains closer to earth, exploiting the market niche of LEO—low earth orbit. At my first SATWG meeting in Washington, DC, in 1994, a presentation by Ken Cureton of Rockwell on "International Space Competitiveness Issues" identified four primary areas in the international commercial space market: communications satellites and services, weather satellites, earth observation satellites, and the vehicles needed to launch them. For example, although at the time space communications only accounted for 5% per year of the total worldwide communications industry ($40 billion/year in 1993), Cureton pointed out that space communications were expected to continue as the largest potential growth space market, constituting a tremendous opportunity for commercial competition. Thus, the key to increased competitiveness in the satellite communications market was launch vehicle capacity. Moans and groans were heard when Cureton noted that in the 1970s the US had held 100% of the commercial launch vehicle market, a percentage that dropped to 51% in the 1980s as the French gained a corner on the market (40% European Space Agency [ESA], 9% others) through their Ariane program; and to 34% in the 1990s, as ESA's market share climbed to 52%, and China's new program took 8%, with 6% split between the Russians and the Japanese. Concurrently, the US had lost its edge in the commercial satellite market as well (87% in the 1970s, 71% in the 1980s, 63% in the 1990s). SATWG as a group was dedicated in part to helping the US aerospace industry reclaim as much as possible of that lost market share. The more launch vehicles we can produce, they said, the more satellites we can put into LEO, and the more money we can make.

The Big Picture: Satellites, Space Debris, and Planet Earth as a Cyborg

At that point it occurred to me to look at the big picture, and I began to wonder how many satellites were presently in orbit all together. Every time I asked one of the guys, he would look at me funny, because that is not the kind of question aerospace engineers ask. Nobody knew exactly, but here is what I learned at that meeting:

Numbers of communications satellites:

- Ellipso (MCHI) 20
- Odyssey (TRW) 20
- Globalstar (Lora) 48
- Iridium (Motorola and Sprint) 66
- Teledesic (Gates and the cable companies) 840

That makes 994 communications satellites that were in orbit in the late 1990s, not to mention the weather, earth monitoring, and spy satellites up there. By 2017 the total number of satellites in orbit was 3,671; 1,071 of them were functional—half of those were in LEO while the rest were higher up.[1] Around 2,600 satellites that no longer function are still in orbit, not to mention space

[1] https://www.google.com/search?q=satellites+in+low+earth+orbit&rlz=1C2EODB_enUS509US518&biw=1166&bih=638&tbm=isch&imgil=dGPgoD_7fXvXQM%253A%253B45; see also http://talkingpointsmemo.com/idealab/satellites-earth-orbit

debris, which, according to writer Fraser Cain (2015), includes spent booster rockets, dead satellites, and even misplaced gloves. Cain states, "According to the United States Space Surveillance Network, there are more than 21,000 objects larger than 10 cm orbiting the Earth. It's estimated there are a further 500,000 bits and pieces between 1 and 10 cm in size." And he continues:

> Near Earth orbit is so polluted with junk that the International Space Station is often moved to avoid impact with dangerous chunks of space debris. Many of these objects are created through collisions, and some scientists are worried that future space travel might be too risky if we get too much junk orbiting the planet. We might seal ourselves inside a shield of shrieking metal moving at 29,000 km/hour. (http://www.universetoday.com/42198/how-many-satellites-in-space/)

If you have seen the Disney movie *Wall-E*, you know exactly what he is talking about.

So what do all the working satellites do? They ensure that anyone with a cellular phone (defined by Google as "a telephone with access to a cellular radio system so it can be used over a wide area, without a physical connection to a network") can call anyone else, anywhere in the world, through the interaction of signals bounced between satellites and terrestrial systems. They let somebody on top of a mountain or in the middle of the Amazon pinpoint his exact location on the map on GPS or send an email or text. They allow TV stations to send a clear signal through their very own satellite systems, and almost any home anywhere to receive it. They track weather patterns with high efficiency, and take extraordinarily detailed photographs of toxic waste dumps, soil erosion patterns, and the effects of acid rain, help to pinpoint possible archaeological sites for excavation, and can also show the armaments, military training sites, aircraft capabilities, and so forth, of other nations and of terrorist groups.

Back at those SATWG meetings, I discovered that, including satellites, there were at the time (the late 1990s) 7,000 objects bigger than 10 cm in LEO that were being tracked by the North American Aerospace Defense Command. So I started to wonder, how many satellites can be tracked? And how many would fit in LEO before they start running into each other? No one could give me a clear answer about that—it depends on type and altitude of orbit, etc., but the overall message was, in effect, the sky's the limit—they were talking *tens of thousands*. I woke up that night dreaming about the planet ringed by thousands and thousands of satellites, all sucking information up from the earth, zinging that information back and forth to each other, and beaming it back down. My *American Heritage Dictionary* defines symbiosis as "a close, prolonged association between two or more different organisms of different species that may, but does not necessarily, benefit each member." *A cyborg is a techno-organic system, a symbiotic fusion of organism and machine,* and so I believe that the system created by the organic earth orbited

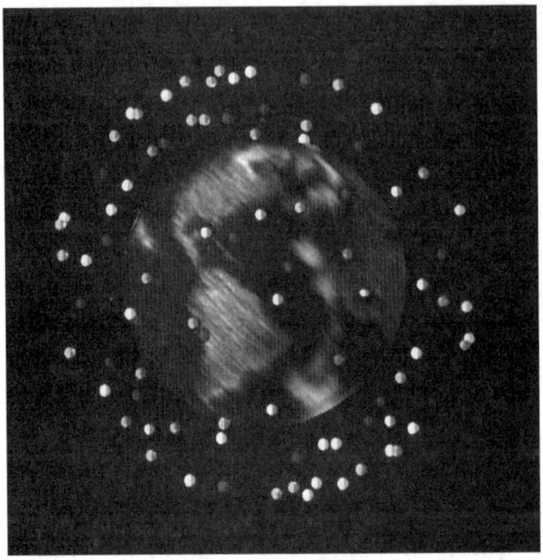

Graphic image of the earth surrounded by orbiting satellites. Drawing by Robert N. Floyd

by technological artifacts and in constant interaction with many of those artifacts is a cyborg—and that is a happening thing.

As Haraway might point out, there is much that is positive in this symbiotic fusion. For example, warnings of weather shifts can save thousands of lives. Earth monitoring satellites are showing us extremely detailed and impressive photographs of the environmental degradation that is only visible in its full ugliness from way up high. We can see the effects of the toxins leaking out of the barrels near Niagara, the massive soil erosion of the Everglades, the silt pileup in the Mississippi Delta, the changes in ocean color from pollution, and the dying of the coral reefs. Such information is enormously useful to environmentalists, to legislators, to all those who are trying to get us to clean ourselves up. Communications satellites increase human contact—it is surely useful to reach out and touch someone, anyone, anywhere on a cell phone—in fact, the wide, often grant-funded distribution of cell phones in developing countries has already prevented countless maternal and fetal mortalities, reminding us that we are all cybernetically connected in the vast web of technolife. In this limitless market, the opportunities for profit, for jobs, for the continued growth of our service- and information-based economy are truly awesome.

But what about the dangers in those cyborgian "dangerous possibilities"? At SATWG meetings, I heard only unreflexive enthusiasm about the good things that are coming from this techno-growth. The only price these engineers and industry leaders see that will have to be paid is the cost of developing new and more efficient launch vehicles to compete for market share with the Russians, the French, the Chinese, and the Japanese. This price at the time was so enormous—more than $15 billion to develop one new rocket—that the American government was not willing to fund the development of the needed launch capability, and no one company was capable of doing so. Consequently, at SATWG meetings, there was much discussion about how to share that price between industry and government, and even between nations.

What was never discussed is the other price—the environmental price. No one asked what will be the effects on humans, animals, the ecosystem of vastly increasing the number of satellite signal waves passing through our bodies, through our food, through the body of the planet. No one proposed studies on what effects the ever-increasing number of rockets taking off to launch those satellites might have on the ozone layer every time they punch a hole through it. What about the exhaust chemicals? the space debris? Instead, they talked about poking more and more holes—they wanted to add to the satellites in orbit (and to the thousands of pieces of space trash also in orbit), passenger vehicles so tourists can take a spin into outer space at $50,000 a pop, planes that can circle the globe in two hours by penetrating to outer space, going halfway around the world, penetrating the atmosphere again, then landing. They were green with envy over Japanese plans to build earth-orbiting hotels and a lunar outpost by 2020, a full-fledged lunar-orbiting hotel by 2030, an outpost on Mars and a Mars orbiting hotel by 2040, and a colony on Mars by 2050, and especially over the fact that those plans were being laid by a consortium of Japanese corporations who could afford to carry them out.

Cyborg Birth and a Holistic Story

It must be obvious to my readers that this sort of fieldwork was a real departure for me, as my primary focus as long been on the other topics covered in this volume—women, childbirth, midwifery, and medicine. Oddly enough, it was my birth research that brought me to a newer interest in cyborgs.

In my first book, *Birth as an American Rite of Passage* (2003 [1992]), I analyzed obstetrical procedures as ritual enactments of the technocratic myth of ultimate control of and transcendence over nature. As I have often stated in the preceding chapters, through hospital routines, organic childbirth is deconstructed into identifiable and controllable segments and reconstructed as a mechanistic process for the production of new social members. At first shocked by women's complicity with such a system, I ultimately came to understand how it serves women's felt needs to be full partners in the technocracy. When I asked professional women, "What is your body?" I was told, "My body is a vehicle that carries me around, a tool for my success in the world." They insisted that they did not want to "drop into biology," that they preferred to be intellectual and emotional women, but would just as soon leave the biology behind (see Chapter 3). I came to see the epidurals they were demanding as the perfect lived expression of Cartesian mind/body dualism—a dualism that these women experienced as real and actually valued, for in the separation of intellect from biology, they felt they achieved a degree of freedom from both the biological and the psychological constraints of womanhood that their predecessors would have envied.

I came finally to understand the American obstetric system as the co-creation of women and obstetricians who profoundly distrust nature and the human body, and just as profoundly trust the technological manifestations produced by human bodies. So when I first read Donna Haraway on cyborgs, I felt the shock of recognition—the most graphic example of a cyborg that I personally could think of was a laboring woman belted to a fetal monitor, especially when her consciousness became interlinked with that monitor.

My readers will remember this quote from Chapter 2, "Once I was hooked up, no one even looked at me any more—they all just stared at the machine. So I started staring at it too, and pretty soon I got the feeling that *it* was having the baby, not me." Was she horrified by this psychic techno-takeover, this cybernetic co-option of her birth experience? Not really. Her response was to demand a cesarean. Through the further cyborgification of her body and the technological production of her fetus, she found both release from bothersome biology and a way to regain a measure of personal control—she lived, in other words, Haraway's optimistic scenarios of "dangerous possibilities and infinite expansions." As an anthropologist, my job was to not to judge but to understand and speak for her, showing the correspondences between her attitudes and those of the wider culture, which I have done, I hope successfully, in a number of publications, including those revised and updated for this volume. Personally, I could not relate. I found the measure of my own subjectivities in the unadulterated organicity of the homebirthers I both interviewed and emulated.

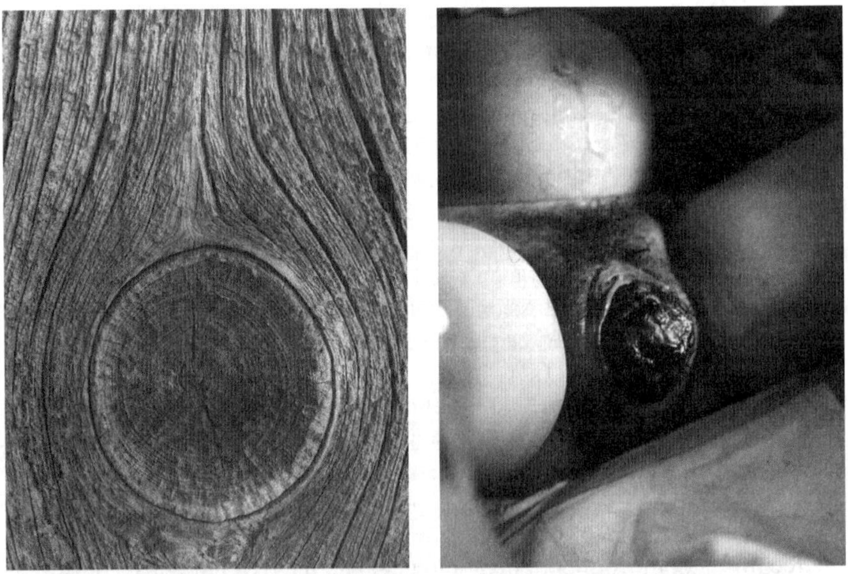

The photograph of the tree was taken by renowned birth photographer Harriette Hartigan, and is called "The Crowning." The birth photo, taken by homebirth midwife Faith Gibson, illustrates why.

I could simultaneously study and identify with ecofeminism; I could both interview and become an active supporter of the homebirth midwives who supported women to live out their organic embodiedness.

I plunged into research on homebirth midwifery and soon completed an article on midwives' astonishing willingness to sometimes rely solely on intuition—embodied inner knowing—even in this technocratic society that officially respects only information obtained from external diagnostic technologies (Chapter 7). But, in my ideological alignment with the Goddess these midwives re-present and my growing understanding of the degree to which this Goddess was excised from hospital technobirth, I was left with the dichotomies of mechanicity and holism, and I longed for a bridge. I found such a bridge in Haraway's cyborg visions, but I am uncomfortable standing on it, as the tensions between the dangers and the possibilities fill me with profound anxiety. That bridge does, however, allow me a hopeful and even heartful way of dealing with the thorough technologization of reproduction; that is, it provides a useful third perspective on the mechanistic/holistic dichotomy in which my birthwork had me stuck.

For example, my previous interpretations of the image below had to do with the symbolic messages of mechanicity sent to the mother through her attachment to the monitor—the message that her body is a defective machine that cannot give birth without the assistance of more perfect machines. In contrast, the cyborgian perspective enables me to look at this photo from multiple points of view. From the point of view of the woman, I know that the symbiosis between her body and the machine makes her feel reassured that everything is under control. She can see or be told when a contraction is coming, can prepare herself mentally, and can feel certain that the baby is

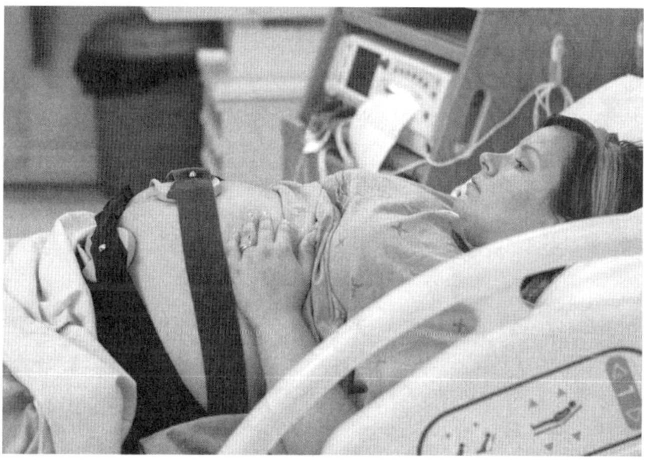

A laboring mother hooked up to the electronic fetal monitor.
Photo by Tyler Olson/Shutterstock.com

fine when it is over, because of her faith in the authority of the machine and those who interpret its squiggles to her. They engage her mind, the part she most values, in the enterprise of controlling a biological process of which she is somewhat afraid. From the point of view of the hospital staff, as long as the monitor is in place, so is the woman. They don't have to try to track her as she wanders the halls. They, too, can feel safe, in control, on top of the situation, because they have continuous access to the information they want—information that also enhances their authority.

From the point of view of the woman's body and the baby inside—well, that's a different story. This machine has her imprisoned in a position that is dysfunctional for labor. It compresses the blood vessels flowing to the baby and cuts down on the baby's oxygen supply, suppressing the bodily movements she might make that would correct this problem, and making the baby's active descent into the vagina more difficult because the compression of her pelvic bones from lying flat on her back gives the baby less room. These conditions often lead to cesarean section for fetal distress caused by the machine. Or the machine may give faulty readouts that lead to an unnecessary cesarean. Or it may diagnose real danger, real distress, and lead to a cesarean that is lifesaving. So we can see how this prosthetized human, this temporary cyborg, is fraught with ambiguity—the dangerous possibilities and infinite expansions of Haraway's vision.

Interestingly enough, I can apply that cyborgian perspective with far less anxiety to the cyborgification of the planet than to the cyborgification of the unborn child. There, my holism haunts me. I am only too aware of how a holistic perspective conceptualizes a child—as a conscious being, with intelligence, emotions, memory, awareness (see Chamberlain 1998). Midwives treat newborns that way—asking the baby's permission, explaining the procedure, and then weighing the baby in a soft cloth hanger. Contrast that with the mechanistic approach that sees the baby as product, unaware, without memory:

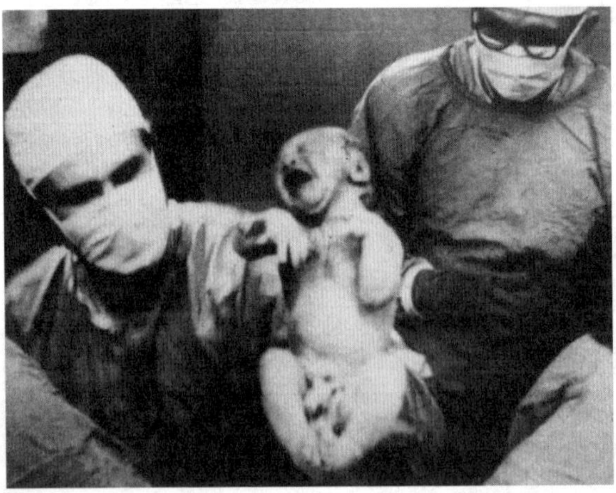

Baby as product.

I cannot forget or ignore the holistic assertion that conscious babies are damaged, wounded, traumatized by technobirth. Holistic homebirthers and midwives often reject amniocentesis; they feel that it is an invasion of the sacred space of the womb that disturbs the child's cocooned sense of safety. They reject repeated ultrasounds as harmful sonic disturbance. A very few of them might be aware, as I have just learned from a book called *OverPowered: What Science Tells Us about the Dangers of Cell Phones and other WiFi-Age Devices* (Blank 2014), that even a little overexposure to the electromagnetic forces generated by cell phones, the bases of cordless landline phones, microwave ovens, hair dryers, etc., have been correlated with higher rates of miscarriage (not to mention cancer), especially when the woman lives near power transformers and cell towers—all powerful generators of the electromagnetic fields and electromagnetic radiation that now practically blankets us all. They say that babies talked to in the womb via "prega-phones,"[2] stored in nurseries, and raised in cribs, plastic carriers, and playpens instead of being held in human arms will grow up bonded to technology instead of people (see Croissant 1998; Turkle 1998), as the photo at right suggests.

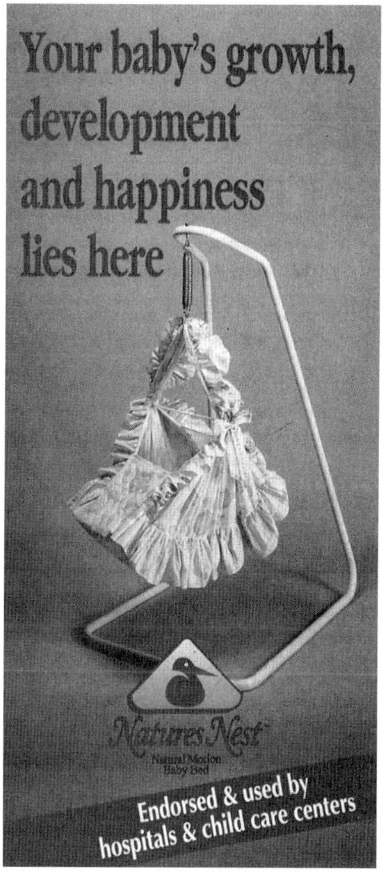

The implications of this are, of course, that we are creating a closed system—that the more we technologize birth and child raising, the more the adults so raised will want to technologize their environments, the more they will extend those technologies to conception, pregnancy, birth, and child raising. And so the notion of the cyborg becomes the only hopeful way of interpreting this process, because at least, even as cyborgification mechanizes humans, it also anthropomorphizes machines. And maybe that will get us somewhere good. I mean, if *Star Trek*'s Data is any kind of model, there may be benefits to this process that we have not foreseen. I don't see them yet. Instead, I see technocratic forces focused like

[2] For information about prega-phones, see https://news.google.com/newspapers?nid=1291&dat=19881221&id=GVpUAAAAIBAJ&sjid=l40DAAAAIBAJ&pg=2265,7823071&hl=en

lasers on babies, too often in lieu of human touch. We can grow them younger and younger now. Will the day come when we grow them from scratch?

And what happens if we can? I once saw a cartoon showing a couple getting an ultrasound; as they stare at their baby's image on the screen, the technician says, "Your baby is developing nicely; would you like to send him an email?" Funny, right? Well maybe not so much. What does thinking about sending our unborn child an email preclude us from thinking? In partial answer to that question, I will share a very personal story with you.

When my son was close to birth, he was facing the wrong way and the midwives wanted him to turn so that the birth would be easier. So I did a visualization with my doula Rima Star (now my best friend of 33 years). She asked me to imagine myself as a tiny being entering my body through my nose, going down through my esophagus into my tummy, then visualizing a window or door opening into my uterus. She went slowly, so I could fully hold that picture in my mind. Then she had me open the door and swim through. I swam around my baby, noting with satisfaction that he was in fact the boy I had intuitively known he would be (I never had an ultrasound during that pregnancy). When I got near his face, he cocked a sleepy eye at me and asked me silently, "What are you doing, here in my space?" I responded, equally silently, that he was a big baby and might be hard to birth, and that he was facing the wrong way and that would make the birth harder for both of us, so I asked him to turn around facing the other way.

In response I felt a wave of fear from him that if he turned, the umbilical cord would cut across his neck and choke him. I verbalized this fear to Rima, who quietly suggested that he could hold the cord in his hand before he turned and pull it down off his shoulder so it would not choke him. I silently made that suggestion to him, and received a wave of relief from him. I told him we were partners in this process, and that we both were going to have to work hard to get him born. Feeling his acceptance of that responsibility, I ended the visualization by telling him I loved him and could hardly wait to hold him in my arms. A few days later he turned, and two weeks later he was born holding the cord in his hand. That amazing experience taught me that as we expand into the infinite possibilities of our cyborgian future, we must also expand into the infinite possibilities of holism, which include those invisible forces we call energy, spirit, and soul.

Limitless Possibilities

It seems quite clear, at least for now, that the limits to the cyborgification of womb and world will not come from technology. I often asked techies at Motorola, at Draper, at the Johnson Space Center: Can we really send faxes from the beach? (Remember, this was 1994–1998; today that question is as anachronistic as: "Can machines ever fly?"). Can we make watches into phones? (Already done.) Can we design our genes? (A happening thing.) The future questions include: Can we grow babies in artificial wombs? (Not yet, thank goodness.) Build launch vehicles that are safe, fast, and cheap? (Already happening via private companies.) Put a hotel into LEO? (Such plans exist.) What are the limits to this technology? I always got the same answer to such questions: "*There are no limits. We can do anything.* All we need is the money." So I am left to wonder, will the organisms set the limits? Will sinkholes in the ozone layer put an end not only to spaceflight but also to airplane flights, as Starhawk predicted in her futuristic book *The Fifth Sacred Thing* (1993)? Will babies grown artificially turn out to be monsters incapable of love? Will the electromagnetic radiation fields buzzing around the earth—also generated by the smartphones glued to our ears—give us all cancer when they reach some critical mass? (According to Martin Blank in *Over-Powered,* their effect is cumulative—for instance, never stand in front of a microwave while using your cell phone—in fact, you should leave the kitchen entirely when the microwave is on.) Or will we, as the quotation at the beginning of this chapter assures us, find a cure for cancer via technology? In his final chapter, Blank notes that electromagnetic radiation at very low and specific dose has many healing applications. Yet he also stresses throughout his book that babies and young children are the most vulnerable to the actual changes in DNA that overexposure to electronic devices can generate, with potentially huge implications for their overall health and well-being. Particularly concerned about the installation of WiFi in schools, he notes:

> Children go to school at least 6 hours a day, 5 days a week, for about 36 weeks a year for approximately 12 years (until the child reaches college, where they will also be exposed to ubiquitous WiFi). This equates to 12,960 hours of exposure to WiFi microwave radiation, for each child, by the time that child graduates from high school—12,960 hours of exposure that could be avoided if the WiFi networks in schools are simply turned off and instead connected by cable. (Blank 2014:218)

Will we break through the dangers and expand into the very real possibilities? Or will the public make the paradigm shift so dear to the hearts of New Agers, alternative healers, and environmentalists, and go back to a more organic way of life? I doubt it.

After four days at the first SATWG meeting I attended in Washington, DC—four days of intense interaction with aerospace engineers and managers, intense effort to learn their language (which mostly consisted of dozens of acronyms) and see the world through their eyes, I was sufficiently on the inside to find myself accompanying them to a reception on Capitol Hill, to watch them lobby members of Congress to fund government support for a commercial space program. They were lobbying because they were nervous. The *Challenger* disaster had severely shaken public enthusiasm for the space program, and continuing cost overruns had eroded congressional support. Funding for the International

Space Station had survived by the thinnest of margins—two votes the other way could have killed it. There were many who felt that the money that was feeding NASA would be far better spent on feeding the homeless—including the wife of one of the prime movers at SATWG, who sat next to me on the subway on the way back to the hotel, confiding that she simply did not understand why the government should be encouraged to spend billions on space when there was so much that needed to be done right here on earth, even in this country.

I opened my mouth to agree, but what came out wasn't what I'd planned. What did I, the staunch defender of organic childbirth, of women's bodies, of the environment, say to this woman who was espousing what no doubt should have been my own position? I told her that I thought that the space program was essential to the future of our species, that we had to reach toward the stars in order to improve life on earth—NASA's own quintessential position! I cannot even plead co-option by the engineers I was studying as my excuse—rather, I blame it all on Captains Kirk, Picard, Sisko, and Janeway.

Okay fine, I admit it—Hi, I'm Robbie and I'm a Trekkie! I've seen every single episode of *Star Trek: Next Generation, Deep Space Nine,* and *Voyager* at least three times, and my personal vision of humans in space is permanently shaped by *Star Trek*'s ongoing enactment of Roddenberry's vision that space travel will help us improve ourselves, to rise above our imperfections to create a paradisiacal earth without war, pollution, racial or gender or even species hierarchies—or capitalist greed—and that space technologies will solve our physical and environmental problems.

My faith was intensified during the last SATWG meeting I attended in 1998, when John Hines from NASA began to talk about a program they were developing at Ames Research Center called Sensors 2000—a system of remote medical monitoring devices. When Hines got to the part about remote monitoring of the fetus during labor, and whipped out a model of a *Star Trek* tricorder, saying this was what they were developing to scan the laboring woman's body for the same information they now have to hook her up to the fetal monitor to provide, I thought that maybe my prayers would be answered—the techies were going to save us after all! The data hospital personnel crave would be available, yet the mother herself would be completely free to move around (again, movement during labor is the essence of a healthy birth).

Well, as of this writing (2017), so far there are still no tricorders in the labor and delivery rooms. Remote fetal monitoring does exist, and when it's used, women *can* move around as much as they like, but it has not so far proved popular with doctors and hospitals, most likely because they prefer the woman to be tethered to the machine that keeps her "in her place."[3] *As*

[3] For thoughtful discussions of whether cyborgs can be holistic too, see Davis-Floyd and Dumit 1998, *Cyborg Babies: From Techno-Sex to Techno-Tots*—in particular the chapters by Davis-Floyd ("From Technobirth to Cyborg Babies: Reflections on the Emergent Discourse of a Holistic Anthropologist"), Steven Mentor ("Witches, Nurses, Midwives, and Cyborgs"), and Anne Hill ("Children of Metis: Beyond Zeus the Creator").

above, so below. Let me conclude with a quote from a friend I ran into as I was writing the first iteration of this Epilogue back in 1994. She said that for her birthday, she had been invited to Florida to watch a shuttle launch, and it was one of the greatest thrills of her life. "It's just like—you're not going to believe this," she said, "but it's so big a thrill, it's better than sex. The only way I can describe it is that it's just like—giving birth!"

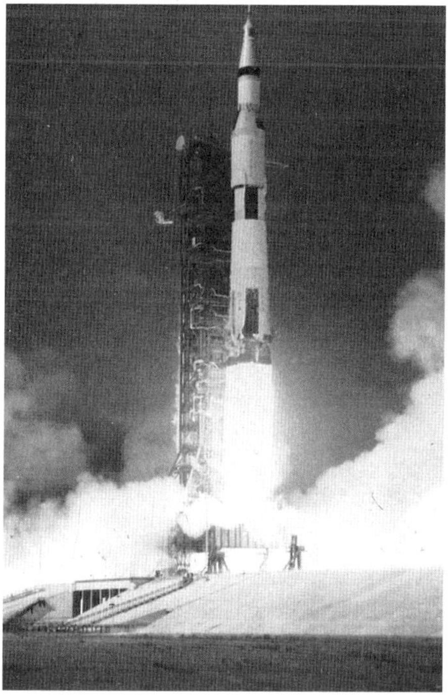

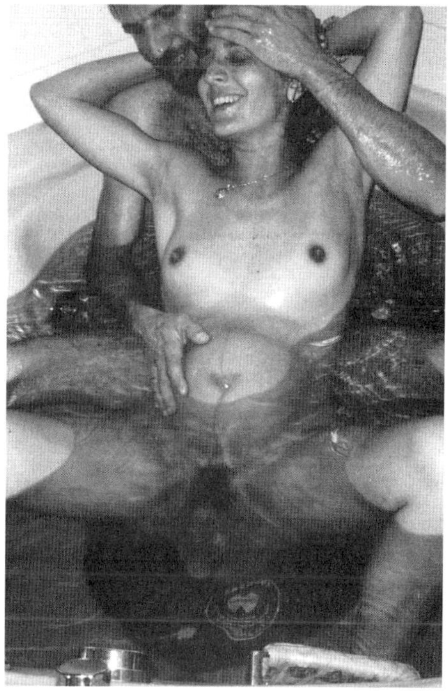

Questions for Thought and Discussion

1. Why does the author suggest that the Earth has become a cyborg?
2. What are some of the pros and cons of the cyborgification of humans and the planet we live on?
3. Why is Davis-Floyd, an advocate of natural childbirth and of midwifery care, so intrigued by the notion of the cyborg?
4. How do you feel about cyborgs?
5. Can cyborgs—cybernetic organisms—be holistic too? (Clue: see footnote 3.)

Recommended Film

Wall-E: 2008. After hundreds of years alone on an abandoned Earth, the curious and lovable robot WALL-E discovers a new purpose in life when he meets a sleek search robot named EVE. The film is premised on the possible notion that humans will so destroy their planetary environment that nothing more will grow on Earth, so the entire human species takes off for 700 years of space flight (first passing in their gigantic spaceship through miles and miles of space debris) before returning to a refreshed planet that is habitable once again. (http://movies.disney.com/wall-e)

Appendix

Applying Anthropology

What You Can Learn from This Book to Help You Achieve the Birth You Want

Dear Readers,

I am being as honest as I can with you in the following section. So sometimes my words may seem harsh. Please know that is not my intent. I just want you to be as fully informed as I personally can help you to be. Everything I say below is based on solid evidence and fully described in the preceding chapters in this volume. I wish you to have the kind of birth experience you want, one that will leave you feeling empowered, valued, respected, and joyful. Please take my words in that light, and know that I really care about women, babies, families, and birth—these have been the subjects of a lifetime of study for me, and I trust that my passion for supporting all women in their birthing choices is clear!

With my best wishes for happy birthing,
— Robbie

Here are my suggestions to you, written with love in my heart:

Read and fully inform yourself about pregnancy, labor, and birth. Childbirth Connection's website (www.childbirthconnection.org) contains a great deal of valuable information. And my favorite childbirth preparation book is still Sheila Kitzinger's *The Complete Book of Pregnancy and Childbirth*—it is older but gives you much more workable information than *What to Expect When You're Expecting*, the authors of which tend to refer you to your doctor for answers rather than provide them themselves.

I also highly recommend Sarah Buckley's fantastically informational book *Gentle Birth, Gentle Mothering* (2009). The author is an Australian physician, world-famous as a birth activist and international speaker, and also a very gentle and lovely person herself. Her book covers everything from the advantages and disadvantages of technocratic birth to yoga, orgasmic birth, attachment parenting, extended breastfeeding, co-sleeping, and elimination communication (EC)—or "diaper-free communication." Sarah refers to the diversity of women's birthing experiences as a "birth crystal" in which differences and dialogues are essential. Thus I'm sure this book will be of most interest and help to my more holistically inclined readers.

No matter what kind of birth you want, from a scheduled cesarean section to a homebirth, **have a doula with you.** The evidence is incontrovertible: the continuous presence of a doula shortens labor length and improves outcomes, even when your partner and family members are also present. Interview various doulas during pregnancy, pick the one who resonates with you the most, and meet with her prenatally to establish a firm relationship before labor begins (most doulas offer between two and six prenatal visits depending on your needs).

Yet even if you meet your doula for the first time during labor (some hospitals provide doula care), you will find that the bond between you can develop quickly and intensely. Your doula will know lots of pain-relieving and relaxation techniques, as well as movement techniques to facilitate labor, and can provide emotional and psychological support. So her presence can be invaluable, even during a scheduled cesarean. Note that her presence should be continuous—the "doula effect" does not work as well if you two are separated for long periods during labor.

Know yourself and your personal ideology and beliefs in terms of the 3 paradigms I present in Chapter 1. Where do you place yourself on the technocratic-humanistic-holistic spectrum? Your ideology has huge implications for the kind of birth you will want.

How do you feel about the **standard obstetric procedures** I analyzed as rituals in Chapter 2? Will their routine performance irritate and annoy you, causing your adrenaline levels to rise? Or will they comfort and calm you, making you feel safe and cared for, generating endorphins instead? (Please do not expect that you can "beat the system" and have a hospital birth without them; that is almost impossible to achieve. Only about 5% of women in the US and many other countries achieve fully normal, physiologic, nonintervened-with birth in the hospital.)

Which group of women in Chapter 3 do you relate to the most? **What do you believe about your body?** Is it a vehicle for your soul, a tool with which to do your work in the world? If so, you may find yourself inclined to a more technocratic/humanistic approach. Or do you feel that you *are* your body? If so, humanism/holism in birth will likely have more appeal to you.

Once you have figured out your own ideology, values, and beliefs about your body and birth, **search for a practitioner that shares the same ideology as you.** It is a proven fact that *the ideology of the practitioner is the most important determinant in the outcome of the birth*, especially its psychological and emotional results. So to have the birth you want, you must pick a practitioner *who wants you to have that kind of birth.* If you really want an epidural, don't pick a nurse-midwife who hates epidurals and will try to talk you out of having one; likewise, if you want an unmedicated physiologic birth where birth unfolds through the power of your own body, don't pick an obstetrician who laughs at you and tells you that you will be begging for an epidural shortly into labor.

If you want a **vaginal birth with an epidural,** as most women do, then *please wait until you are at least 6 cm dilated to have the epidural.* Before that, you are not really in labor (though it can certainly feel like you are), and having an epidural too early can slow labor and lead to the "cascade of interventions" I describe in Chapters 1 and 2. If you and the baby are healthy at the onset of labor (as the vast majority of women in high-resource countries are) and you arrive at the hospital and are told that you are only 4 cm dilated or less, I strongly suggest going back home! The latent phase of labor—up to 6 cm—can last for many hours or even days, especially if it is your first birth. If your hospital truly practices evidence-based care, it will have a policy in place that laboring women should not be admitted until they are in active labor, so its practitioners themselves will send you home.

While at home in early (latent) labor, have your doula with you to support you. Eat protein, drink electrolyte balancing liquids like Recharge (sold at Whole Foods—not Gatorade, which will spike and then suddenly drop your blood sugar level). Eating protein—meat, fish, tofu, miso, nuts, etc., will keep your blood sugar levels stable and give you the energy you need.

If you are hungry, that's a sign that you are indeed in early labor and will need nutrition for the long haul. Take walks, if your water has not broken, make love (the very best and most pleasurable way to stimulate and enjoy labor), dance to rock music, get in the bath or shower and let the water relax you. Perform some rituals if you wish (see Chapter 2 on the rituals of homebirth). Sing, clean house, bake a cake—*upright movement is the essence of a healthy labor*—or simply rest while you can if you are tired.

If your water *has* broken and you are not Group B strep positive, you can still stay at home for latent labor—take simple precautions like monitoring your temperature, not putting anything in your vagina (no sex, for example), and no tub baths—showers are OK. The point is to protect yourself from getting an infection (indicated by a fever), since the sac that protected the baby is now broken and open. Note that if your waters break very early, before you are due, and you do not go into labor, instead of rushing to the hospital you can simply wait, taking the precautions mentioned above. The amniotic sac will often reseal. Midwives are the providers most familiar with helping you through this occurrence.

Once you are truly in active labor, your doula will tell you when it is time to head for the hospital, and if you are admitted there at 6 cm or more, and still want that epidural, go ahead and enjoy being pain-free. Ask the anesthesiologist to turn down the epidural as you are getting ready to push (this is called "laboring down") so you can feel what you are doing, and thus, push more effectively.

If you choose to stay at the hospital anyway and have that epidural at 1–4 cm, you will be strapped to an electronic fetal monitor (EFM) and likely given a synthetic (or human-made) hormone called pitocin, which can and often does cause very strong contractions that are nonphysiologic, meaning that they may come more closely together with less recovery time in between, or build more quickly than is usual with an unmedicated labor. This can and often does cause the baby to become distressed. Know that you or your doula can initiate a conversation about *how* the pitocin is used if you choose to have it (or it is forced upon you). It may be turned up slowly and it may also be discontinued if there are any signs the baby is not tolerating the type of contractions it is causing.

When interventions are recommended, it is often helpful to ask: "Is this an emergency? What will happen if I choose to wait and give my body more time to birth?" Many times these questions help break providers out of their "standard operating procedures" mode of thinking or what is "normal" for them (which is to offer interventions that speed delivery). Often there is no emergency; it is simply that medical providers have been socialized into an overuse of procedures that can be life-saving when used appropriately but that are harmful when overused.

Overall, you must prepare yourself and please *do not be shocked or surprised if by accepting a series of interventions you end up with a cesarean,* which is a common result of having an epidural too soon and/or having your labor induced before the baby has indicated that it is ready to be born. Instead, be psychologically prepared for a surgical birth.

Please keep in mind that **even with the EFM, you can get out of the bed** and sit on a ball near it (if the tubes are long enough) and rock your pelvis, and put the bed upright, turn around, and kneel with your arms over the top of the bed to help gravity bring the baby down and widen your pelvic outlet. **If you have an epidural, you will be much more limited** in the positions you can assume, though as you begin to "labor down," more upright positioning may become available to you. Again, *movement and frequent position changes are the essence of a healthy labor*. Don't lie flat on your back for long, keep the birthing bed and yourself upright most of the time, and do your best to push your baby out in upright, knees to chest, or side-lying positions. Pick the position(s) that feels best to you and don't worry about it if the one(s) you pick makes it more difficult or status-challenging for your attendant(s).

If the thought of labor truly terrifies you, then you might want to **schedule a cesarean,** or if you are determined to control the timing of your birth, then you will want to **schedule an**

induction. In either case, *I beg you not to have a cesarean or an induction before your baby is completely and without doubt full-term,* meaning 40–42 weeks. Ultrasounds and due dates can be wrong by *multiple days or weeks* in terms of the baby's actual developmental stage. The best way for you to know if your baby is ready to come is for you to actually go into labor spontaneously. Many thousands of babies around the world are born prematurely, which can cause death or lifelong complications, because of inductions and cesareans scheduled too soon. If you do choose to schedule in advance, please be as certain as possible that you are past 40 weeks.

Do not accept a diagnosis of "failure to progress" as a valid reason for a cesarean if you are not yet in fully active labor (6 cm or more). How can you be "failing to progress" if you are not even in active labor? Go home and wait, unless you really want a cesarean or at least are OK with having one.

If hospitals make you feel safer than homes or birth centers, yet you want a normal **vaginal birth in the hospital without an epidural**, *bring a doula and choose a midwife to be your primary attendant.* Interview those available to pick the right personality and ideological fit for you. Some hospital-based midwives are extremely holistic and fully practice the Midwifery Model of Care (Chapter 11). Others can be extremely medicalized, which might be exactly what you want because even medically-oriented CNMs tend to spend far more time with their clients than obstetricians during prenatal visits, and to take a more relationship-based approach. They also have lower cesarean rates overall. **In fact, any mother who wants truly humanistic care in any setting should choose a midwife as her primary provider if at all possible.**

If there are no hospital midwives in your area, then search for the most humanistic or holistic obstetrician you can find. You can judge his or her level of commitment to humanistic, woman-centered practice by asking about his or her cesarean rate (if it is well above 15% for women having their first babies, that tells you that he or she is way too interventive), as well as by the amount of time he or she spends with you during prenatal visits. You can also evaluate how thoroughly he or she answers your questions and shares decision making (and your chart) with you. Seek out practitioners who do "Centering Pregnancy" group prenatal care, which is far more fun and more informative than one-on-one short office visits—Google it and you will see why. *To find the most humanistic obstetricians in your city, ask the doulas and the midwives practicing there—they always know!*

If you fully ground yourself in the holistic model, and truly desire an **unmedicated**, untrammeled, fully natural birth, do not be fooled into thinking you can achieve that in a technocratic hospital where the midwifery model does not prevail. No matter what promises are made, or how prepared you are or what birth plan you bring in, the system will suck you in—unless you have a truly holistic midwife who will hold the space for you. That may be very possible to achieve in midwife-friendly countries, but if you live in the US, remember that American midwives only attend around 13% of births so can be hard to find—and even they often cannot "beat the system." If you fight the system during labor, your birth, which should be a peaceful and loving experience, may become a battleground full of tension. Tension and anxiety during labor produce adrenalin, which interferes with the flow of oxytocin and can inhibit your ability to labor productively. Labor is not the best time to fight for your rights. Follow your instincts and choose a homebirth or birth center birth with a midwife (see Chapters 6 and 11), so that the birth space itself will shelter and nurture you. Find and interview all those in your area who are less than an hour away—perhaps more if you live in a rural area. If so, be fully prepared to do the birth on your own in case your midwife can't arrive in time—she can talk you or your partner through it on her cell phone—and know your options for transport.

If you are planning a midwife-attended homebirth, see Chapter 10 and prepare yourself for the possibility of **transport**, which occurs in around 10% of such births. Make sure your midwife has good relationships with at least one hospital and some of its practitioners; if that is not possible, have a backup obstetrician who at least thinks he or she is your primary practitioner—you don't have to tell the obstetrician you are planning a homebirth if you think he or she will respond punitively to that information. Ideally you can be honest with him or her, and know he or she will be there for you if you end up having to transport.

Make sure your hospital, your midwife or midwives, and your backup obstetrician if you have one, all have copies of the **Best Practice Guidelines for Transfers** described in Chapter 10. Remember that only 3 out of those 10 transports occur in emergency situations. If your transport is an emergency, be sure that your midwife follows those protocols by calling ahead to notify the hospital and ask them to have the OR ready. If your hospital does have the Best Practice for Transfer Guidelines, they should be prepared to respond appropriately.

Have at least one talk with your care provider about the **possibility of baby death**. Regardless of place and manner of birth, in high resource countries at least one or two babies out of every 1,000 will die. That is the natural order of things. These rates are much higher in low-resource countries, and for high-risk babies everywhere. It is highly unlikely that your baby will be one of those, but every pregnant mother should spend at least a bit of time contemplating that possibility, so that you will not be completely unprepared should that happen to you. The few women I have interviewed who had prepared for this eventuality and whose babies did die said that the advance preparation helped them greatly to cope with their loss. Those who had not prepared themselves were more completely shocked and had a harder road to recovery.

Before labor begins, work on cultivating your **intuition** (see Chapter 7) and if that still, small voice speaks to you before, during, or after labor, pay attention to what it says and act on its advice. Check with your midwife about her own intuitions about your labor—if you two are in sync, all should be well, but if your intuitions do not match, then it is likely there is something off and you should take action, such as talking with your midwife between contractions and embracing her during them to see if you two can get in sync, and if not, consider a hospital transport or possibly bring in another midwife. (Most homebirth midwives have others they can call for backup.)

Be aware of the energy field in your labor space and, for example, don't hesitate to send someone away if you feel that their energy is negatively affecting your labor, or to ask someone to come in because you need their positive energy in that moment. Check your emotional state: do you feel safe and secure, protected and loved? If not, take measures to get there, which can range from changing your own attitude to asking those around you to change theirs, or leave—as Michel Odent often points out, too many people in the labor space can negatively affect the mother's sense of privacy and safety. Perhaps you need time to labor alone. Perhaps intimate, private, even sexual time with your partner will do the trick—again, making love during labor is the best kept secret about how to make it most enjoyable—it enhances your oxytocin and endorphin levels, making labor more effective and much more pleasurable as the contractions become orgasms too.

Or perhaps, if you are at home, you need to head for the hospital—some women who *think* they want to give birth at home find out that their labors pick up when they walk through the hospital door, because that's where they really feel safe. Others tense up in fear at the thought of hospitals, so clearly they are most likely to find their sense of safety and security in a birth center or at home.

If you wish to have a homebirth yet cannot find a nearby midwife to attend you because you are **out of protocols** but not necessarily high-risk (e.g., past 42 weeks, a baby in breech position, one or two previous cesareans), I have fully described **"renegade midwives"** in Chapter 12, and so you can make your own decisions about whether to access that option. To find a renegade midwife who will go outside of protocols to assist you to achieve the birth you want, simply ask your local midwifery community—just as they always know which doctors are the most supportive of normal birth and midwives, they also will know who the renegades are. Some renegade midwives will even travel to you from other areas of the country. Inform yourself and your partner about the risks you may be taking, then follow your intuition and your heart.

Some women choose to give birth **unassisted by any care provider**. I do not recommend this option yet feel that I should mention it, as such women have written about the amazing birth experiences they have had, and I trust that birth works well the vast majority of the time. Marilyn Moran and Laura Kaplan Shanley have written about unassisted birth; you might want to Google their works to find out more. Know that if you choose this option, you (and your partner) are taking full responsibility for the outcome of your birth. For full information, simply Google "unassisted birth" or go to http://www.unassistedhomebirth.com/.

In any labor in any setting, DO NOT FIGHT THE CONTRACTIONS. If you try to stand up against a powerful ocean wave, it will knock you down. But if you dive into it head-on, it will carry you back up. A book I love called *Water Dancer* describes a woman determined to be the first to swim from Florida to Cuba. On her first try, all she could think about was "how much farther?" And when her guardians in the boat nearby would tell her, she would think, "I can never make it that far." So that attempt failed. On her next attempt, she gave no thought at all to how far she had to go; she knew she probably could not go that far, but *she always knew that she could take one more stroke*. So she entered what athletes and laboring women call "the zone," a timeless space in which all that matters is that next stroke, and the next, and was actually surprised when she hit sand—in Cuba.

Contractions only last about 45–60 seconds, though you can sometimes feel them building or relaxing for longer. Don't think about how many cm dilated you are or how long you have to go, or wonder how you are going to stand all the pain that is coming. *Dive deep into the present contraction, surrendering to it fully.* You may not believe that you can possibly make it to the end of labor, but you do know that *you can get through just that next contraction*. If you get into that **"zone,"** which some midwives call **"laborland,"** just stay in it, ignoring all outside distractions—that is a time when your doula and your other supporters, if you have them, should become your watchdog guardians, not letting anyone interfere or try to snap you out of that blessed state, during which many women have intense spiritual experiences and/or of profound connection with their bodies, their babies, and the universe itself.[1,2]

Once the baby is born, if possible, make sure (this should be planned in advance), that **you be the first one to touch him or her** besides the person (who might be your partner) who

[1] This happened to me during the last few hours of my three-day home labor. When I finally stopped separating myself from the pain by trying to do something about it (breathe with it, chant with it, resist it, fight it, resent it) and completely surrendered to the pain, saying silently, "I give up. Take me, I'm yours," I magically somehow became one with the pain, and then there was no more pain. I found myself floating above my body in a state of pure bliss and unity that lasted until my waters finally broke and pushing contractions kicked in. Having experienced that bliss gave me the energy and trust in myself and the Universe to push out my 10-pound baby. And the oxytocin/endorphin rush I got right after the birth was truly amazing—it was like being surrounded by golden light—I guess that's why they call it "the Golden Hour."

[2] In a 2016 study by Patty Van Cappellen, Baldwin May, Susanna Isgett, and Barbara L. Fredrickson, called "Effects of Administration on Spirituality and Emotional Responses to Meditation," published in *Social Cognitive and Affective Neuroscience* 11(10): 1579–1587, and in another by Christopher Bergland in *Psychology Today* called "Oxytocin, Spirituality, and the Biology of Feeling Connected" (2016), the research showed a strong connection between oxytocin and spirituality, bringing together the mystical and the scientific. High levels of oxytocin can generate a strong feeling of spirituality, a sense of awe, and of connection to a higher source or power. The administration of pitocin (a synthetic form of oxytocin) cuts off your natural supply of oxytocin, "the hormone of love" that floods your body during lovemaking, birth, and breastfeeding, denying you those possibilities. Many of you, my readers, may not care one bit about spirituality during birth; others might, therefore I include this information.

is catching the baby. The baby's passage through the birth canal began the colonization of his gut with your internal flora; holding her naked, skin-to-skin is the final step in that process and the first step in the process of what is called "external gestation"—growing the baby through ongoing mother–baby contact and breastfeeding.

Seconds or minutes after birth, your body (if you have not had the artificial hormone pitocin) will receive **the greatest oxytocin and endorphin rush you will ever experience**. This hormonal rush will facilitate your falling in love with your baby and greatly enhance your ability to breastfeed. Don't worry if he doesn't latch on immediately—he may not be hungry just then and he, like you, may need some time to recover from this very intense process of being born.

If you are upright for the birth, you can birth the baby onto the bed and **take your time to breathe and recuperate for a moment, then reach down and touch your baby little by little**, picking him up when you are fully ready. If you are lying down, your practitioner can gently lay the baby on your belly or chest. **A healthy baby should not be bathed immediately, or taken away from you for any reason**, before a long period of skin-to-skin contact, called the "Golden Hour" has unfolded. Don't allow anyone to take that precious time away from you to perform "routine procedures."

A small percentage of babies need **some help breathing** after birth. They may be taken to a bassinet/resuscitation table for assistance, but your partner or doula can always go with and touch and talk to the baby as he or she comes around. At home and in some birth centers and hospitals, babies who need help taking their first breaths are assisted right next to Mom where she can talk to and comfort her baby during the process. **Under no circumstances should the cord be cut until it stops pulsating. CALL THE BABY to help her soul decide to come through the gateway** (see the box, "Calling the Baby," in Chapter 1). Call her name and ask her to breathe and live and come and share your lives together. Doing so can do no harm, can empower you and your partner to do something to help while the baby is being resuscitated, and might just work!

Finally, in rare instances for healthy women, a **cesarean section can be lifesaving** for a mother and/or baby. Whether you choose a cesarean or find yourself facing one after having tried everything else, be aware that some providers have started offering what is called **"gentle," "family-centered" or sometimes "natural" cesarean sections.** As described in Chapter 2, these involve essentially treating the cesarean like a vaginal birth with an epidural. The surgical team is quiet and respectful, using the same kinds of language and encouragements they would use for a vaginal birth. Soft music is played. The anesthesiologist places the leads for vital signs monitoring on the sides rather than top of the mother's chest so that the baby can go skin-to-skin on her chest after birth.

After the incision is made and the baby is ready to emerge, **the drape** is lowered so that you can watch the baby be born gently and slowly. The drape itself can be made of clear plastic so you can watch the whole operation—see the photos in Chapter 2. Or, if your obstetrician is really willing to think outside the box, you too can wear a mask and your head can be inside the drapes that demarcate the sterile field. (You would have to plan this in advance,) The physician may even ask you to push lightly as though you are having a vaginal birth. The baby goes immediately to you, the cord is allowed to complete its pulsing before being cut to ensure maximum blood, oxygen, and nutrient supply to the newborn, and nursing can be initiated while the incisions are being repaired. Consider having this "gentle cesarean" option as part of your birth plan should a surgical birth become your last resort, or is your initial plan. Talk with your provider beforehand to make clear that this is an option you would like to have available if needed. If your care providers are not familiar with gentle cesarean, bring them these articles to read:

Magee, Susanna R., et al. 2014. "Promotion of Family-centered Birth with Gentle Cesarean Delivery." *The Journal of the American Board of Family Medicine* 27(5). 690–693.

Smith, J., F. Plaat, and Nicholas M. Fisk. 2009. "The Natural Caesarean: A Woman-centred Technique." *BJOG: An International Journal of Obstetrics & Gynaecology* 115(8): 1037–1042.

Know your rights to informed consent and refusal and respectful, compassionate care during labor and birth. Insist on having them honored. *It's your body, your baby, your birth!*

Acknowledgement

I wish to sincerely thank Missy Cheyney for her helpful edits and suggestions for this Appendix.

References

Abrahams, Roger D. 1973. "Ritual for Fun and Profit (or The Ends and Outs of Celebration)." Paper delivered at the Burg Wartenstein Symposium on Ritual: Reconciliation in Change. New York: WennerGren Foundation for Anthropological Research.

ACOG and the Society for Maternal Fetal Medicine. 2014. "Obstetric Care Consensus: Safe Prevention of the Primary Cesarean Delivery." http://www.acog.org/Resources-And-Publications/Obstetric-Care-Consensus-Series/Safe-Prevention-of-the-Primary-Cesarean-Delivery

ACNM (American College of Nurse-Midwives). 2012. *Issue Brief: Where Midwives Work.* Silver Spring, MD: American College of Nurse- Midwives. http://www.midwife.org/ACNM/files/

———. 2014. Position Statement. "Principles for Licensing and Regulating Midwives in the United States in Accordance with the Global Standards of the International Confederation of Midwives." http://www.midwife.org/ACNM/files/ACNMLibraryData/UPLOADFILENAME/000000000287/Principles-for-Licensing-and-Regulating-Midwives-in-US-According-to-ICM-Global-Standards-March-2014.pdf

———. 2016. Home Birth Clinical Bulletin. http://www.midwife.org/acnm/files/ccLibraryFiles/Filename/000000005842/Home_Birth_Clinical_Bulletin_Press-Release_Final.pdf

Alfirevic, Z., D. Devane, and G. M. Gyte. 2013. "Continuous Cardiotocography (CTG) as a Form of Electronic Fetal Monitoring (EFM) for Fetal Assessment during Labour." *Cochrane Database of Systematic Reviews* May 31; 5: CD006066. doi:10.1002/14651858.CD006066.pub2. http://www.ncbi.nlm.nih.gov/pubmed/23728657

Allen, Denise Roth. 2002. *Managing Motherhood, Managing Risk: Fertility and Danger in West Central Tanzania.* Ann Arbor: University of Michigan Press.

Alvarez, S. E., E. Dagnino, and A. Escobar. 1998. "Introduction: The Cultural and Political in Latin American Social Movements." In *Cultures of Politics/Politics of Cultures: Re-Visioning Latin American Social Movements*, edited by S. E. Alvarez, S. E. Dagnino, and A. Escobar, pp. 1–32. Boulder, CO: Westview Press.

American College of Obstetricians and Gynecologists (ACOG). 2007. "ACOG Committee Opinion No. 394, December 2007. Cesarean delivery on maternal request." *Obstetrics and Gynecology* 110(6): 1501.

American Heritage Dictionary. 1993. In Microsoft Word for Windows 6.0, Windows 3.1.

Anderson, David A., Betty-Anne Daviss, and Kenneth C. Johnson. forthcoming. "What If 10% More Women Delivered at Home or in a Birth Center? The Economics and Politics of Out-of-Hospital Birth in the U.S." In *Speaking Truth to Power: Birth Models on the Human Rights Frontier*, edited by Betty-Anne Daviss and Robbie Davis-Floyd. Berkeley: University of California Press.

APHA (American Public Health Association). 2002. "Increasing Access to Out-of-Hospital Maternity Care Services through State-Regulated and Nationally-Certified Direct-Entry Midwives (Policy Statement)." *American Journal of Public Health* 93(3): 453–455.

Appadurai, A. 1996. *Modernity at Large: Cultural Dimensions of Globalization*. Minneapolis: University of Minnesota Press.

Appiah, K. A. 1997. "Is the 'Post-' in 'Postcolonial' the 'Post-' in 'Postmodern'?" In *Dangerous Liaisons: Gender, Nation, and Postcolonial Perspectives*, edited by A. McClintock, A. Mufti, and E. Shohat, pp. 420–444. Minneapolis: University of Minnesota Press.

Arms, Suzanne. 1981 [1975]. *Immaculate Deception*. New York: Bantam Books.

Babcock, Barbara (ed.). 1978. *The Reversible World: Symbolic Inversion in Art and Society.* Ithaca, NY: Cornell University Press.

Barclay, Leslie M. 1998. "Midwifery in Australia and Surrounding Regions: Dilemmas, Debates, and Developments." *Reproductive Health Matters* 6(11): 149–155.

———. 2009. "Samoan Midwives' Stories: Joining Social and Professional Midwives in New Models of Birth." In *Birth Models That Work*, edited by R. Davis-Floyd, L. Barclay, B. A. Daviss, and J. Tritten, pp. 119–140. Berkeley: University of California Press.

Barnes, Patricia M., Barbara Bloom, and Richard L. Nahin. 2008. "Complementary and Alternative Medicine Use among Adults and Children: United States, 2007." *Natl Health Stat Report* 10(12): 1–23.

Barnes-Josiah, Debora, C. Myntti, and A. Augustin. 1998. "The Three Delays as a Framework for Examining Maternal Mortality in Haiti." *Social Science and Medicine* 46: 981–993.

Bastick, Tony. 1982. *Intuition: How We Think and Act*. New York: Wiley.

Bauman, Zymunt. 1997. *Postmodernity and Its Discontents*. New York University Press, New York.

Berman, Morris. 1989. *Coming to Our Senses: Body and Spirit in the Hidden History of the West*. New York: Simon and Schuster.

Benoit, Cecilia, Robbie Davis-Floyd, Edwin R. van Teijlingen, Jane Sandall, and Janneli F. Miller. 2001. "Designing Midwives: A Comparison of Educational Models." In *Birth by Design: Pregnancy, Maternity Care, and Midwifery in North America and Europe*. New York: Routledge.

Beth, Easton, and Jean Piaget. 1966. *Mathematical Epistemology and Psychology*. Dordrecht, Holland: D. Reidel.

Bhutta, Z. A., R. A. Salam, Z. S. Lassi, A. Austin, and A. Langer. 2014. "Approaches to Improve Quality of Care (QoC) for Women and Newborns: Conclusions, Evidence Gaps and Research Priorities." *Reprod Health* 11 (Suppl 2): S5.

Blank, Martin. 2014. *Over-Powered: What Science Tells Us about the Dangers of Cell Phones and Other Wifi-Age Devices*. New York: Seven Stories Press.

Block, Jennifer. 2007. *Pushed: The Painful Truth about Childbirth and Modern Maternity Care*. Boston: Da Capo Press.

Boyle, A., U. M. Reddy, H. J. Landy, C. C. Huang, R. W. Driggers, and S. K. Laughon. 2013. "Primary Cesarean Delivery in the United States." *Obstet Gynecol* 122(1): 33–40.

Brodie, P., and C. Homer. 2009. "Transforming the Culture of a Maternity Service: St George Hospital, Sydney, Australia." In *Birth Models That Work*, edited by R. Davis-Floyd, L. Barclay, B. A. Daviss, and J. Tritten, pp. 187–212. Berkeley: University of California Press.

Bryden, M. P. 1982. *Laterality: Functional Asymmetry in the Intact Brain*. New York: Academic Press.

Bryers, Helen MacKenzie, and Edwin Van Teijlingen. 2010. "Risk, Theory, Social and Medical Models: A Critical Analysis of the Concept of Risk in Maternity Care." *Midwifery* 26(5): 488–496.

Buckley, Sarah J. MD. 2009. *Gentle Birth, Gentle Mothering: A Guide to Natural Childbirth and Gentle Early Parenting Choices*. Berkeley, CA: Celestial Arts.

Byford, Julia. 1999. *Dealing with Death Beginning with Birth: Women's Health and Childbirth on Misima Island, Papua New Guinea*. PhD dissertation, Dept. of Anthropology, Australian National University.

Cain, Fraser. 2015. "How Many Satellites are in Space?" *The Universe Today: Space and Astronomy News*. http://www.universetoday.com/42198/how-many-satellites-in-space/

Carleto de Paulo, Gabrielle. 2016. "Renegades or Untouchables? Values, Ideology and Politics of Midwives in Austin, Texas." Unpublished ms. written during an internship with Robbie Davis-Floyd.

Camann, MD, William, and Robert L. Barbieri, MD. 2013. "Mother-, Baby-, and Family-Centered Cesarean Delivery: It Is Possible." *OBG Management* 25(3): 10–15.

Carver, Cynthia. 1981. "The Deliverers: A Woman Doctor's Reflections on Medical Socialization." In *Childbirth: Alternatives to Medical Control*, edited by Shelly Romalis. Austin: University of Texas Press.

Castaneda, Angela N., and Julie J. Searcy (eds.). 2015. *Intimate Labour: Boundaries, Bodies, and Birth*. Bradford, Ontario: Demeter Press.

Castro, Arachu, Angela Heimburger, and Ana Langer. 2001. "Iatrogenic Epidemic: How Health Care Professionals Contribute to the High Proportion of Cesarean Sections in Mexico." Unpublished ms.

Chamberlain, David. 1998. "'Babies Don't Feel Pain': A Century of Denial in Medicine." In *Cyborg Babies: From Techno-Sex to Techno-Tots*, edited by Robbie Davis-Floyd and Joseph Dumit, pp.168–191. New York: Routledge.

Charon, Rita. 2004. "Narrative and Medicine." *New England Journal of Medicine* 350(9): 862–864.

Chen, P. C. Y. 1977. "Incorporating the Traditional Birth Attendant in the Health Team: The Malaysian Example." *Tropical and Geographical Medicine* 29: 192–196.

Chester, Penfield. 1997. *Sisters on a Journey: Portraits of American Midwives*. New Brunswick, NJ: Rutgers University Press.

Cheyney, Melissa. 2011. "Reinscribing the Birthing Body: Homebirth as Ritual Performance." *Medical Anthropology Quarterly* 25(4): 519–537.

Cheyney, Melissa, Marit Bovbjerg, Courtney Everson, W. Gordon, D. Hannibal, and Saraswathi Vedam. 2014a. "Development and Validation of a National Data Registry for Midwife-Led Births: The Midwives Alliance of North America Statistics Project 2.0 Dataset." *Journal of Midwifery & Women's Health* 59: 8–16.

———. 2014b. "Outcomes of Care for 16,924 Planned Home Births in the United States: The Midwives Alliance of North America Statistics Project, 2004 to 2009." *J Midwifery Women's Health* 59(1): 17–27. doi:10.1111/jmwh.12172

Cheyney, Melissa, Courtney Everson, and Paul Burcher. 2014c. "Homebirth Transfers in the United States: Narratives of Risk, Fear and Mutual Accommodation." *Qualitative Health Research* 24(4): 443–456. doi:10.1177/104973231452

Cheyney, Melissa, Bahareh Goodarzi, and Therese Wiegers. forthcoming. "Midwifery Care as Integrated Option or Contested Privilege? Giving Birth in the United States and the Netherlands." In *Birth in Eight Cultures: A Cross-Cultural Investigation*, edited by Robbie Davis-Floyd and Melissa Cheyney. Long Grove, IL: Waveland Press.

Cheyney, Melissa, Christine Olsen, Marit Bovbjerg, Courtney Everson, Ida Darragh, and Brynne Potter. 2015. "Practitioner and Practice Characteristics of Certified Professional Midwives in the United States: Results of the 2011 North American Registry of Midwives Survey." *Journal of Midwifery and Women's Health*. doi:10.1111/jmwh.12367

Clifford, James, and George E. Marcus (eds.). 1986. *Writing Politics: The Poetics and Politics of Ethnography*. Berkeley: University of California Press.

Comité Promotor por una Maternidad sin Riesgos. 1997. "Cesáreas: Tendencias actuales y perspectivas." Secretaría de Salud, Mexico.

Contreras, Doña Queta. 2009. *Medicina Tradicional: Doña Queta y El Legado de Los Habitantes de las Nubes*. Aida Guerra Falcón and Hamalgama Editorial. ISBN #978-84-935100-0-8.

Corea, Gena. 1985. *The Mother Machine: Reproductive Technologies from Artificial Insemination to Artificial Wombs*. New York: Harper and Row.

Cosminsky, Sheila. 1977. "Childbirth and Midwifery on a Guatemalan Finca." *Medical Anthropology* 6(3): 69–104.

———. 1983. "Traditional Midwifery and Contraception." In *Traditional Medicine and Health Care Coverage*, edited by Robert Bannerman, John Burton, and Ch'en Wen-Chieh, pp. 143–162. Geneva: World Health Organization.

Cox, K. J., R. Schlegel, P. Payne, D. Teaf, and L. Albers. 2013. "Outcomes of Planned Home Births Attended by Certified Nurse-Midwives in South-Eastern Pennsylvania, 1983–2008." *J Midwifery Women's Health*. 58(2): 145–149. doi:10.1111/j.1542-2011.2012.00217.x

Craven, Christa. 2010. *Pushing for Midwives: Homebirth Mothers and the Reproductive Rights Movement*. Philadelphia: Temple University Press.

Croissant, Jennifer. 1998. "Growing Up Cyborg: Developmental Stories for Postmodern Children." In *Cyborg Babies: From Techno-Sex to Techno-Tots*, edited by Robbie Davis-Floyd and Joseph Dumit, pp. 285–300. New York: Routledge.

Cunningham F. G., P. C. Macdonald, and N. F. Gant. 1989. *Williams Obstetrics* (18th ed.). Norwalk CT: Appleton and Lange.

Curtin, S. C. 1999. "Recent Changes in Birth Attendant, Place of Birth, and the Use of Obstetric Interventions." *Journal of Nurse-Midwifery* 44(4): 349–354.

Dahlen, Hanna. 2006. "Midwifery: At the Edge of History." *Women and Birth* 19(1): 3–10.

Darragh, Ida. 2004. *North American Registry of Midwives Newsletter,* Vol. VI, Issue 1, winter, p. 3.

Davis, Elizabeth. 1987. *A Guide to Midwifery: Heart and Hands*. New York: Bantam Books.

———. 1988. *Energetic Pregnancy*. Berkeley, CA: Celestial Arts.

———. 1989. *Women's Intuition*. Berkeley, CA: Celestial Arts.

———. 1994. *Women's Sexual Cycles*. London: Little, Brown, and Co.

———. 1995. *Woman, Sex, and Desire*. Alameda, CA: Hunter House.

———. 1997. *Heart and Hands: A Midwife's Guide to Pregnancy and Birth* (3rd ed.). Berkeley, CA: Celestial Arts.

———. 2012. *Heart and Hands: A Midwife's Guide to Pregnancy and Birth* (5th ed.). Berkeley, CA: Celestial Arts.

———. 2013. *The Rhythms of Women's Desire*. Alameda, CA: Hunter House

Davis, Elizabeth, and Carol Leonard. 2012. *The Women's Wheel of Life*. Berkeley, CA: Celestial Arts.

Davis, Elizabeth, and Debra Pascali-Bonaro. 2010. *Orgasmic Birth*. New York: Rodale Books.

Davis-Floyd, Robbie. n.d. "Knowing: A Story of Two Births." Unpublished ms.

———. 1987a. "Pregnancy and Cultural Confusion: Contradictions in Socialization." In *Cultural Constructions of Woman*, edited by P. Kolenda, pp. 9–71. Salem, WI: Sheffield Press.

———. 1987b. "The Technological Model of Birth." *Journal of American Folklore* 100: 479–495.

———. 1987c. "Obstetric Training as a Rite of Passage." *Medical Anthropology Quarterly* 1(3): 288–318.

———. 1994. "The Technocratic Body: American Childbirth as Cultural Expression." *Social Science & Medicine* 38(8): 1125–1140.

———. 1998a. "From Technobirth to Cyborg Babies: Reflections on the Emergent Discourse of a Holistic Anthropologist." In *Cyborg Babies: From Techno-Sex to Techno-Tots*, edited by R. Davis-Floyd and J. Dumit, pp. 255–283. New York: Routledge.

———. 1998b. "Types of Midwifery Training: An Anthropological Overview." In *Paths to Becoming a Midwife: Getting an Education*, edited by Jan Tritten and Joel Southern, pp. 119–133. Eugene, OR: Midwifery Today. Also available at www.davis-floyd.com

———. 2000. "Technologies of the Exterior, Technologies of the Interior: Can We Expand the Discourse of Reproductive Studies?" Afterword to *Body Talk: Rhetoric, Technology, Reproduction*, edited by Mary M. Lay, Laura J. Gurak, Clare Gravon, and Cynthia Myntti. Madison: University of Wisconsin Press, pp 277–300.

———. 2000a. "Commercializing Outer Space: The SATWG Stories." In *Late Editions VII: Para-Sites*, edited by George Marcus. Chicago: University of Chicago Press.

———. 2000b, March. "Global Issues in Midwifery: Mutual Accommodation or Biomedical Hegemony?" *Midwifery Today* 12-17: 68–69.

———. 2001a. "*La Partera Profesional*: Articulating Identity and Cultural Space for a New Kind of Midwife in Mexico." In "Daughters of Time: The Shifting Identities of Contemporary Midwives," edited by Robbie Davis-Floyd, Sheila Cosminsky, and Stacy L. Pigg, [special issue] *Medical Anthropology* 20(2-3): 185–244.

———. 2001b, November. "*Las parteras de Morelos*: The Strategic Negotiation of Knowledge Systems by Postmodern Midwives in Mexico." Paper presented at the meeting of the American Anthropological Association, Washington, DC.

———. 2001c. "The Technocratic, Humanistic, and Holistic Models of Birth." *International Journal of Gynecology & Obstetrics* 75, Supplement No. 1, pp. S5–S23.

———. 2002. "Southern Discomfort: American Midwifery as a Cautionary Tale." In *Reconceiving Midwifery: The New Canadian Model of Care*, edited by I. Bourgeault, C. Benoit, and R. Davis-Floyd. Ann Arbor: University of Michigan Press.

———. 2003a. "Home Birth Emergencies in the U.S. and Mexico: The Trouble with Transport." In *Reproduction Gone Awry*, [special issue] *Social Science and Medicine* 56(9): 1913–1931.

———. 2003b. "Windows in Space/Time: A Personal Perspective on Birth and Death." *Birth: Issues in Perinatal Care* 30(4): 272–277.

———. 2003 [1992]. *Birth as an American Rite of Passage*. Berkeley and London: University of California Press

———. 2004a. "Qualified Commodification: Consuming Midwifery Care." In *Consuming Motherhood*, edited by Janelle Taylor, Danielle Wozniack, and Linda Layne. New Brunswick NJ: Rutgers University Press.

———. 2004b. "Ways of Knowing: Open and Closed Systems." *Midwifery Today* 69: 9–13.

———. 2005. "Daughter of Time: The Postmodern Midwife." *MIDIRS Midwifery Digest* 15(1): 32–39.

———. 2006. "Qualified Commodification: The Creation of the Certified Professional Midwife." In *Mainstreaming Midwives: The Politics of Change*, edited by Robbie Davis-Floyd and Christine Barbara Johnson, pp. 163–204. New York: Routledge.

———. 2007. "Changing Childbirth: The Latin American Example." *Midwifery Today* 84: 9–13, 64–65.

———. 2010. "The Ups, Downs, and Interlinkages of Nurse- and Direct-Entry Midwifery: Status, Practice, and Education." In *Paths to Becoming a Midwife: Getting an Education*, edited by J. Tritten and J. Southern. Eugene, OR: Midwifery Today. Available: www.midwiferytoday.com

Davis-Floyd, Robbie, Lesley Barclay, Betty-Anne Daviss, and Jan Tritten (eds.). 2009. *Birth Models That Work*. Berkeley: University of California Press.

Davis-Floyd, R., S. Cosminsky, and S. L. Pigg (eds.). 2001. "Daughters of Time: The Shifting Identities of Contemporary Midwives," [special issue] *Medical Anthropology* 20(2-3).

Davis-Floyd, Robbie, Kenneth J. Cox, and Frank White. 2012. *Space Stories: Oral Histories from the Pioneers of America's Space Program.* Kindle E-Book.

Davis-Floyd, Robbie, and Elizabeth Davis. 1997. "Intuition as Authoritative Knowledge in Midwifery and Home Birth." In *Childbirth and Authoritative Knowledge: Cross-Cultural Perspectives*, edited by Robbie Davis-Floyd and Carolyn Sargent, pp. 315–349. Berkeley: University of California Press.

Davis-Floyd, Robbie E., and Joseph Dumit. 1998. *Cyborg Babies: From Techno-Sex to Techno-Tots*. New York: Routledge.

Davis-Floyd, R., and C. B. Johnson (eds.). 2006. *Mainstreaming Midwives: The Politics of Change*. New York: Routledge.

Davis-Floyd, Robbie, and Charles Laughlin. 2016. *The Power of Ritual*. Brisbane, Australia: Daily Grail Press.

Davis-Floyd, Robbie, and Carolyn Sargent. 1997. *Childbirth and Authoritative Knowledge: Cross-Cultural Perspectives*. Berkeley: University of California Press.

Davis-Floyd, R., and G. St. John. 1998. *From Doctor to Healer: The Transformative Journey*. New Brunswick, NJ: Rutgers University Press.

Daviss, Betty-Anne. 1997. "Heeding Warnings from the Canary, the Whale, and the Inuit: A Framework for Analyzing Competing Types of Knowledge about Birth." In *Childbirth and Authoritative Knowledge: Cross-Cultural Perspective*, edited by Robbie Davis-Floyd and Carolyn Sargent, pp. 441–473. Berkeley: University of California Press.

———. 2006. "From Calling to Career: Keeping the Social Movement in the Professionalization Project." In *Mainstreaming Midwives: The Politics of Change*, edited by Robbie Davis-Floyd and Christina Barbara Johnson, pp. 413–446. New York: Routledge.

Daviss, Betty-Anne, and Andrew Biskits. forthcoming. "Bringing Back Breech." In *Speaking Truth to Power: Birth Models on the Human Rights Frontier*, edited by Betty-Anne Daviss and Robbie Davis-Floyd. Berkeley: University of California Press.

de Jonge, A., et al. 2009. "Perinatal Mortality and Morbidity in a Nationwide Cohort of 529,688 Low-Risk Planned Home and Hospital Births." *BJOG: An International Journal of Obstetrics & Gynaecology* 116 (9): 1177–1184. http://onlinelibrary.wiley.com/doi/10.1111/j.1471-0528.2009.02175.x/full

———. 2015. "Perinatal Mortality and Morbidity up to 28 Days after Birth among 743,070 Low-Risk Planned Home and Hospital Births: A Cohort Study Based on Three Merged National Perinatal Databases." *BJOG* 122(5): 720–728.

Declerq, Eugene. 2015. "Midwife-Attended Births in the U.S., 1990–2012: Results from Revised Birth Certificate Data." *Journal of Midwifery and Women's Health* 60(1): 10–15.

Declerq, E., R. DeVries, K. Viisainen, H. B. Salvesen, and S. Wrede. 2001. "Where to Give Birth? Politics and the Place of Birth." In *Birth by Design: Pregnancy, Maternity Care and Midwifery in North America and Europe*, edited by R. DeVries, E. van Teijlingen, S. Wrede, and C. Benoit, pp. 7–27. New York: Routledge.

Declerq, Eugene R., et al. 2006. *Listening to Mothers II*. New York: Childbirth Connection. (Also see www.childbirthconnection.org.)

Dekker, Rebecca. 2017. "Evidence on Friedman's Curve and Failure to Progress: A Leading Cause of Unplanned Cesareans." https://evidencebasedbirth.com/friedmans-curve-and-failure-to-progress-a-leading-cause-of-unplanned-c-sections/

Department of Consumer Affairs, State of California. 1999 (August 16–20). *In the Matter of the Accusation Against Alison Osborn*, Case No. 1M-98-83794.

DeVries, R., T. Weigers, B. Smulders, and E. van Teijlingen. 2009. "The Dutch Obstetrical System: Vanguard of the Future in Maternity Care." In *Birth Models That Work*, edited by R. Davis-Floyd, L. Barclay, B. A. Daviss, and J. Tritten, pp. 31–54. Berkeley: University of California Press.

DeVries, R., E. van Teijlingen, S. Wrede, and C. Benoit (eds.). 2001. *Birth by Design: Pregnancy, Maternity Care and Midwifery in North America and Europe*. New York: Routledge.

Diamond, Irene. 1994. *Fertile Ground: Women, Earth, and the Limits of Control*. Boston: Beacon Press.

Diamond, Irene, and Gloria Feman Orenstein. 1990. *Rewaving the World: The Emergence of Ecofeminism*. San Francisco: Sierra Club Books.

Diamantis, Peter H., and Steven Kotler. 2014. *Abundance: The Future Is Better than You Think.* New York: Free Press.

Diener, Ed, and Micaela Y. Chan. 2011. "Happy People Live Longer: Subjective Wellbeing Contributes to Health and Longevity." *Applied Psychology: Health and Wellbeing* 3(1): 1–43.

Dietiker, Marianne. n.d. "The Construction of Urban Midwife Identities in Popular Neighborhoods in Mexico City." In *Midwives in Mexico: Continuity, Controversy, and Change*, edited by Marcia Good Maust, Miguel Guëmez Piñeda, and Robbie Davis-Floyd. Austin: University of Texas Press.

Dixon, Lydia Z., Vania Smith Oka, and Mouni El Kotni. forthcoming. "Teaching about Childbirth in Mexico: Working across Birth Models." In *Birth in Eight Cultures: A Cross-Cultural Investigation*, edited by Robbie Davis-Floyd and Melissa Cheyney. Long Grove, IL: Waveland Press.

Duncan, David. 1993. "Is This Any Way to Train a Doctor? Medical Residencies: The Next Health Care Crisis." *Harper's* 286 (1715): 61–66.

Durrin, Ginny. 1982. *Daughters of Time: The Classic Film on Nurse-Midwives Today.* Washington, DC: Durrin (1-800-536-6843 durrinprod@aol.com).

Ehrenreich, Barbara, and Deirdre English. 1973a. *Complaints and Disorders: The Sexual Politics of Sickness*. Old Westbury, NY: The Feminist Press.

———. 1973b. *Witches, Midwives, and Nurses: A History of Women Healers*. Old Westbury, NY: Feminist Press.

Eisenberg, David M. 1996. "The Invisible Mainstream." *Harvard Medical Alumni Bulletin* 70(1): 20–25.

Eisenberg, David M., et al. 1998. "Trends in Alternative Medicine Use in the United States, 1990–1997: Results of a Follow-Up National Survey." *Journal of the American Medical Association* (280)18: 1569–1575.

Eisenberg, David M., R. C. Kessler, C. Foster, F. E. Norlock, D. R. Calkins, and T. L. Delbanco. 1993. "Unconventional Medicine in the United States: Prevalence, Costs, and Patterns of Use." *New England Journal of Medicine* 328: 246–252.

Eisler, Rianne. 1988. *The Chalice and the Blade*. New York: HarperCollins.

———. 1995. *Sacred Pleasure: Sex, Myth, and the Politics of the Body.* San Francisco: HarperSanFrancisco.

Ellul, Jacques. 1964. *The Technological Society.* Translated by John Wilkinson. New York: Vintage Books. (First published in French in 1954.)

Enkin, Murray, Marc J. N. C. Keirse, James Neilson, Caroline Crowther, Lelia Duley, Ellen Hodnett, and Justus Hofmeyr. 2000. *A Guide to Effective Care in Pregnancy and Childbirth* (3rd ed.). New York: Oxford University Press.

Ettinger, Laura E. 2006. *Nurse-Midwifery: The Birth of a New American Profession.* Columbus: Ohio State U Press.

Farrer, Ginger. 1980. "Singing for Life: The Mescalero Apache Girls' Puberty Ceremony." In *Southwestern Indian Ritual Drama,* edited by Charlotte Frisbie. Albuquerque: University of New Mexico Press.

Flint, Janna. 1996. "Residents: From Students to Physicians." Student term paper, Medical Anthropology, Dept. of Anthropology, Rice University, Spring.

Foucault, M. 1973. *The Birth of the Clinic: An Archaeology of Medical Perception.* Translated by A. M. Sheridan. London: Tavistock.

———. 1978. *The History of Sexuality: An Introduction* (Vol. 1). Translated by R. Hurley. New York: Random House.

Fox, Renee C., 1957. "Training for Uncertainty." In *The Student Physician*, edited by R. Merton, G. Reader, and P. L. Kendall. Cambridge MA: Harvard University Press.

———. 1980. "The Evolution of Medical Uncertainty." *Milbank Quarterly* 58: 1–49.

Fraser, G. 1995. "Modern Bodies, Modern Minds: Midwifery and Reproductive Change in an African American Community." In *Conceiving the New World Order: The Global Politics of Reproduction*, edited by F. Ginsburg and R. Rapp. Berkeley: University of California Press.

Freeman, Roger K., T. J. Garite, M. P. Nageotte, and L. A. Miller. 2012. *Fetal Heart Rate Monitoring*. Philadelphia: Lippincott Williams & Wilkins.

Freidson, Elliot. 1967. "'Review Essay': Health Factories: The New Industrial Sociology," *Social Problems* 14(Spring): 493–500.

Friedl, Ernestine. 1990 [1978]. "Society and Sex Roles." In *Anthropology: Contemporary Perspectives*, edited by Peter Whitten and D. Hunter, pp. 215–219. Glenview IL: Scott Foresman.

Frye, A. 1995. Holistic Midwifery: *A Comprehensive Textbook for Midwives in Home Birth Practice Vol. I: Care during Pregnancy.* Portland, OR: Labyrs Press.

Fullerton, J. (ed.). 2000. *Skilled Attendance at Delivery: A Review of the Evidence.* New York: Family Care International.

Gaby, Alan. 2017. *Nutritional Medicine* (2nd ed.). Self published: https://doctorgaby.com/

Gaines, Atwood, and Robbie Davis-Floyd. 2003. Entry on "Biomedicine." In *Encyclopedia of Medical Anthropology*, edited by Carol and Melvin Ember. New Haven, CT: Human Relations Area Files.

Garsten, Christine. 2001. "Trust, Control and Post-bureaucracy." *Organizational Studies.* March.

Gaskin, Ina May. 1990 [1977]. *Spiritual Midwifery* (3rd ed.). Summertown TN: The Book Publishing Co.

———. 2002 [1975]. *Spiritual Midwifery* (4th ed.). Summertown TN: Book Publishing Company.

Geertz, Clifford. 2000 [1973]. *The Interpretation of Cultures*. New York: Basic Books.

Georges, Eugenia, and Robbie Davis-Floyd. 2016. "Humanistic Obstetrics in Brazil: A Revolution in Maternity Care." In *The Routledge Handboook of Medical Anthropology*, edited by Lenore Manderson, Anita Hardon, and Elizabeth Cartwright, pp. 240–345. London and New York: Routledge.

Georges, Eugenia, and Rea Dallenbach. forthcoming. "Birth in Greece and New Zealand: A Comparative Analysis." In *Birth in Eight Cultures: A Cross-Cultural Investigation*, edited by Robbie-Davis Floyd and Melissa Cheyney. Long Grove, IL: Waveland Press.

Geurts, Kathryn. 2001. "Childbirth and Pragmatic Midwifery in Rural Ghana." In "Daughters of Time: The Shifting Identities of Contemporary Midwives," edited Robbie Davis-Floyd, Sheila Cosminsky, and Stacy L. Pigg, [special issue] *Medical Anthropology* 20(2-3).

Gilligan, Carol. 1993. *In a Different Voice: Psychological Theory and Women's Development* (2nd ed.). Cambridge: Harvard University Press.

Goer, Henci. 1995. *Obstetric Myths versus Research Realities*. Westport CT: Bergin and Garvey.

———. 1999. *The Thinking Woman's Guide to a Better Birth.* New York: Penguin Putnam/Perigree.

Goldberg, Phillip. 1983. *The Intuitive Edge*. Los Angeles: Jeremy P. Tarcher.

Good Maust, M. 2000. "Making Bodies: Cesarean Narratives in Merida, Yucatan." Unpublished doctoral dissertation, University of Florida, Gainesville.

Good, Byron, and Mary-Jo Delvecchio Good. 1993. "'Learning Medicine': The Construction of Medical Education at Harvard Medical School." In *Knowledge, Power, and Practice: The Anthropology of Medicine and Everyday Life*, edited by Shirley Lindenbaum and Margaret Lock, pp. 81–107. Berkeley: University of California Press.

Good, Mary-Jo Delvecchio. 1995. *American Medicine: The Quest for Competence*. Berkeley: University of California Press.

Goodman, Nadine. forthcoming. "Update on the Development of Professional Midwifery in Mexico." In *Speaking Truth to Power: Birth Models on the Human Rights Frontier*, edited by Betty-Anne Daviss and Robbie Davis-Floyd. Berkeley: University of California Press.

Graham, S. 1999. "Traditional Birth Attendants in Karamoja, Uganda." Unpublished doctoral dissertation, South Bank University, London.

Greenhalgh, Trisha, et al. 2008. *Diffusion of Innovations in Health Service Organisations: A Systematic Literature Review*. Hoboken, NJ: John Wiley & Sons.

Grol, Richard, and Jeremy Grimshaw. 2003. "From Best Evidence to Best Practice: Effective Implementation of Change in Patients' Care." *The Lancet* 362(9391): 1225–1230.

Grol, Richard, and Michel Wensing. 2004. "What Drives Change? Barriers to and Incentives for Achieving Evidence-Based Practice." *Medical Journal of Australia* 180(6): S57.

Grossberg, L. 1992. *We Gotta Get outa This Place: Popular Conservatism and Postmodern Culture*. New York: Routledge.

Guilliland, Karen. forthcoming. "Update on the New Zealand Model." In *Speaking Truth to Power: Birth Models on the Human Rights Frontier*, edited by Betty-Anne Daviss and Robbie Davis-Floyd. Berkeley: University of California Press.

Haire, Doris. 1972. "The Cultural Warping of Childbirth." *ICEA News* 11(1): 5–35.

Hamilton, Brady E., Joyce A. Martin, Michelle J. K. Osterman, Sally C. Curtin, and T. J. Mathews. 2015. "Births: Final Data for 2014." *National Vital Statistics Reports* 6(12): 1 63. http://www.cdc.gov/nchs/data/nvsr/nvsr64/nvsr64_12.pdf

Haraway, Donna. 1991. *Simians, Cyborgs, and Women: The Reinvention of Nature*. New York: Routledge.

Harris, P. E., et al. 2012. "Prevalence of Complementary and Alternative Medicine (CAM) Use by the General Population: A Systematic Review and Update." *International Journal of Clinical Practice* 66(10): 924–939.

Harrison, Michelle. 1982. *A Woman in Residence*. New York: Random House.

Harmon, Toni, and Alex Wakeford. 2016. *Your Baby's Microbiome: The Critical Role of Vaginal Birth and Breastfeeding for Lifelong Health*. White River Junction, VT: Chelsea Green Publishing.

Harwood, Michael. 1984. "The Ordeal: Life as a Medical Resident." *The New York Times Magazine*, 3 June, pp. 38–46, 70–82.

Hayward, John. 1984. *Perceiving Ordinary Magic*. Boston: Shambala.

Hazzell, Lester D. 1976 [1969]. *Commonsense Childbirth*. New York: Berkeley Medallion Books.

Hendry, C. 2009. "The New Zealand Maternity System: A Midwifery Renaissance." In *Birth Models That Work*, edited by R. Davis-Floyd, L Barclay, B. A. Daviss, and J. Tritten, pp. 55–88. Berkeley: University of California Press.

Hill, Anne. 1998. "Children of Metis: Beyond Zeus the Creator." In *Cyborg Babies: From Techno-Sex to Techno-Tots*, edited by Robbie Davis-Floyd and Joseph Dumit, pp. 330–344. New York: Routledge.

Hodnett E. D. 2002a. "Pain and Women's Satisfaction with the Experience of Childbirth: A Systematic Review." *American Journal of Obstetrics and Gynecology* 186.5: S160–S172.

———. 2002b. "Caregiver Support for Women during Childbirth." *The Cochrane Library*, Issue 4. Cochrane Database Syst Rev. 2002(1): CD000199.

Hodnett, E. D., S. Gates, G. J. Hofmeyr, and Carol Sakala. 2003. "Continuous Support for Women during Childbirth" (Cochrane Review). *The Cochrane Library*, Issue 3. Oxford: Update Software. http://www.maternitywise.org/pdfs/continuous_support.pdf

Hopkins, Kristine. 2000. "Are Brazilian Women Really Choosing to Deliver by Cesarean?" *Social Science and Medicine* 51(5): 725–740.

Houston, J., J. Foster, A. Davenport, A. Anderson, A. Romano, V. Lamprecht, and G. Frenkel. n.d. "Weaving Traditional and Professional Midwifery: Midwives for Midwives in Guatemala." Unpublished manuscript.

Houghton, P., and K. Windom. 1996a. *1995 Job Analysis of the Role of Direct-Entry Midwives*. North American Registry of Midwives. www.mana.org/NARM

———. 1996b. *Executive Summary of the 1995 Job Analysis of the Role of Direct-Entry Midwives. North American Registry of Midwives*. www.mana.org/NARM

Hsu, C. 2001. "Making Midwives: The Logics of Midwifery Training in St. Lucia." In "Daughters of Time: The Shifting Identities of Contemporary Midwives," edited by R. Davis-Floyd, S. Cosminsky, and S. L. Pigg, [special issue] *Medical Anthropology* 20(2-3).

Hunt, Katherine Jane, et al. 2010. "Complementary and Alternative Medicine Use in England: Results from a National Survey." *International Journal of Clinical Practice* 64(11): 1496–1502.

Hunt, L. M., M. G. Namino, and D. Halperin. 2002. "Childbirth Care-Seeking Behavior in Chiapas." *Health Care for Women International* 23(1): 98–118.

Hunt, Lauren. 2013. "Literature Review: Eating and Drinking in Labour." *British Journal of Midwifery* 21(7): 499–502.

Hutton, E. K., A. H. Reitsma, and K. Kaufman. 2009. "Outcomes Associated with Planned Home and Planned Hospital Births in Low-Risk Women Attended by Midwives in Ontario, Canada, 2003–2006: A Retrospective Cohort Study." *Birth* 36(3): 180–189.

INEGI (Instituto Nacional de Estadistica, Geografia e Informatica). 1999. "Encuesta Nacional de la Dinamica Demografica 1997." *INEGI, Aguascalientes*. Available: www.inegi.gob.mx

IMBCI (International MotherBaby Childbirth Initiative). 2008. Created by the International MotherBaby Childbirth Organization in collaboration with the Coalition for Improving Maternity Services and Childbirth Connection. www.imbci.org.

Inhorn, Marcia, and Gwynne Jenkins (eds.). 2003. "Reproduction Gone Awry," [special edition] *Social Science and Medicine* 56(9).

International Federation of Gynecology and Obstetrics (FIGO) et al. 2014. "Mother-Baby Friendly Birthing Facilities." *International Journal of Gynecology and Obstetrics*. http://dx.doi.org/10.1016/j.jigo.2014.10.013

Irwin, Susan, and Brigitte Jordan. 1987. "Knowledge, Practice, and Power: Court-Ordered Cesarean Sections." *Medical Anthropology Quarterly* 1(3): 319–334.

Iskandar, M., B. Atom, T. Hull, N. Dharmaputra, and Y. Azwa. 1996. *Unraveling the Mysteries of Maternal Death in West Java: Reexamining the Witnesses*. Depok: Center for Health Research, Research Institute University of Indonesia.

Jackson, D. J., J. M. Lang, W. H. Swartz, et al. 2003. "Outcomes, Safety, and Resource Utilization in a Collaborative Care Birth Center Program Compared with Traditional Physician-Based Perinatal Care." *Am J Public Health* 93(6): 999–1006.

Janssen, P. A., et al. 2002. "Outcomes of Planned Home Births versus Planned Hospital Births after Regulation of Midwifery in British Columbia." *CMAJ* 166(3): 315–323. http://www.cmaj.ca/content/166/3/315.short

———. 2009. "Outcomes of Planned Home Birth with Registered Midwife versus Planned Hospital Birth with Midwife or Physician." *CMAJ* 181(6-7): 377–383. http://www.cmaj.ca/content/181/6-7/377.short.

Janssen, Patricia A., Angela D. Henderson, and Saraswathi Vedam. 2009. "The Experience of Planned Home Birth: Views of the First 500 Women." *Birth* 36(4): 297–304. http://onlinelibrary.wiley.com/doi/10.1111/j.1523-536X.2009.00357.x/abstract?userIsAuthenticated=false&deniedAccessCustomisedMessage=

Jeffery, Roger, and Patricia M. Jeffery. 1993. "Traditional Birth Attendants in Rural North India: The Social Organization of Childbearing." In *Knowledge, Power, and Practice: The Anthropology of Medicine in Everyday Life*, edited by S. Lindenbaum and M. Lock, pp. 7–31. Berkeley and London: University of California Press.

Jenkins, Gwynne. 2001. "Changing Roles and Identities of Midwives in Rural Costa Rica." In "Daughters of Time: The Shifting Identities of Contemporary Midwives," edited by Robbie Davis-Floyd, Sheila Cosminsky, and Stacy L. Pigg, [special issue] *Medical Anthropology* 20(2-3).

Johantgen, M., L. Fountain, G. Zangaro, R. Newhouse, J. Stanik-Hutt, and K. White. 2012. "Comparison of Labor and Delivery Care Provided by Certified Nurse-Midwives and

Physicians: A Systematic Review, 1990 to 2008." *Women's Health Issues Off Publ Jacobs Inst Women's Health* 22(1): e73–e81. doi:10.1016/j.whi.2011.06.005

Johnson, K. C., and B. A. Daviss. 2001, October. "Results of the CPM Statistics Project 2000: A Prospective Study of Births by Certified Professional Midwives in North America." Abstract presented at the annual meeting of the American Public Health Association, Atlanta, GA.

———. 2005. "Outcomes of Planned Home Births with Certified Professional Midwives: Large Prospective Study in North America." *BMJ* 330(7505): 1416. http://www.bmj.com/content/330/7505/1416.full.pdf+html

Jones, Ricardo. 2009. "Teamwork: An Obstetrician, a Midwife, and a Doula." In *Birth Models That Work*, edited by Robbie Davis-Floyd, Lesley Barclay, Betty-Anne Daviss, and Jan Tritten, pp. 271–304. Berkeley: University of California Press.

———. 2010. *Memoirs of a Man Made of Glass*. Porto Alegre, Brazil: Editora Ideias a Granel.

———. 2012. *Entre as Orelhas—Histórias de Parto* (*Between the Ears: Birth Stories*). Porto Alegre, Brazil: Editora Ideias a Granel.

———. forthcoming. "Update on the Teamwork Model in Brazil." In *Speaking Truth to Power: Birth Models on the Human Rights Frontier*, edited by Betty-Anne Daviss and Robbie Davis-Floyd. Berkeley: University of California Press.

Jordan, Brigitte. 1992. "Technology and Social Interaction: Notes on the Achievement of Authoritative Knowledge." *IRL Technical Report #92-0027*. Palo Alto, CA: Institute for Research on Learning.

———. 1993. *Birth in Four Cultures: A Crosscultural Investigation of Childbirth in Yucatan, Holland, Sweden and the United States* (4th ed., rev. and updated by Robbie Davis-Floyd). Long Grove, IL: Waveland Press.

———. 1997. "Authoritative Knowledge and Its Construction." In *Childbirth and Authoritative Knowledge: Cross-Cultural Perspectives*, edited by Robbie Davis-Floyd and Carolyn Sargent, pp. 55–79. Berkeley: University of California Press.

Jordan, Brigitte, and Susan Irwin. 1989. "The Ultimate Failure: Court-Ordered Cesarean Section." In *New Approaches to Human Reproduction*, edited by Linda Whiteford and M. Poland. Boulder: Westview Press.

Joseph, Jennie. forthcoming. "There's Something Wrong Here: African-American Women and Their Babies Are at Greatest Risk in the USA." In *Speaking Truth to Power: Birth Models on the Human Rights Frontier*, edited by Betty-Anne Daviss and Robbie Davis-Floyd. Berkeley: University of California Press.

Jung, Carl G. 1971. *Psychological Types*. Princeton NJ: Princeton University Press.

Kelly, Kevin. 2016. *The Inevitable: Understanding the 12 Technological Forces That Will Shape Our Future*. New York: Penguin.

Kennedy, Holly. 2009. "'Orchestrating Normal': The Conduct of Midwifery in the United States." In *Birth Models That Work*, edited by R. Davis-Floyd, L. Barclay, B. A. Daviss, and J. Tritten, pp. 415–440. Berkeley: University of California Press.

———. 2010. "The Problem of Normal Birth." *Journal of Midwifery and Women's Health* 51(2): 71–77.

Kennell, John. 1982. "The Physiologic Effects of a Supportive Companion (Doula) During Labor." In *Birth: Interaction and Attachment*, edited by Marshall H. Klaus and Martha O. Robertson, pp. 92–105. New Jersey: Johnson and Johnson.

Kennell, John, Marshall Klaus, Susan McGrath, Steven Robertson, and Clark Hinckley. 1988 "Medical Intervention: The Effect of Social Support during Labor." *Pediatric Research* April: 211 (Abstract #61).

Kennell, John, Marshall Klaus, Susan McGrath, et al. 1991. "Continuous Emotional Support during Labor in a US Hospital: A Randomized Controlled Trial." *JAMA* 265: 2197–2201.

Kim, Hyun Kyoung. 2011. "Impact Factors of Korean Women's Cesarean Section According to an Ecological Approach." *Korean Journal of Women's Health Nursing* 17(2): 109–117.

Kitzinger, Sheila. 1991. *Homebirth: The Essential Guide to Giving Birth Outside the Hospital*. New York: Dorling Kindersley.

Klaus, Marshall H., John Kennell, and Phyllis Klaus. 1993. *Mothering the Mother: How a Doula Can Help You Have a Shorter, Easier, and Healthier Birth*. Boston: Addison Wesley.

Klassen, Pamela. 2001. *Blessed Events: Religion and Home Birth in America*. Princeton NJ: Princeton University Press.

Kleinman, Arthur. 1988. *The Illness Narratives: Suffering, Healing, and the Human Condition*. New York: Basic Books.

Kolenda, Pauline. 1998. "Fewer Deaths, Fewer Births." *Manushi* 105: 5–13.

Kroeger, Mary. 1996. "Final Consultant Report." CHN 3 Project, Provincial Department of Health Central Java, Indonesia.

Kunisch, Judith. 1989. "Electronic Fetal Monitors: Marketing Forces and the Resulting Controversy." In *Healing Technology: Feminist Perspectives*, edited by Kathryn Strother Ratcliff, pp. 41–60. Ann Arbor: University of Michigan Press.

Kwast, Barbara. 1992. "Midwives Role in Safe Motherhood." *GRMA News: A Publication of the Ghana Registered Midwives Association* 16: 6.

Laughlin, Charles D. 1992. *Brain, Symbol, and Experience: A Neurophenomenology of Human Consciousness*. New York: Columbia University Press.

———. 1997. "The Nature of Intuition: A Neuropsychological Approach." In *Intuition: Interdisciplinary Perspectives*, edited by R. Davis-Floyd and P. S. Arvidson. New York: Routledge.

Lay, Mary M. 2000. *The Rhetoric of Midwifery: Gender, Knowledge, and Power*. New Brunswick, NJ: Rutgers University Press.

LeBaron, Charles. 1981. *Gentle Vengeance: An Account of the First Year at Harvard Medical School*. New York: Richard Marek.

Lee, Peter R. 1976. *Symposium on Consciousness*. New York: Penguin.

Ley, R. G. 1983. "Cerebral Laterality and Imagery." In *Imagery: Current Theory, Research, and Application*. New York: Wiley.

Life magazine. 1989, February. "Visions of Tomorrow," pp. 50–94.

Litoff, Judy Barrett. 1978. *American Midwives: 1860 to the Present*. Westport, CT: Greenwood Press.

MacDonald, M., and I. Bourgeault. 2009. "The Ontario Midwifery Model of Care." In *Birth Models That Work*, edited by R. Davis-Floyd, L. Barclay, B. A. Daviss, and J. Tritten, pp. 89–118. Berkeley: University of California Press.

MacDorman, M. F., E. Declerq, and T. J. Mathews. 2013. "Recent Trends in Out-of-Hospital Births in the United States." *Journal of Midwifery and Women's Health* 58(5): 494–501.

MacDorman, M. F., T. J. Matthews, and E. Declerq. 2014. "Trends in Out-of- Hospital Births in the United States, 1990–2012." *NCHS Data Brief* 144: 1–8.

MacDorman, M. F., F. Menacker, and E. Declerq. 2010. "Trends and Characteristics of Home and Other Out-of-Hospital Births in the United States, 1990–2006." *National Vital Statistics Reports from the Centers for Disease Control and Prevention, National Center for Health Statistics, National Vital Statistics System* 58(11): 1–14, 16. http://europepmc.org/abstract/med/20575315

MacDorman, M., and G. Singh. 1998. "Midwifery Care, Social and Biomedical Risk Factors, and Birth Outcomes in the USA." *Journal of Epidemiology and Community Health* 52: 310–317.

Macones, George A., et al. 2008. "The 2008 National Institute of Child Health and Human Development Workshop Report on Electronic Fetal Monitoring: Update on Definitions, Interpretation, and Research Guidelines." *Journal of Obstetric, Gynecologic, & Neonatal Nursing* 37(5): 510–515.

Malloy, M. H. 2010. "Infant Outcomes of Certified Nurse-Midwife Attended Home Births: United States 2000 to 2004." *J Perinatal Off J Calif Perinat Assoc*. 30(9): 622–627. doi:10.1038/jp.2010.12

MANA (Midwives' Alliance of North America). 1992. "MANA Statement of Values and Ethics." *MANA News* 10(4): 10–12.

———. 1994. "MANA Core Competencies." *MANA News* 12(1): 24–27.

Manahan, Bill. 2011. "The Whole Systems Medicine of Tomorrow: A Half-Century Perspective." *Explore: The Journal of Science and Healing* 7(4): 212–214.

Marcus, George E. 1993. "What Comes (Just) After 'Post'? The Case of Ethnography." In *The Handbook of Qualitative Social Science*, edited by N. Denzin and Y. Lincoln. Beverly Hills, CA: Sage Publications.

Marcus, George E. 1998. *Ethnography through Thick and Thin*. Princeton NJ: Princeton University Press.

Marcus, George E., and Michael J. Fischer. 1986. *Anthropology as Cultural Critique: An Experimental Moment in the Human Sciences*. Chicago: University of Chicago Press.

Martin, J. A., B. E. Hamilton, M. J. K. Osterman, et al. 2015. "Births: Final Data for 2013." *National Vital Statistics Reports* (64)1. Hyattsville, MD: National Center for Health Statistics.

Martin, Emily. 1987. *The Woman in the Body*. Boston: Beacon Press.

———. 1990. "The Ideology of Reproduction: The Reproduction of Ideology." In *Uncertain Terms: Negotiating Gender in American Society*, edited by Faye Ginsburg and Anna L. Tsing, pp. 300–314. Boston: Beacon Press.

Matsuoka, Etsuko. 2001. "The Postmodern Midwife in Japan." In "Daughters of Time: The Shifting Identities of Contemporary Midwives," edited by Robbie Davis-Floyd, Sheila Cosminsky, and Stacy L. Pigg, [special issue] *Medical Anthropology* 20(2-3): 141–184.

Matsuoka E., and F. Hinokuma. 2009. "Maternity Homes in Japan: Reservoirs of Normal Childbirth." In *Birth Models That Work*, edited by R. Davis-Floyd, L. Barclay, B. A. Daviss, and J. Tritten, pp. 213–238. Berkeley: University of California Press.

May, Maureen. 2017. *Epiduralized Birth and Nurse-Midwifery: Childbirth in the United States. A Medical Ethnography*. Visalia, CA: Sampson Book Publishing.

May, Maureen, and Robbie Davis-Floyd. 2006. "Idealism and Pragmatism in the Creation of the Certified Midwife: The Development of Midwifery in New York and the New York Midwifery Practice Act of 1992." In *Mainstreaming Midwives: The Politics of Change*, edited by Robbie Davis-Floyd and Christine Barbara Johnson, pp. 81–162. New York: Routledge.

Mentor, Steven. 1998. "Witches, Nurses, Midwives, and Cyborgs." In *Cyborg Babies: From Techno-Sex to Techno-Tots*, edited by Robbie Davis-Floyd and Joseph Dumit, pp. 40–66. New York: Routledge,

Merchant, Carolyn. 1983. *The Death of Nature: Women, Ecology, and the Scientific Revolution*. San Francisco: Harper & Row.

Merewood, Anne, et al. 2005. "Breastfeeding Rates in US Baby-Friendly Hospitals: Results of a National Survey." *Pediatrics* 116(3). pediatrics.aappublications.org/content/116/3/628.short

Miller, Amy Chasteen, and Thomas E. Shriver. (2012). "Women's Childbirth Preferences and Practices in the United States." *Social Science & Medicine* 75(4): 709–716.

Miller, Suellen, et al. 2016. "Beyond Too Little, Too Late and Too Much, Too Soon: A Pathway towards Evidence-Based, Respectful Maternity Care Worldwide." *The Lancet* 388,10056: 2176–2192.

Miller, Suzanne, and Joan Skinner. 2012. "Are First-Time Mothers Who Plan Home Birth More Likely to Receive Evidence-Based Care? A Comparative Study of Home and Hospital Care Provided by the Same Midwives." *Birth* 39(2): 135–144. http://onlinelibrary.wiley.com/doi/10.1111/j.1523-536X.2012.00534.x/abstract;jsessionid=9DFC636B5B2CAA38B0EA5E6F2998AC49.f03t04?userIsAuthenticated=false&deniedAccessCustomisedMessage

Miller, S., M. Cordero, A. L. Coleman, J. Figueroa, S. Brito-Anderson, R. Dabash, et al. 2003. "Quality of Care in Institutionalized Deliveries: The Paradox of the Dominican Republic." *Int J Gynecol Obstet* 82(1): 89–103.

Mills, L., and R. Davis-Floyd. 2009. "The CASA Hospital and Professional Midwifery School: An Education and Practice Model That Work." In *Birth Models That Work*, edited by R. Davis-Floyd, L. Barclay, B. A. Daviss, and J. Tritten, pp. 305–336. Berkeley: University of California Press.

Mondal, Sambhu Charan, Anuradha Verma, Shiv Kumar Gupta, and Babita Kumar. 2012. "Genetic and Gestational Surrogacy: an Overview." *Walailak Journal of Science and Technology* 9(3): 189–193.

Moore, Sally Falk, and Barbara Myerhoff (eds.). 1977. *Secular Ritual*. Assen, The Netherlands: Van Gorcum.

Moran, Marilyn A. 1981. *Birth and the Dialogue of Love*. Leawood KS: New Nativity Press.

Morris, Theresa. 2013. *Cut It Out: The C-section Epidemic in America*. New York: New York University Press.

Morris, Theresa, and Katherine McInerney. 2010. "Media Representations of Pregnancy and Childbirth: An Analysis of Reality Television Programs in the United States." *Birth* 37(2): 134–140.

Morsy, Soheir. 1995. "Deadly Reproduction among Egyptian Women: Maternal Mortality and the Medicalization of Population Control." In *Conceiving the New World Order: The Global Politics of Reproduction*, edited by F. Ginsburg and R. Rapp, pp. 162–176. Berkeley: University of California Press.

Naisbitt, John. 1980. *Megatrends: Ten New Directions Transforming Our Lives*. New York: Warner.

Nelson, Craig S., et al. 1995. "Residents' Performance before and after Night Call as Evaluated by an Indicator of Creative Thought." *Journal of the American Osteopathic Association* 95(10): 600–603.

Niino, Yoshiko. 2011. "The Increasing Cesarean Rate Globally and What We Can Do about It." *Bioscience Trends* 5(4): 139–150.

Northrup, Christiane. 2010 [1994]. *Women's Bodies, Women's Wisdom*. New York: Bantam Books.

Oakley, Anne. 1984. *The Captured Womb: A History of the Medical Care of Pregnant Women*. New York: Basil Blackwell.

Odent, Michel. 1994. *Birth Reborn*. London: Souvenir Press.

Oparah, Julia C., and Alicia D. Bonaparte (eds.). 2016. *Birthing Justice: Black Women, Pregnancy, and Childbirth*. New York: Routledge.

Osterman, Michelle, and Joyce A. Martin. 2014. "Recent Declines in Induction of Labor by Gestational Age." *NCHS Data Brief No. 155*. Hyattsville, MN: National Center for Health Statistics.

O'Sullivan, Geraldine, et al. 2009. "Effect of Food Intake during Labour on Obstetric Outcome: Randomised Controlled Trial." *British Medical Journal* 338:b784. http://www.bmj.com/content/338/bmj.b784

Paciornik, Moises. 1979. *Learn How to Give Birth with the Indians*. Editora Brasiliense.

Paine, L. L., C. M. Dower, and E. O'Neil. 1999. "Midwifery in the 21st Century: Recommendations from the Pew Health Professions Commission/UCSF Center for the Health Professions 1998 Taskforce on Midwifery." *Journal of Nurse Midwifery* 44(4): 341–348.

Parsons, Myra, John Bidewell, and Rhonda Griffiths. 2007. "A Comparative Study of the Effect of Food Consumption on Labour and Birth Outcomes in Australia." *Midwifery* 23(2): 131–138.

Parvati-Baker, Jeannine. 1978. *Hygeia: A Woman's Herbal*. Copyright Jeannine Parvati-Baker, self-published.

———. 1986a. *Conscious Conception: Elemental Journey through the Labyrinth of Sexuality*. Monroe, UT: Freestone Publishing.

———. 1986b. *Prenatal Yoga and Natural Childbirth*. Monroe, Utah: Freestone Publishing.

———. 1992. "The Shamanic Dimensions of Childbirth." *Journal of Pre- and Perinatal Psychology* 7(1): 5–21.

Pascali-Bonaro, Debra. 2005. "Shedding Light in Brazil." *International Journal of Childbirth Education* 20(1): 22–26.

Perez, Paulina, and Cheryl Snedeker. 2000. *Special Women: The Role of the Professional Labor Assistant* (3rd ed.). Johnson, VT: Cutting Edge Press.

Pert, Candace. 1993. "The Chemical Communicators." In *Healing and the Mind*, edited by Bill Moyers and Betty Sue Flowers, pp. 177–194. New York: Doubleday.

Peterson, Caroline. 2010. "Midwifery and the Crowning of Health Care Reform." *Journal of Midwifery and Women's Health* 55(1)5–8.

Peterson, Gayle. 1981. *Birthing Normally: A Personal Growth Approach to Childbirth.* Berkeley: Mindbody Press.

Pigg, S. L. 1997. "Authority in Translation: Finding, Knowing, Naming, and Training 'Traditional Birth Attendants' in Nepal." In *Childbirth and Authoritative Knowledge: Cross-Cultural Perspectives*, edited by R. Davis-Floyd and C. Sargent, pp. 233–262. Berkeley: University of California Press.

Poincare, Howard. 1913. *The Foundations of Science.* New York: Science Press.

Potter, Joe C., Elza Berquo, Ignez H. O. Perpetuo, et al. 2001. "Unwanted Cesarean Sections among Public and Private Patients in Brazil." Unpublished ms.

Quinn, Daniel. 1993. *Ishmael.* New York: Bantam and Turner.

Reed, Rebecca, and Cathy Walton. 2009. "The Albany Birth Practice." In *Birth Models that Work,* edited by Robbie Davis-Floyd, Lesley Barclay, Betty-Anne Daviss, and Jan Tritten, pp. 119–186. Berkeley: University of California Press.

Rensselaer Polytechnic Institute. 2011, July 26. "Minority Rules. Scientists Discover Tipping Point for the Spread of Ideas." *Science Daily.* Available: https://www.sciencedaily.com/releases/2011/07/110725190044.htm

Reynolds, Peter C. 1991. *Stealing Fire: The Atomic Bomb as Symbolic Body.* Palo Alto CA: Iconic Anthropology Press.

Richards, L. 1987. *The Vaginal Birth after Cesarean Experience.* South Hadley, MA: Bergin and Garvey.

Romalis, Shelley (ed.). 1981. *Childbirth: Alternatives to Medical Control.* Austin: University of Texas Press.

Romano, Amy M., and Judith A. Lothian. 2008. "Promoting, Protecting, and Supporting Normal Birth: A Look at the Evidence." *Journal of Obstetric, Gynecologic, & Neonatal Nursing* 37(1): 94–105.

Roncalli, Lucia. 1997. "Standing by Process: A Midwife's Notes on Storytelling, Passage, and Intuition." In *Intuition: The Inside Story*, edited by Robbie Davis-Floyd and P. Sven Arvidson, pp. 177–200. New York: Routledge.

Rooks, Judith. 1997. *Midwifery and Childbirth in America.* Philadelphia: Temple University Press.

———. 1999. "The Midwifery Model of Care." *Journal of Nurse-Midwifery* 44(4): 370–374.

Rosario, Santi. 1998. "The Dai and the Doctor: Discourses on Women's Reproductive Health in Rural Bangladesh." In *Maternities and Modernities: Colonial and Post-Colonial Experiences in Asia and the Pacific*, edited by Kalpana Ram and Margaret Jolly, pp. 144–176. Cambridge, UK: Cambridge University Press.

Roth, Denise. 2000. *Bodily Risks, Spiritual Risks: Contrasting Discourses on Pregnancy in a Rural Tanzanian Community.* Ann Arbor: University of Michigan Press.

Rothman, Barbara Katz. 1982. *In Labor: Women and Power in the Birthplace.* New York: Norton. (Reprinted in paperback under the title *Giving Birth: Alternatives in Childbirth.* New York: Penguin Books, 1985.)

———. 1989. *Recreating Motherhood: Ideology and Technology in Patriarchal Society.* New York: W.W. Norton.

———. 1992. Plenary Address, Midwives Alliance of North America Conference, New York City, November.

———. 1998. "Daughters of Time." In *Paths to Becoming a Midwife: Getting an Education*, edited by Jan Tritten and Joel Southern. Eugene, OR: Midwifery Today.

Rubinstein, Robert A., Charles D. Laughlin, Jr., and John McManus. 1984. *Science as Cognitive Process: Toward an Empirical Philosophy of Science*. Philadelphia: University of Pennsylvania Press.

Sadler, Michelle, Mario J. D. S. Santos, Dolores Ruiz-Berdun, Gonzalo Leiva Rojas, Elena Skoko, Patricia Gillen, and Jette A. Clausen. 2016. "Moving beyond Disrespect and Abuse: Addressing the Structural Dimensions of Obstetric Violence." *Reproductive Health Matters* 24: 47–55.

Sargent, Carolyn. 1989. *Maternity, Medicine, and Power: Reproductive Decisions in Urban Benin*. Berkeley: University of California Press.

Schaef, A. 1992. *Women's Reality* (Rev. ed.). San Francisco: Harper.

Schild, Veronica. 1998. "New Subjects of Rights? Women's Movements and the Construction of Citizenship in the 'New Democracies.'" In *Cultures of Politics/Politics of Cultures: Re-Visioning Latin American Social Movements*, edited by S. E. Alvarez, E. Dagnino, and A. Escobar, pp. 93–117. Boulder, CO: Westview Press.

Schuiling, K. D., T. A. Sipe, and J. Fullerton. 2013. "Findings from the Analysis of the American College of Nurse-Midwives' Membership Surveys 2009–2011." *Journal of Midwifery and Women's Health* 58(4): 404–415.

Scott, K. D., G. Berkowitz, and M. Klaus. 1999. "A Comparison of Intermittent and Continuous Support During Labor: A Meta-Analysis." *Am J Obstet Gynecol* 180(5): 1054–1059.

Scott, K. D., Phyllis H. Klaus, and Marshall Klaus. 1999. "The Obstetrical and Postpartum Benefits of Continuous Support during Childbirth." *Journal of Women's Health and Gender Based Medicine* 8(10): 1257–1264.

SSA (Secretaria de Salud). 1994. *La partera tradicional en la atencion materno infantil en Mexico*. Available: www.ssa.gob.mx

Shanley, Laura Kaplan. 1994. *Unassisted Childbirth*. Westport CT: Bergin and Garvey.

Shaw, Nancy S. 1974. *Forced Labor: Maternity Care in the United States*. New York: Pergamon Press.

Shearer, Elizabeth L. 1989. "Commentary: Does Cesarean Delivery Affect the Parents?" *Birth* 16(2): 57–58.

Shen, C., and John B. Williamson. 1999. "Maternal Mortality, Women's Status, and Economic Dependency in Less Developed Countries: A Cross-National Analysis." *Social Science and Medicine* 49: 197–214.

Sieglin, Veronica. n.d. "The Integration of Traditional Midwives into the State Health Care System: A Case Study in Northeastern Mexico." Unpublished ms.

Singata, M., J. Tranmer, and G. M. L. Gyte. 2013. "Eating and Drinking in Labour." *Cochrane Database of Systematic Reviews*. http://www.cochrane.org/CD003930/PREG_eating-and-drinking-in-labour

Singata, M., J. Tranmer, et al. 2010. "Restricting Oral Fluid and Food Intake during Labour." *Cochrane Database of Systematic Reviews* (1): CD003930.

Singer, Linda. 1992. "Feminism and Postmodernism." In *Feminists Theorize the Political*, edited by J. Butler and J. W. Scott. New York: Routledge.

Slaatte, Harold A. 1983. *The Creativity of Consciousness: An Empirico-Phenomenological Psychology*. New York: University Press of America.

Smith, Linda. 2010. *The Impact of Birth Practices on Breastfeeding* (2nd ed.). Sudbury, MA: Jones and Bartlett Publishers.

Smith, Robert C. 1996. *The Patient's Story: Integrated Patient-Doctor Interviewing*. Boston: Little, Brown and Co.

Sorokin, Pitirim A. 1941. *The Crisis of Our Age*. New York: E. P. Dutton.

Sosa, R., J. Kennell, M. Klaus, S. Robertson, and J. Urrutia. 1980. "The Effect of a Supportive Companion on Perinatal Problems, Length of Labor, and Mother-Infant Interaction." *New England Journal of Medicine* 303: 597–600.

Spallone, P. 1989. *Beyond Conception: The New Politics of Reproduction*. Granby MA: Bergin and Garvey Publishers.

Sperry, Roger W. 1974. "Lateral Specialization in Surgically Separated Hemispheres." In *The Neurosciences: Third Study Program*, edited by P. J. Vinken and G. W. Bruyn. Cambridge MA: MIT Press.

———. 1982. "Some Effects of Disconnecting the Cerebral Hemispheres." *Science* 217: 1223–1226.

Spiegel, David. 1993. "Social Support: How Friends, Family, and Groups Can Help." In *Mind-Body Medicine: How To Use Your Mind for Better Health*, edited by Daniel Goleman and Joel Gurin, pp. 331–349. Yonkers, New York: Consumer Reports Books.

Spiegel, David, J. R. Bloom, H. C. Kramer, and E. Gottheil. 1989. "Effect of Psychosocial Treatment on Survival of Patients with Metastatic Breast Cancer." *Lancet* 2: 888–891.

Spong, Catherine Y., et al. 2012. "Preventing the First Cesarean Delivery: Summary of a Joint Eunice Kennedy Shriver National Institute of Child Health and Human Development, Society for Maternal-Fetal Medicine, and American College of Obstetricians and Gynecologists Workshop." *Obstetrics and Gynecology* 120(5): 1181.

Sprenger, Jally, and George Deutsch. 1981. *Left Brain Right Brain*. San Francisco: W. H. Freeman.

Stapleton, S. R., C. Osborne, and J. Illuzzi. 2013. "Outcomes of Care in Birth Centers: Demonstration of a Durable Model." *J Midwifery Women's Health* 58(1): 3–14. doi:10.1111/jmwh.12003

Starhawk. 1988. *Dreaming the Dark: Magic, Sex, and Politics*. Boston: Beacon Press.

———. 1989. *The Spiral Dance: A Rebirth of the Ancient Religion of the Great Goddess*. San Francisco: HarperSanFrancisco.

———. 1993. *The Fifth Sacred Thing*. New York: Bantam Books.

Stein, Howard F. 1990. *American Medicine as Culture*. Boulder CO: Westview.

SUS. n.d. *Manual Pratico para Implementacao da Rede Cegonha*. www.saude/mt/gov.br/arquivo/3062

Susie, Deborah Ann. 1988. *In the Way of Our Grandmothers: A Cultural View of Twentieth-Century Midwifery in Florida*. Athens: University of Georgia Press.

Temel, Jennifer S., et al. 2010. "Early Palliative Care for Patients with Metastatic Non–Small-Cell Lung Cancer." *New England Journal of Medicine* 363(8): 733–742.

TenHouten, Warren. 1978–1979. "Hemispheric Interaction in the Brain and the Propositional, Compositional, and Dialectical Modes of Thought." *Journal of Altered States of Consciousness* 4(2): 129–140.

Toan, Tran Khanh, et al. 2013. "Technology Preference in Choices of Delivery Care Utilization from User Perspective–A Community Study in Vietnam." *American Journal of Public Health* 1(1): 10–17.

Tornquist, C. 2004. "Parto e Poder: O movimento pela humanização do parto no Brasil." PhD dissertation. Florianopolis, Brazil: Universidad Federal de Santa Catarina.

Tresolini, Carol P., and the Pew-Fetzer Task Force on Advancing Psychosocial Health Education. 1994. *Health Professions Education and Relationship-Centered Care*. San Francisco CA: Pew Health Professions Commission.

Tritten, Jan, and Kelley Meyer (eds.). 2010. *Paths to Becoming a Midwife: Getting an Education*. Eugene, OR: Midwifery Today.

Turkle, Sherry. 1998. "Cyborg Babies and Cy-Dough-Plasm." In *Cyborg Babies: From Techno-Sex to Techno-Tots*, edited by Robbie Davis-Floyd and Joseph Dumit, pp. 317–329. New York: Routledge.

Turner, Victor W. 1979. "Betwixt and Between: The Liminal Period in *Rites de Passage*." In *Reader in Comparative Religion* (4th ed.), edited by W. Lessa and E. Z. Vogt, pp. 238–239. New York: Harper and Row.

Tyler, Terry, and Gloria St. John. 1989. *MetaPhysicians Tales*. Unpublished ms.

Vallejo, Manuel C., et al. 2013. "Maternal Outcomes in Women Supplemented with a High-Protein Drink in Labour." *Australian and New Zealand Journal of Obstetrics and Gynaecology* 53(4): 369–374.

van Gennep, Arnold. 1966. *The Rites of Passage*. Chicago: University of Chicago Press.

Van Teijlingen, Edwin, Sirpa Wrede, Cecilia Benoit, Jane Sandall, and Raymond DeVries. 2009. "Born in the USA: Exceptionalism in Maternity Care Organisation among High-Income Countries." *Sociological Research Online* 14(1): 5. Retrieved from http://www.socresonline.org.uk/14/1/5.html

Varney, Helen, and Joyce Thompson. 2016. *A History of Midwifery in the United States: The Midwife Said "Fear Not."* Thompson. NY: Springer.

Vaughn, Francis E. 1979. *Awakening Intuition*. Garden City, NY: Anchor Books.

Vedam, S., L. Leemam, M. Cheyney, T. Fisher, S. Myers, L. Low, and C. Ruhl. 2014. "Transfer from Planned Home Birth to Hospital: Improving Inter-Professional Collaboration." *Journal of Midwifery and Women's Health* 59(6): 624–634.

Victora, Cesar G., et al. 2011. "Maternal and Child Health in Brazil: Progress and Challenges." *The Lancet* 377(9780): 1863–1876.

Wagner, Marsden. 1994. *Pursuing the Birth Machine*. Australia: Ace Graphics.

———. 1997. "Confessions of a Dissident." In *Childbirth and Authoritative Knowledge: Cross-Cultural Perspectives*, edited by Robbie Davis-Floyd and Carolyn Sargent, pp. 366–396. Berkeley: University of California Press.

Walsh, Denis. 2006. "'Nesting' and 'Matrescence' as Distinctive Features of a Freestanding Birth Center in the UK." *Midwifery* 22(3): 228–239.

———. *Evidence-Based Care for Normal Labour and Birth: A Guide for Midwives*. New York: Routledge.

———. 2009. "Small Really Is Beautiful: Tales from a Freestanding Birth Center in England." In *Birth Models That Work*, edited by R. Davis-Floyd, L. Barclay, B. A. Daviss, and J. Tritten, pp. 159–186. Berkeley: University of California Press.

Weil, Andrew. 1972. *The Natural Mind*. Boston: Houghton-Mifflin.

Wertz, Richard, and Dorothy Wertz. 1989. *Lying-In: A History of Childbirth in America* (2nd ed.). New York: Free Press.

Westcott, Alan. 1968. *Toward a Contemporary Psychology of Intuition*. New York: Holt, Rinehart, and Winston.

Wheatley, Margaret. 1992. *Leadership and the New Science: Learning about Organization from an Orderly Universe*. San Francisco: Berrett-Koehler Publishers.

Whittaker, Andrea. 1999. "Birth and the Postpartum in Northeast Thailand: Contesting Modernity and Tradition." *Medical Anthropology* 183: 215–242.

Wiseman, R., and Marilyn Schlitz. 1996. "Experimenter Effects and the Remote Detection of Staring." Annual Proceedings of the Parapsychological Convention, San Diego, California.

Wooten, Lynn Perry, and Patricia Crane. 2004. "Generating Dynamic Capabilities through a Humanistic Work Ideology: The Case of a Certified-Nurse Midwife Practice in a Professional Bureaucracy." *American Behavioral Scientist* 47(6): 848–866.

Yang, Tony, Laura Attanasio, and Katy Kozhimammil. 2016. "State Scope of Practice Laws, Nurse-Midwifery Workforce, and Childbirth Procedures and Outcomes." *Women's Health Issues* May/June.

Zhang, Jun, et al. 2010. "Contemporary Cesarean Delivery Practice in the United States." *American Journal of Obstetrics and Gynecology* 203(4): 326.e1–326.e10.

Contributors

Robbie Davis-Floyd PhD, Senior Research Fellow, Dept. of Anthropology, University of Texas Austin and Fellow of the Society for Applied Anthropology, is a well-known cultural/medical anthropologist, international speaker, and researcher in transformational models in childbirth, midwifery, and obstetrics. She is author of over 80 articles and of *Birth as an American Rite of Passage* (1992, 2003), soon to be revised and updated with Melissa Cheyney; coauthor (with Gloria St. John) of *From Doctor to Healer: The Transformative Journey* (1998) and *The Power of Ritual* with Charles Laughlin (2016); and lead editor of 10 collections, including *Childbirth and Authoritative Knowledge: Cross-Cultural Perspectives* (1997); *Cyborg Babies: From Techno-Sex to Techno-Tots* (1998); *Intuition: The Inside Story*; *Mainstreaming Midwives: The Politics of Change* (2006); and *Birth Models That Work* (2009), which highlights optimal models of birth care around the world. *Speaking Truth to Power: Birth Models on the Human Rights Frontier*, coedited with Betty-Anne Daviss, is in process, as is *Sustainable Birth*, coedited with Kim Gutschow and Betty-Anne Daviss, and *Birth in Eight Cultures: A Cross-Cultural Investigation*, coedited with Melissa Cheyney. Davis-Floyd serves as editor for the *International MotherBaby Childbirth Initiative (IMBCI): 10 Steps to Optimal Maternity Care* (www.imbci.org), board member of the International MotherBaby Childbirth Organization (IMBCO), senior advisor to the Council on Anthropology and Reproduction, and associate editor of *Medical Anthropology Quarterly*. She is listed in *Who's Who in America, Who's Who in American Women, Who's Who in the World, and Who's Who in Science and Technology,* and can be found on Wikipedia as well. She can be reached at davis-floyd@austin.utexas.edu and www.davis-floyd.com.

Elizabeth Davis CPM has been a midwife since 1977 and a Holistic Maternity Care Midwifery Educator since 1982. She is a founding member of MANA, a past-president of MEAC, and a former Pacific regional representative to MANA. She is cofounder and codirector of the MEAC-accredited National Midwifery Institute, a three-year midwifery educational program that qualifies graduates for national certification and California licensure. A popular international lecturer and activist, she serves as academic advisor to many midwifery programs throughout Europe. Her books have been translated into 11 languages and include *The Rhythms of Women's Desire: How Female Sexuality Unfolds at Every Stage of Life, The Women's Wheel of Life, Orgasmic Birth: Your Guide to a Safe, Satisfying, and Pleasurable Birth Experience* (with Debra Pascali-Bonaro), and the world-renowned introductory midwifery textbook *Heart and Hands: A Midwife's Guide to Pregnancy and Birth*, now in its 5th edition. She can be reached at elizabeth@elizabethdavis.com.

COURTNEY L. EVERSON PHD is a medical anthropologist and Dean of Graduate Studies at the Midwives College of Utah, Salt Lake City, UT. Dr. Everson's research and teaching focus on cultural humility and collaborative care models, examining doula and midwifery care for reducing health inequities among underserved communities. Dr. Everson is also the director of research education for the Midwives Alliance of North America (MANA) Division of Research (DOR); an Accreditation Review Committee (ARC) member for the Midwifery Education Accreditation Council (MEAC); and serves on the boards of directors for the Australasian Professional Doula Regulatory Association (APDRA), the Association of Midwifery Educators (AME), and the Academic Collaborative for Integrative Health (ACIH). She also serves families in her local community as a perinatal health educator and doula. (ceverson@gmail.com)

EUGENIA (NIA) GEORGES PHD, Professor and Chair of the Department of Anthropology at Rice University in Houston, has conducted research on the implications of transnational migration for gender and class hierarchies in the Dominican Republic and on the political mobilization of Dominican immigrants in New York City. Her research in Greece examines the medicalization of reproduction, with a focus on the historical processes through which pregnancy and Greek obstetrical practice have been shaped in interaction with a range of reproductive technologies. Her research in Brazil examines the ethical and political strategies of a network of obstetricians-activists who have organized to demedicalize childbirth on the national level and redefine a range of choices in maternity care as a woman's human right. She is the author of *Bodies of Knowledge: The Medicalization of Reproduction in Greece* (Vanderbilt University Press) and *The Making of a Transnational Community: Migration, Development and Cultural Change in the Dominican Republic* (Columbia University Press). Her articles have appeared in *Medical Anthropology Quarterly*, *Social Science and Medicine*, *Feminist Studies*, *Journal of Mediterranean Studies* and other journals. (nia@rice.edu)

HOLLY HORAN MA is a doctoral candidate in Oregon State University's (OSU's) Applied Anthropology Program with a concentration in biocultural, applied medical anthropology. Horan specializes in using a community-led research framework and applies this framework to her research on maternal stress and gestational outcomes in Puerto Rico. Horan is also currently involved in four community-led research projects in Puerto Rico in addition to various other maternal and infant health research projects in the continental United States. She has been a birth and postpartum doula since 2012. (horanh@onid.orst.edu)

CHRISTINE BARBARA JOHNSON PHD is a sociologist, a midwifery advocate for over 30 years, and a national speaker who has presented numerous papers on normalizing birth. She has been an adjunct professor at Boston University and Boston College teaching medical sociology, and a research consultant on a National Library of Medicine study that included a key component on midwives. She sat on the board of directors of the Massachusetts Friends of Midwives for many years and has been an active participant on many committees supporting the midwifery model of care. Presently, Christine offers change management and conflict resolution seminars as well as executive and leadership coaching. In 2005 she was selected for inclusion in *Who's Who in Executives and Professionals.*

ETSUKO MATSUOKA PHD, Professor, Faculty of Human Life and Environment, Nara Women's University, Japan, is an anthropologist specializing in childbirth and midwifery studies in different parts of the world. Her works in English cover such topics as "The Interpretation of Fox-Possession: Illness as Metaphor" (*Culture, Medicine and Psychiatry* 1991), "Is Hospital the Safest Place for Birth? (*Curare* 1995), "Postmodern Midwives in Japan: The Offspring of Modern Hospital Birth (*Medical Anthropology* 2001), "Maternity Homes in Japan: Reservoirs of Normal Childbirth" (coauthored with Fumiko Hinokuma, in *Birth Models that Work* 2009), *Challenges to Women's Reproductive Health and Rights in Asia* (coedited by Pande Made Kutanegara, Gadjah Mada University Press 2015). She is an associate editor of the *International Journal of Childbirth*. Currently she is conducting research in Asia comparing different patterns of the modernizing process with regard to childbirth and midwifery. (matsuokae1@gmail.com)

Bonnie Ruder CPM, MPH, MA is a doctoral student in biocultural anthropology at Oregon State University. In 2012, she received a dual Master's Degree in Anthropology and Public Health. Her research examined the causes and lived experience of women suffering from obstetric fistulas in eastern Uganda. She also examined traditional birth attendants' understanding of obstetric fistula and the impact of international policies on local maternity care. Bonnie is a Certified Professional Midwife and has attended births in Oregon since 1997. She has also had the privilege of attending births internationally, working at a birth center in Haiti six months post-earthquake and in the maternity ward of a referral hospital in Soroti, Uganda. She served as a researcher for the MANA Division of Research in 2010–2014. (bonnieruder@gmail.com)